Clinical Dilemmas in

Viral Liver
Disease

T0176559

Clinical Dilemmas in
Viral Liver Disease

SECOND EDITION

EDITED BY

Graham R. Foster, PhD, FRCP
Professor of Hepatology
The Blizard Institute
Barts and The London School of Medicine
Queen Mary University of London
London, UK

K. Rajender Reddy, MD, FACP, FACG, FRCP, FAASLD
Ruimy Family President's Distinguished Professor of Medicine
Professor of Medicine in Surgery
Director of Hepatology
Director of Viral Hepatitis Center
Medical Director of Liver Transplantation
University of Pennsylvania
Philadelphia, PA, USA

WILEY Blackwell

This edition first published 2020
© 2020 by John Wiley & Sons Ltd

Edition History [1e, 2010]

All rights reserved. No part of this publication may be reproduced, stored in a retrieval system, or transmitted, in any form or by any means, electronic, mechanical, photocopying, recording or otherwise, except as permitted by law. Advice on how to obtain permission to reuse material from this title is available at http://www.wiley.com/go/permissions.

The rights of Graham R. Foster and K. Rajender Reddy be identified as the authors of editorial work has been asserted in accordance with law.

Registered Office(s)
John Wiley & Sons, Inc., 111 River Street, Hoboken, NJ 07030, USA
John Wiley & Sons Ltd, The Atrium, Southern Gate, Chichester, West Sussex, PO19 8SQ, UK

Editorial Office
9600 Garsington Road, Oxford, OX4 2DQ, UK

For details of our global editorial offices, customer services, and more information about Wiley products visit us at www.wiley.com.

Wiley also publishes its books in a variety of electronic formats and by print-on-demand. Some content that appears in standard print versions of this book may not be available in other formats.

Limit of Liability/Disclaimer of Warranty
The contents of this work are intended to further general scientific research, understanding, and discussion only and are not intended and should not be relied upon as recommending or promoting scientific method, diagnosis, or treatment by physicians for any particular patient. In view of ongoing research, equipment modifications, changes in governmental regulations, and the constant flow of information relating to the use of medicines, equipment, and devices, the reader is urged to review and evaluate the information provided in the package insert or instructions for each medicine, equipment, or device for, among other things, any changes in the instructions or indication of usage and for added warnings and precautions. While the publisher and authors have used their best efforts in preparing this work, they make no representations or warranties with respect to the accuracy or completeness of the contents of this work and specifically disclaim all warranties, including without limitation any implied warranties of merchantability or fitness for a particular purpose. No warranty may be created or extended by sales representatives, written sales materials or promotional statements for this work. The fact that an organization, website, or product is referred to in this work as a citation and/or potential source of further information does not mean that the publisher and authors endorse the information or services the organization, website, or product may provide or recommendations it may make. This work is sold with the understanding that the publisher is not engaged in rendering professional services. The advice and strategies contained herein may not be suitable for your situation. You should consult with a specialist where appropriate. Further, readers should be aware that websites listed in this work may have changed or disappeared between when this work was written and when it is read. Neither the publisher nor authors shall be liable for any loss of profit or any other commercial damages, including but not limited to special, incidental, consequential, or other damages.

Library of Congress Cataloging-in-Publication Data

Names: Foster, Graham R., editor. | Reddy, K. Rajender, editor.
Title: Clinical dilemmas in viral liver disease / edited by, Graham R. Foster, K. Rajender Reddy.
Description: Second edition. | Hoboken, NJ, USA : Wiley-Blackwell, 2020. | Includes bibliographical references and index.
Identifiers: LCCN 2019057711 (print) | LCCN 2019057712 (ebook) | ISBN 9781119533399 (paperback) | ISBN 9781119533436 (adobe pdf) | ISBN 9781119533443 (epub)
Subjects: MESH: Hepatitis, Viral, Human–diagnosis | Hepatitis, Viral, Human–therapy | Hepatitis, Chronic–diagnosis | Hepatitis, Chronic–therapy | Liver Cirrhosis–diagnosis | Liver Cirrhosis–therapy | Diagnostic Techniques, Digestive System
Classification: LCC RC848.H43 (print) | LCC RC848.H43 (ebook) | NLM WC 536 | DDC 616.3/623–dc23
LC record available at https://lccn.loc.gov/2019057711
LC ebook record available at https://lccn.loc.gov/2019057712

Cover Design: Wiley
Cover Images: Doctor on the ward © sturti /Getty Images, Human liver with hepatitis © ALFRED PASIEKA/SCIENCE PHOTO LIBRARY/Getty Images, Hepatitis C virus © JUAN GAERTNER/SCIENCE PHOTO LIBRARY, Liver with Hepatitis B © Kateryna Kon/Shutterstock, Medical of human tumour © Pan Xunbin / Getty Images

Set in 8.75/12pt Minion by SPi Global, Pondicherry, India

Printed and bound in Singapore by Markono Print Media Pte Ltd

10   9   8   7   6   5   4   3   2   1

Contents

List of Contributors, vii

Preface, xi

Part I: Investigating the Liver

1 Noninvasive markers of fibrosis: how reliable
are they?, 3
Laurent Castera

2 Liver biopsy in chronic viral hepatitis: is there still
life left in it?, 9
Jaspreet Suri and Michael P. Curry

3 Screening for hepatocellular carcinoma in viral liver
disease: any new biomarkers on the horizon?, 15
Saroja Bangaru, Jorge A. Marrero, and Amit G. Singal

4 Realistic estimates of hepatitis C virus and
hepatitis B virus disease burden, 19
Homie Razavi

PART II: Today's Therapies

Section 1: HCV
5 Acute hepatitis C: treat immediately or give a chance
to spontaneously clear?, 29
David E. Kaplan

6 Is ribavirin alive or dead in the current
era of HCV therapy?, 35
Vijay Prabhakar and Paul Y. Kwo

7 Hepatitis C virus genotype and viral testing, and
on-treatment monitoring: necessary or overkill?, 41
Sirina Ekpanyapong and K. Rajender Reddy

8 Treatment of hepatitis C virus in renal disease:
can we use all the drugs without additional
monitoring?, 48
Stanislas Pol

9 Does directly acting antiviral therapy improve
quality of life?, 54
Daniel M. Forton

10 Morbid obesity and hepatitis C: treat as normal
or are there additional issues to consider?, 59
*María Fernanda Guerra, Javier Ampuero,
and Manuel Romero-Gómez*

11 Generic direct-acting antiviral agents: do they
work well?, 66
Omar Salim Al Siyabi and Seng-Gee Lim

12 Impact and management of patients with multiple
hepatitis C virus genotypes, 74
Peter Ferenci

13 Hepatitis C virus and injecting drug use:
what are the challenges?, 78
Olav Dalgard

14 Hepatitis B virus reactivation while on hepatitis C virus
direct-acting antiviral therapy: is that a real concern and
when is it a concern?, 82
Marina Serper

15 Drug–drug interactions with direct-acting antivirals:
when do we need to care?, 86
Fiona Marra and David Back

16 Treatment of hepatitis C in children, 94
Maureen M. Jonas

17 While direct-acting antivirals are effective,
are there any unique safety considerations?, 97
Olivia Pietri, Félix Trottier-Tellier, and Marc Bourlière

18 Harm reduction strategies to prevent new infections
and reinfections among people who inject drugs:
how effective are they?, 106
Jason Grebely and Marianne Martinello

19 Hepatitis C virus therapy in advanced liver disease: treat or transplant and treat?, 112
Chalermrat Bunchorntavakul and K. Rajender Reddy

20 Hepatocellular carcinoma and hepatitis C virus: which should be treated first?, 117
Mario U. Mondelli, Andrea Lombardi, and Massimo Colombo

21 Should we incentivize patients to take hepatitis C virus therapy?, 122
Ed Gane

22 Treating prisoners with hepatitis C: should we do it and how?, 125
Seth Francis-Graham and William Rosenberg

23 Use of hepatitis C virus-positive organs for uninfected recipients in the era of effective and safe direct-acting antivirals: pros and cons, 132
Sirina Ekpanyapong and K. Rajender Reddy

24 Is real-life hepatitis C virus therapy as effective as in clinical trials?, 138
Jessica Su and Joseph K. Lim

Section 2: HBV, HDV, and HEV
25 Management of acute hepatitis B infection: when should we offer antiviral therapy?, 145
Emma Hathorn and David J. Mutimer

26 Rethinking the inactive carrier state: management of patients with low-replicative HBeAg-negative chronic hepatitis B and normal liver enzymes, 150
María Buti, Mar Riveiro-Barciela, and Rafael Esteban

27 Hepatitis B e antigen-positive chronic hepatitis B infection with minimal changes on liver biopsy: what to do next, 156
Apostolos Koffas and Patrick T. Kennedy

28 The management of hepatitis B virus in pregnancy, 160
Henry L.Y. Chan

29 Treatment of hepatitis B in children, 164
Maureen M. Jonas

30 Hepatitis B vaccine failures: how do we handle them?, 169
Daniel Shouval

31 The stopping rules in hepatitis B virus therapy: can we provide any guidance?, 175
Florian van Bömmel and Thomas Berg

32 Hepatitis C and hepatitis B coinfection, 182
Chun-Jen Liu and Jia-Horng Kao

33 Chronic hepatitis E virus infection: is it reality or hype and where does it matter?, 189
Nassim Kamar and Jacques Izopet

34 Hepatitis E virus vaccines: have they arrived – when, where and for whom?, 193
Amit Goel and Rakesh Aggarwal

PART III: Clinical Set-up and the Future

35 Do we need expert hepatitis C virus treaters or are amateur treaters good enough?, 203
Shyamasundaran Kottilil and Poonam Mathur

36 Hepatitis C vaccines: how close are we to the promised land?, 208
Timothy Donnison, Senthil Chinnakannan, Paola Cicconi, and Eleanor Barnes

37 Elimination of hepatitis C virus in high-prevalence, low-income countries: is it feasible?, 216
Mahmoud Abdo and Hadeel Gamal Eldeen

38 Hepatitis B virus diagnostics: anything new?, 220
Dina Ginzberg, Robert J. Wong, and Robert G. Gish

PART IV: Ongoing Controversies

39 Is hepatocellular carcinoma risk impacted favorably or unfavorably by hepatitis C virus therapy with direct-acting antivirals?, 233
Giuseppe Cabibbo, Calogero Cammà, and Antonio Craxì

40 Global elimination of hepatitis C virus by 2030: the optimistic view, 238
Gregory J. Dore and Marianne Martinello

41 Global elimination of hepatitis C virus by 2030: the pessimistic view, 244
Thomas G. Cotter and Michael Charlton

Index, 250

List of contributors

Mahmoud Abdo
Department of Endemic Medicine and
  Hepatology
Faculty of Medicine, Cairo University
Cairo, Egypt

Rakesh Aggarwal
Jawaharlal Institute of Postgraduate Medical
  Education & Research
Puducherry, India

Omar Salim Al Siyabi
Division of Gastroenterology and Hepatology
Department of Medicine
Royal Hospital, Oman

Javier Ampuero
UCM Digestive Diseases and CIBEREHD
Virgen del Rocío University Hospital
Institute of Biomedicine of Seville
University of Seville
Sevilla, Spain

David Back
Department of Molecular and Clinical
  Pharmacology
University of Liverpool
Liverpool, UK

Saroja Bangaru
Division of Digestive and Liver Diseases
UT Southwestern Medical Center
Dallas, TX, USA

Eleanor Barnes
Peter Medawar Building for Pathogen
  Research
University of Oxford
Oxford, UK

Thomas Berg
Section of Hepatology
University of Leipzig
Leipzig, Germany

Marc Bourlière
Hepato-gastroenterology Department
Hospital Saint Joseph
Marseilles, France

Chalermrat Bunchorntavakul
Division of Gastroenterology and Hepatology
Department of Internal Medicine
Rajavithi Hospital, College of Medicine
Rangsit University
Bangkok, Thailand

María Buti
Liver Unit, Department of Internal Medicine
Hospital Universitari Vall d'Hebron
Universitat Autònoma de Barcelona
Barcelona;
Centro de Investigación Biomédica en Red de
  Enfermedades Hepáticas y Digestivas
  (CIBERehd)
Instituto de Salud Carlos III
Madrid, Spain

Giuseppe Cabibbo
Section of Gastroenterology and Hepatology
Dipartimento di Promozione della Salute
Materno Infantile, Medicina Interna e
  Specialistica di Eccellenza (PROMISE)
University of Palermo, Palermo, Italy

Calogero Cammà
Section of Gastroenterology and Hepatology
Dipartimento di Promozione della Salute
Materno Infantile, Medicina Interna e
  Specialistica di Eccellenza (PROMISE)
University of Palermo, Palermo, Italy

Laurent Castera
Department of Hepatology
Hôpital Beaujon
Assistance Publique-Hôpitaux de Paris
INSERM UMR 1149-CRI
University Denis Diderot Paris-7
Clichy, France

Henry L.Y. Chan
Department of Medicine and
  Therapeutics
The Chinese University of
  Hong Kong
Hong Kong SAR, China

Michael Charlton
Center for Liver Diseases
University of Chicago Medicine
Chicago, IL, USA

Senthil Chinnakannan
Peter Medawar Building for Pathogen
  Research
University of Oxford
Oxford, UK

Paola Cicconi
Peter Medawar Building for Pathogen
  Research;
Jenner Vaccine Trials
Nuffield Department of Medicine
University of Oxford
Oxford, UK

Massimo Colombo
Department of Internal Medicine
Center for Translational Research
  in Hepatology
Humanitas, Rozzano, Italy

Thomas G. Cotter
Center for Liver Diseases
University of Chicago Medicine
Chicago, IL, USA

Antonio Craxì
Section of Gastroenterology and Hepatology
Dipartimento di Promozione della Salute
Materno Infantile, Medicina Interna e
Specialistica di Eccellenza (PROMISE)
University of Palermo, Palermo, Italy

Michael P. Curry
Division of Gastroenterology and Hepatology
Department of Medicine
Beth Israel Deaconess Medical Center
Harvard Medical School
Boston, MA, USA

Olav Dalgard
Akershus University Hospital;
University of Oslo
Oslo, Norway

Timothy Donnison
Peter Medawar Building for Pathogen
Research
University of Oxford
Oxford, UK

Gregory J. Dore
The Kirby Institute
UNSW Sydney
Sydney, Australia

Sirina Ekpanyapong
Department of Medicine
Division of Gastroenterology and
Hepatology
University of Pennsylvania
Philadelphia, PA, USA

Hadeel Gamal Eldeen
Department of Endemic Medicine and
Hepatology
Faculty of Medicine, Cairo University
Cairo, Egypt

Rafael Esteban
Liver Unit, Department of Internal Medicine
Hospital Universitari Vall d'Hebron
Universitat Autònoma de Barcelona
Barcelona;

Centro de Investigación Biomédica en Red
de Enfermedades Hepáticas y Digestivas
(CIBERehd)
Instituto de Salud Carlos III
Madrid, Spain

Peter Ferenci
Department of Internal Medicine III
Division of Gastroenterology and
Hepatology
Medical University of Vienna
Vienna, Austria

Daniel M. Forton
St George's University Hospitals NHS
Foundation Trust
London, UK

Seth Francis-Graham
Institute for Liver and Digestive Health
Division of Medicine
University College London
London, UK

Ed Gane
University of Auckland
Auckland
New Zealand

Dina Ginzberg
Department of Medicine
Alameda Health System – Highland
Hospital
Oakland, CA, USA

Robert G. Gish
Division of Gastroenterology and
Hepatology
Stanford Health Care
Palo Alto, CA, USA

Amit Goel
Department of Gastroenterology
Sanjay Gandhi Postgraduate Institute of
Medical Sciences
Lucknow, India

Jason Grebely
The Kirby Institute
UNSW Sydney
Sydney, Australia

María Fernanda Guerra
Digestive Diseases Department
Virgen Macarena University Hospital
Sevilla, Spain

Emma Hathorn
Liver Unit
University Hospitals NHS Foundation
Trust
Birmingham, UK

Jacques Izopet
Department of Virology
University Paul Sabatier
Toulouse, France

Maureen M. Jonas
Children's Hospital Boston
Division of Gastroenterology
Boston, MA, USA

Nassim Kamar
Department of Nephrology
Dialysis and Organ Transplantation
CHU Rangueil
University Paul Sabatier
Toulouse, France

Jia-Horng Kao
Graduate Institute of Clinical Medicine
National Taiwan University College of
Medicine;
Department of Internal Medicine and
Hepatitis Research Center
National Taiwan University Hospital;
Taiwan Liver Disease Consortium
Taipei, Taiwan

David E. Kaplan
Division of Gastroenterology
Department of Medicine
Perelman School of Medicine
University of Pennsylvania;
Corporal Michael J. Crescenz
Veterans Affairs Medical Center;
Philadelphia, PA, USA

Patrick T. Kennedy
Barts Liver Centre
The Blizard Institute
Queen Mary University of London
London, UK

Apostolos Koffas
Barts Liver Centre
The Blizard Institute
Queen Mary University of London
London, UK

Shyamasundaran Kottilil
Institute of Human Virology
University of Maryland School of
  Medicine
Baltimore, MD, USA

Paul Y. Kwo
Gastroenterology/Hepatology Division
Stanford University School of Medicine
Stanford, CA, USA

Joseph K. Lim
Yale Liver Center, Section of Digestive Diseases
Yale University School of Medicine
New Haven, CT, USA

Seng-Gee Lim
Division of Gastroenterology and
  Hepatology, Department of Medicine
National University Health System;
Faculty of Medicine, Yong Loo Lin School
  of Medicine
National University of Singapore, Singapore

Chun-Jen Liu
Graduate Institute of Clinical Medicine
National Taiwan University College of
  Medicine;
Department of Internal Medicine and
  Hepatitis Research Center
National Taiwan University Hospital;
Taiwan Liver Disease Consortium
Taipei, Taiwan

Andrea Lombardi
Division of Infectious Diseases II and
  Immunology
Department of Medical Sciences and
  Infectious Diseases
Fondazione IRCCS Policlinico San
  Matteo di Pavia;
Department of Internal Medicine
  and Therapeutics
University of Pavia
Pavia, Italy

Fiona Marra
Department of Molecular and Clinical
  Pharmacology, University of Liverpool
  Liverpool, UK;

NHS Greater Glasgow and Clyde
Glasgow, Scotland, UK

Jorge A. Marrero
Division of Digestive and Liver Diseases
UT Southwestern Medical Center
Dallas, TX, USA

Marianne Martinello
The Kirby Institute
UNSW Sydney
Sydney, Australia

Poonam Mathur
Institute of Human Virology
University of Maryland School of
  Medicine
Baltimore, MD, USA

Mario U. Mondelli
Division of Infectious Diseases II and
  Immunology
Department of Medical Sciences and
  Infectious Diseases
Fondazione IRCCS Policlinico San
  Matteo di Pavia;
Department of Internal Medicine
  and Therapeutics
University of Pavia
Pavia, Italy

David J. Mutimer
Liver Unit
University Hospitals NHS Foundation
  Trust
Birmingham, UK

Olivia Pietri
Hepato-gastroenterology Department
Hospital Saint Joseph
Marseilles, France

Stanislas Pol
Université Paris Descartes
Hepatology Department
Cochin Hospital, APHP;
INSERM U1223, UMS-20 and
Center for Translational Science
Institut Pasteur
Paris, France

Vijay Prabhakar
Department of Medicine
Stanford University School of Medicine
Stanford, CA, USA

Homie Razavi
Center for Disease Analysis Foundation
  (CDAF)
Lafayette, CO, USA

K. Rajender Reddy
Department of Medicine
Division of Gastroenterology and
  Hepatology
University of Pennsylvania
Philadelphia, PA, USA

Mar Riveiro-Barciela
Liver Unit, Department of Internal
  Medicine
Hospital Universitari Vall d'Hebron
Universitat Autònoma de Barcelona
Barcelona;
Centro de Investigación Biomédica en Red
  de Enfermedades Hepáticas y Digestivas
  (CIBERehd)
Instituto de Salud Carlos III
Madrid, Spain

Manuel Romero-Gómez
UCM Digestive Diseases and CIBEREHD
Virgen del Rocío University Hospital
Institute of Biomedicine of Seville
University of Seville
Sevilla, Spain

William Rosenberg
Institute for Liver and Digestive Health
Division of Medicine
University College London
London, UK

Marina Serper
Division of Gastroenterology and
  Hepatology
Perelman School of Medicine
University of Pennsylvania
Philadelphia, PA, USA

Daniel Shouval
Liver Unit
Hadassah-Hebrew University Hospital
Jerusalem, Israel

Amit G. Singal
Division of Digestive and Liver Diseases
UT Southwestern Medical Center
Dallas, TX, USA

Jessica Su
Department of Internal Medicine
Yale University School of Medicine
New Haven, CT, USA

Jaspreet Suri
Division of Gastroenterology and
    Hepatology
Department of Medicine
Beth Israel Deaconess Medical Center
Harvard Medical School
Boston, MA, USA

Félix Trottier-Tellier
Hepato-gastroenterology Department
Hospital Saint Joseph
Marseilles, France;
Gastroenterology Department
Hôtel-Dieu de Lévis
Lévis, Quebec, Canada

Florian van Bömmel
Section of Hepatology
University of Leipzig
Leipzig, Germany

Robert J. Wong
Division of Gastroenterology and
    Hepatology
Alameda Health System – Highland
    Hospital
Oakland, CA, USA

Preface

Viral hepatitis is a global problem of enormous magnitude and the consequences of chronic liver disease due to hepatitis B virus (HBV) and hepatitis C virus (HCV) have significant economic implications. However, effective therapies are now available and the WHO has recognized that elimination of these infections over the next few years is achievable. We are now approaching a transformative moment in the epidemiology of these infections, with healthcare interventions radically altering the natural history of these diseases. The massive changes that have taken place since the first edition of *Clinical Dilemmas* have revolutionized our approach to the diagnosis and management of these conditions, with new treatments, new diagnostic approaches, and new understanding of the complexities of these diseases. It is therefore timely to launch the second edition of *Clinical Dilemmas* which looks at the new areas of contention that have emerged over the last few years and which will, we hope, contribute to the WHO goals of viral elimination.

This book, the second edition of *Clinical Dilemmas in Viral Liver Diseases*, has been compiled to address the existing controversial understudied questions that arise in day-to-day clinical practice and some of the challenging issues around the global elimination programs. As previously, the book is not intended to be an exhaustive review of a specific topic but to be a focused approach, supported by literature and expert opinion, covering controversial questions and topics where there is divergence of opinion. We have assembled a team of globally recognized investigators and clinicians to address these issues and readers will find the issues tackled to be unique and not readily accessed in standard textbooks or online literature. The style remains simple, with key learning points and practical guidance. We hope you enjoy the book and learn as much as we have while assembling it.

Graham R. Foster, PhD, FRCP
K. Rajender Reddy, MD, FACP, FACG, FRCP, FAASLD

PART I
Investigating the Liver

1 Noninvasive markers of fibrosis: how reliable are they?

Laurent Castera

Department of Hepatology, Hôpital Beaujon, Assistance Publique-Hôpitaux de Paris, INSERM UMR 1149-CRI, University Denis Diderot Paris-7, Clichy, France

LEARNING POINTS

- Noninvasive tests must always be interpreted critically, according to the context of use and setting (primary healthcare or tertiary referral center and clinical context), taking into account the recommended quality criteria for each test and its possible pitfalls.

- Limitations include cost and availability for patented serum markers, and operator experience and obesity for transient elastography.

- The most validated serum markers are APRI and FIB-4 (nonpatented) and FibroTest® (patented).

- Transient elastography is a point-of-care technique and the most validated and accurate for diagnosing cirrhosis (better at ruling out than ruling in), outperforming serum markers.

- Noninvasive tests (transient elastography >> serum markers) are recommended as first line for detection of cirrhosis before antiviral treatment in patients with viral hepatitis.

- In patients with cirrhosis, posttreatment decrease in liver stiffness should not substitute for the recommended, periodic surveillance for hepatocellular carcinoma.

Introduction

Staging of liver fibrosis and early detection of compensated cirrhosis are critical in the management and surveillance of patients with chronic viral liver disease. For many years, liver biopsy has been considered the "gold standard" for evaluation of hepatic fibrosis. However, liver biopsy is an invasive procedure with rare but potentially life-threatening complications and prone to sampling errors. These limitations, as well as the availability of powerful virologic tools and antiviral agents, have rapidly decreased the use of liver biopsy in patients with chronic viral hepatitis and led to the development of noninvasive methods. These methods are now widely used in clinical practice and recommended by international and European Association for the Study of the Liver (EASL) guidelines [1–5].

Currently available noninvasive methods

Among the currently available noninvasive methods, there are two distinct approaches: (i) a "biological" approach based on the dosage of serum markers of fibrosis; (ii) a "physical" approach based on the measurement of liver stiffness, using either ultrasound (US) or magnetic resonance (MR)-based elastography techniques. Although complementary, these two approaches are based on different rationales and conceptions: liver stiffness is related to elasticity, which corresponds to a genuine and intrinsic physical property of liver parenchyma, whereas serum biomarkers are combinations of several, not strictly liver-specific, blood parameters optimized to mimic fibrosis stages as assessed by liver biopsy. The critical endpoint in clinical practice is the detection of cirrhosis as the choice of direct-acting antiviral agents in hepatitis C virus (HCV) patients and the posttreatment prognosis depend on the stage of fibrosis. Finally, treatment with nucleoside analogs should not be stopped in hepatitis B virus (HBV) patients with cirrhosis.

Clinical Dilemmas in Viral Liver Disease, Second Edition. Edited by Graham R. Foster and K. Rajender Reddy.
© 2020 John Wiley & Sons Ltd. Published 2020 by John Wiley & Sons Ltd.

Serum markers of liver fibrosis

Many serum markers have been evaluated for their ability to detect cirrhosis in patients with chronic viral liver disease. Details can be found elsewhere [1]. Their respective advantages and limitations are summarized in Table 1.1. Nonpatented tests are cost-free, easy to calculate, and almost universally available, whereas patented tests are commercially available proprietary formulae.

Liver stiffness measurement

Transient elastography (TE) was the first commercially available ultrasound-based elastography method developed for the measurement of liver stiffness, using a dedicated device (FibroScan®, Echosens, Paris, France). Several other liver elasticity-based imaging techniques challenging TE have been developed, including point shear wave elastography (pSWE), also known as acoustic radiation force impulse imaging (ARFI), (2-D) shear-wave elastography (2D-SWE), and magnetic resonance elastography (MRE) [6]. Their respective advantages and limitations are summarized in Table 1.1. The units and scales are different between the different techniques. The main limitation of TE in clinical practice is its limited applicability in cases of obesity, which is solved with the use of an XL probe. Confounding factors for liver stiffness, whatever the technique, include inflammation (transaminases $>5 \times$ upper limit of normal [ULN]), liver congestion, food intake, and extrahepatic cholestasis. Procedures should be performed using a standardized protocol in fasting patients (for at least two hours).

Diagnostic performance of noninvasive methods for diagnosing cirrhosis

Serum biomarkers of fibrosis

Among nonpatented tests, the AST to Platelet Ratio Index (APRI) and the Fibrosis-4 (FIB-4) are the most extensively studied and validated with evidence based on large metaanalyses [7,8], including several thousands of patients reporting area under the receiver operating characteristic curve (AUROC) for diagnosing cirrhosis ranging from 0.73 to 0.84 (Table 1.2). They all perform better at ruling out than ruling in cirrhosis with high negative predictive value (>90%).

As for patented tests, the FibroTest® is the most extensively studied, mainly in patients with viral hepatitis. However, all patented tests lack external validation, and metaanalyses independent from the developers are very

few [9]. When compared with nonpatented tests, patented tests offer slight improvement in accuracy but their widespread application is limited by cost and availability.

Liver stiffness measurement

The diagnostic accuracy of TE for cirrhosis is based on large metaanalyses including several thousands of patients with viral hepatitis [10,11] and considered excellent with AUROCs of 0.93–0.94, and sensitivities and specificities of 86–87% and 89–91%, respectively (Table 1.2). However, a metaanalysis based on individual data is still awaited. Actually, TE is better at ruling out than ruling in liver cirrhosis (with negative predictive value higher than 90%).

Different cut-offs have been proposed for HBV and HCV but no consensus has been reached. As shown in Table 1.2, cut-offs for cirrhosis ranged from 9.0 to 16.9 kPa in HBV. This may be related to the so-called spectrum bias, depending on the uneven distribution of different fibrosis stages in different cohorts. In that respect, the 2015 Baveno VI consensus workshop recommended a diagnosis of compensated liver cirrhosis in asymptomatic patients using TE, if liver stiffness values are repeatedly (two different days, fasting) >15 kPa [12]. When compared head to head with serum markers, TE outperforms all of them. ARFI performance for diagnosing cirrhosis has been evaluated mainly in viral hepatitis with high accuracy (AUROC 0.91) and cut-off of 2.42 m/sec [13]. When compared with TE, ARFI has equivalent results. 2D-SWE has been evaluated in a single metaanalysis [14], based on individual data in 1340 patients with chronic liver disease, reporting high accuracies (AUROCs 0.93–0.95) for cirrhosis with an optimal cut-off of 13.5 kPa. When compared to TE in this metaanalysis, no significant difference was found, if the quality criteria of TE were respected. As for MRE, evidence is based on a few hundred patients, but with excellent accuracy (97%) for diagnosing cirrhosis [15]. However, widespread use of this method will depend on cost and availability.

Finally, it should be kept in mind that cut-offs for cirrhosis are system specific.

Use in clinical practice

Before starting antiviral treatment

The EASL clinical practice guidelines recommend that all patients with chronic hepatitis B or C should be assessed for liver disease severity before antiviral therapy using noninvasive tests as first line [2,3]. Serum levels of

Table 1.1 Respective advantages and limitations of currently available non-invasive methods in patients with chronic liver disease

Serum markers	Measurement of liver stiffness			
	Transient elastography (TE)	ARFI (pSWE)	2D-SWE	MR elastography
Advantages				
• Good reproducibility • High applicability (95%) • No cost and wide availability (nonpatented) • Well validated • Can be performed in primary healthcare setting	• Most widely used and validated technique: standard to be beaten • Point-of care technique • Can be performed by nurses • High range of values (2–75 kPa) • Quality criteria well defined (IQR/M <30%) • Good reproducibility • High performance for cirrhosis • Quantification of steatosis (CAP) • Low failure rate in obese patients when using XL probe (3%)	• Can be implemented on a regular US machine • ROI smaller than TE but location chosen by the operator • Higher applicability than TE (ascites and obesity) • Performance equivalent to TE for cirrhosis	• Can be implemented on a regular US machine • ROI can be adjusted in size and location and chosen by the operator • High range of values (2–150 kPa) • Good applicability • Performance equivalentto TE for cirrhosis	• Can be implemented on a regular MRI machine • Examination of the whole liver • Higher applicability than TE (ascites and obesity) • High performance for cirrhosis
Limitations				
• Nonspecific for the liver • Unable to discriminate between intermediate stages of fibrosis • Performance not as good as TE for cirrhosis • Cost and limited availability (patented) • Limitations (hemolysis, Gilbert syndrome, inflammation…)	• Requires a dedicated device • ROI cannot be chosen • Unable to discriminate between intermediate stages of fibrosis • Applicability (80%) lower than serum markers (obesity, ascites, operator experience) • False positive in cases of acute hepatitis, cholestasis, liver congestion, food intake, and excessive alcohol intake	• Unable to discriminate between intermediate stages of fibrosis • Units (m/sec) different from that of TE (kPa) • Narrow range of values (0.5–4.4 m/sec) • Quality criteria not well defined • Cannot be perfomed by nurses	• Further validation warranted • Unable to discriminate between intermediate stages of fibrosis • Quality criteria not well defined • Cannot be perfomed by nurses	• Further validation warranted, especially in comparison with TE • Small range of values (2–11 kPa) • Not applicable in case of iron overload • Time-consuming • Limited availability • Costly

Source: Adapted from reference [1].
ROI, region of interest.

Table 1.2 Diagnostic performances (metaanalyses) of serum markers and elastography techniques for cirrhosis taking liver biopsy as reference

	Etiology	Patients (n)	Cut-offs	Area under receiver operating characteristic	Sensitivity (%)	Specificity (%)e
Serum markers						
Nonpatented						
APRI [8]	HBV	8773	1.0–2.0	0.73	66–31	74–89
[7]	HCV	4548	1.0–2.0	0.83	76–46	72–91
FIB-4 [8]	HBV	6068	1.05–2.65	0.84	87–64	65–86
Patented						
FibroTest [9]	HBV	1754	0.74	0.87	62	91
Liver stiffness						
Ultrasound-based elastography						
Transient elastography [11]	HBV	4386	9.0 16.9 kPa	0.93	86	87
[10]	CLD (HCV)	8206	13.0 kPa	0.94	91	89
ARFI [13]	HBV/HCV	2691	2.42 m/sec	0.91	86	84
2D-SWE [14]	HBV	400	11.5 kPa	0.95	80	93
	HCV	379	13.0 kPa	0.93	86	88
Magnetic resonance-based elastography						
[15]	HBV	1470	4.6 kPa	0.97	89	92

CLD, chronic liver disease; HBV, hepatitis B virus; HCV, hepatitis C virus.

aminotransferases should be taken into account in interpreting TE results in patients with hepatitis B. To avoid the risk of false-positive results, some authors have proposed adopting TE cut-offs based on levels of alanine aminotransferase (ALT). In cases of unexplained discordance or suspected additional etiologies of liver disease, a liver biopsy is still recommended [2,3].

Monitoring of fibrosis regression in treated patients

Several studies have reported a significant decrease in liver stiffness and biomarker values, compared with baseline values, in HBV patients treated with analogs and in HCV patients who achieved sustained virologica response (SVR), consistent with significant histologic improvement documented in studies of paired liver biopsies in these patients. It should be stressed, however, that these studies suffer from several methodologic shortcomings: most are retrospective, with small sample size and short follow-up and, most importantly, no paired liver biopsies.

Nevertheless, in a recent metaanalysis based on 24 studies (10 with DAA), including a total of 2934 HCV patients, SVR was associated with a significant decrease in liver stiffness, particularly in patients with high baseline level of inflammation or patients who received direct-acting agents [16]. Almost half the patients considered to have advanced fibrosis, based on TE, before therapy achieved posttreatment liver stiffness levels <9.5 kPa. Similarly, in a recent study in 164 HBV Chinese patients treated with telbivudine and paired with liver biopsies (baseline and week 104), a two-phase decline in liver stiffness was observed: rapid within the first 24 weeks (−2.2 kPa/24 weeks) in parallel with ALT levels, then slower (−0.3 kPa/24 weeks) but continous from week 24 to week 104 while ALT levels remained within the normal range [17]. This pattern suggests that the first phase decline was mostly related to inflammation whereas the second phase could be related to fibrosis improvement. Although this study is the only one to date with paired liver biopsies, only 10 patients had baseline cirrhosis and no information was available regarding the regression of cirrhosis. Finally, in a large cohort of HBV patients (n = 575) treated with tenofovir and baseline liver biopsy, APRI or FIB-4 reduction did not correlate with fibrosis regression after 240 weeks of antiviral therapy [18].

Thus, although it is tempting to use noninvasive tests to assess fibrosis regression in treated patients with chronic hepatitis B or C, no recommendation can be made, given the influence of inflammation on serum biomarkers and liver stiffness. In patients with cirrhosis, posttreatment decrease in liver stiffness should not replace the recommended periodic surveillance for hepatocellular carcinoma, using ultrasound examination and measurement of alpha-fetoprotein levels.

Monitoring of disease progression

In patients with liver stiffness values in the range of liver cirrhosis, screening for portal hypertension and hepatocellular carcinoma (HCC) is also recommended without prior liver biopsy. A metaanalysis based on 17 studies in 7058 patients with chronic liver diseases (mainly related to viral hepatitis) has shown that baseline liver stiffness, measured using TE, was significantly associated with risk of hepatic decompensation (six studies; relative risk [RR] 1.07; 95% confidence interval [CI] 1.03–1.11), hepatocellular carcinoma (nine studies; RR 1.11; 95% CI 1.05–1.18), death (five studies; RR 1.22; 95% CI 1.05–1.43), or a composite of these outcomes (seven studies; RR 1.32; 95% CI 1.16–1.51) [19]. Thus, the potential of liver stiffness values for predicting clinical outcomes seems to be greater than that of liver biopsy, probably because liver stiffness measures chart ongoing pathophysiologic processes and functions that a biopsy cannot. As for other elastography techniques, data are currently lacking in viral hepatitis B or C.

The 2015 Baveno VI consensus recommendations stated that: (i) in patients with viral-related compensated advanced chronic liver disease (cACLD), TE (≥20–25 kPa) alone or combined with platelets and spleen size is sufficient to rule in clinically significant portal hypertension, defining the group of patients at risk of having endoscopic signs of portal hypertension; (ii) in patients with a liver stiffness <20 kPa and a platelet count >150 000, the risk of having varices requiring treatment is very low and screening endoscopy can be avoided [12]. Interestingly, the performance of these criteria has been confirmed independently in various populations and all studies confirmed that about 20% of upper gastrointestinal (GI) endoscopies could be safely avoided, missing less than 4% of patients with varices needing treatment [20]. These recommendations represent a significant advance in the management of patients with viral hepatitis and early cirrhosis and can be confidently applied in everyday practice. Recently, expanded Baveno VI criteria (liver stiffness <25 kPa and

platelet count >110 000) have been proposed [21], allowing avoidance of around 40% of endoscopies and missing less than 5% of patients with varices needing treatment. As for ARFI and 2D-SWE, given the very limited number of studies reporting on their performance for detection of esophageal varices, no recommendation can be made [20].

Conclusions and perspectives

Considerable progress has been made over the past decade in noninvasive assessment of liver disease in patients with hepatitis B and C. Noninvasive tests are now widely used in clinical practice and recommended by national and international guidelines as first-line tools for the management of these patients together with transaminases and serologic and virologic markers. The choice of test may depend on accuracy, reliability and local availability, as well as cost. Importantly, clinicians need to keep in mind the importance of interpreting critically the results of the different noninvasive tests with the risk of false-positive results, given the frequence of flare of necroinflammation in patients with chronic hepatitis B. In doubtful cases or in those with comorbidities, a liver biopsy should still be performed, especially before starting antiviral treatment. TE as a point-of-care technique remains the most widely used and validated method. There is also growing evidence for the prognostic value of liver stiffness in the context of cirrhosis, which can be used to stratify patients at risk of developing complications. There are, however, promising challengers for the measurement of liver stiffness, such as ARFI and 2D-SWE, whose place in practice remains to be better defined. Finally, noninvasive tests may also be used for screening liver fibrosis in populations at risk for hepatitis B and C or in the general population [22]. This is now becoming an area of active research.

References

1. EASL-ALEH Clinical Practice Guidelines. Non-invasive tests for evaluation of liver disease severity and prognosis. *Journal of Hepatology* 2015;63:237–264.
2. EASL. Clinical practice guidelines on the management of hepatitis B virus infection. *Journal of Hepatology* 2017;67: 370–398.
3. EASL. Recommendations on treatment of hepatitis C 2018. *Journal of Hepatology* 2018;69:461–511.

4. Dietrich C, Bamber J, Berzigotti A et al. EFSUMB Guidelines and Recommendations on the Clinical Use of Liver Ultrasound Elastography, Update 2017. *European Journal of Ultrasound* 2017;38:e16–e47.

5. Ferraioli G, Wong VW, Castera L et al. Liver ultrasound elastography: an update to the World Federation for Ultrasound in Medicine and Biology Guidelines and Recommendations. *Ultrasound in Medicine and Biology* 2018;44:2419–2440.

6. Friedrich-Rust M, Poynard T, Castera L. Critical comparison of elastography methods to assess chronic liver disease. *Nature Reviews Gastroenterology and Hepatology* 2016;13: 402–411.

7. Lin ZH, Xin YN, Dong QJ et al. Performance of the aspartate aminotransferase-to-platelet ratio index for the staging of hepatitis C-related fibrosis: an updated meta-analysis. *Hepatology* 2011;53:726–736.

8. Xiao G, Yang J, Yan L. Comparison of diagnostic accuracy of aspartate aminotransferase to platelet ratio index and fibrosis-4 index for detecting liver fibrosis in adult patients with chronic hepatitis B virus infection: a systemic review and meta-analysis. *Hepatology* 2015;61:292–302.

9. Salkic NN, Jovanovic P, Hauser G, Brcic M. FibroTest/ Fibrosure for significant liver fibrosis and cirrhosis in chronic hepatitis B: a meta-analysis. *American Journal of Gastroenterology* 2014;109:796–809.

10. Friedrich-Rust M, Ong MF, Martens S et al. Performance of transient elastography for the staging of liver fibrosis: a meta-analysis. *Gastroenterology* 2008;134:960–974.

11. Li Y, Huang YS, Wang ZZ et al. Systematic review with meta-analysis: the diagnostic accuracy of transient elastography for the staging of liver fibrosis in patients with chronic hepatitis B. *Alimentary Pharmacology and Therapeutics* 2016;43:458–469.

12. de Franchis R, Baveno VIF. Expanding consensus in portal hypertension: report of the Baveno VI consensus workshop: stratifying risk and individualizing care for portal hypertension. *Journal of Hepatology* 2015;63:743–752.

13. Hu X, Qiu L, Liu D, Qian L. Acoustic Radiation Force Impulse (ARFI) Elastography for noninvasive evaluation of hepatic fibrosis in chronic hepatitis B and C patients: a systematic review and meta-analysis. *Medical Ultrasonography* 2017;19: 23–31.

14. Herrmann E, de Lédinghen V, Cassinotto C et al. Assessment of biopsy-proven liver fibrosis by two-dimensional shear wave elastography: an individual patient data-based meta-analysis. *Hepatology* 2018;67:260–272.

15. Xiao H, Shi M, Xie Y, Chi X. Comparison of diagnostic accuracy of magnetic resonance elastography and Fibroscan for detecting liver fibrosis in chronic hepatitis B patients: a systematic review and meta-analysis. *PLoS One* 2017;12: e0186660.

16. Singh S, Facciorusso A, Loomba R, Falck-Ytter YT. Magnitude and kinetics of decrease in liver stiffness after antiviral therapy in patients with chronic hepatitis C: a systematic review and meta-analysis. *Clinical Gastroenterology and Hepatology* 2018;16:27–38 e24.

17. Liang X, Xie Q, Tan D et al. Interpretation of liver stiffness measurement-based approach for the monitoring of hepatitis B patients with antiviral therapy: a 2-year prospective study. *Journal of Viral Hepatology* 2018;25:296–305.

18. Kim WR, Berg T, Asselah T et al. Evaluation of APRI and FIB-4 scoring systems for non-invasive assessment of hepatic fibrosis in chronic hepatitis B patients. *Journal of Hepatology* 2016;64:773–780.

19. Singh S, Fujii LL, Murad MH et al. Liver stiffness is associated with risk of decompensation, liver cancer, and death in patients with chronic liver diseases: a systematic review and meta-analysis. *Clinical Gastroenterology and Hepatology* 2013;11:1573–1584 e1571–1572; quiz e1588–1579.

20. Berzigotti A. Non-invasive evaluation of portal hypertension using ultrasound elastography. *Journal of Hepatology* 2017;67: 399–411.

21. Augustin S, Pons M, Maurice JB et al. Expanding the Baveno VI criteria for the screening of varices in patients with compensated advanced chronic liver disease. *Hepatology* 2017;66: 1980–1988.

22. Gines P, Graupera I, Lammert F et al. Screening for liver fibrosis in the general population: a call for action. *Lancet Gastroenterology and Hepatology* 2016;1:256–260.

2 Liver biopsy in chronic viral hepatitis: is there still life left in it?

Jaspreet Suri and Michael P. Curry

Division of Gastroenterology and Hepatology, Department of Medicine, Beth Israel Deaconess Medical Center, Harvard Medical School, Boston, MA, USA

LEARNING POINTS

- While liver biopsy has been the gold standard tool for the diagnosis and staging of the degree of fibrosis, its role has steadily declined with the advent of disease-specific diagnostic serologic markers and noninvasive markers for evaluation of fibrosis.

- Noninvasive tests and diagnostic modalities can provide us with enough information to assess liver fibrosis and advise patients on the prognosis of their disease, especially in chronic viral hepatitis.

- There may still be a role for liver biopsy in the assessment of liver inflammation in chronic hepatitis B virus (HBV) infection.

- Liver biopsy may additionally be helpful in objective assessment of inflammation, in detecting coexisting steatosis secondary to alternative causes of liver injury such as alcohol, and in assessing hepatic iron distribution in cases of elevated serum ferritin.

Liver biopsy

Liver biopsy has been an important diagnostic tool for the evaluation and management of patients with chronic liver disease. It has been the gold standard by which all other assessments are compared, but it has also been associated with significant morbidity and rare instances of mortality. Thus, with the advent of noninvasive measures for evaluating liver fibrosis in patients with chronic viral hepatitis, the utility of liver biopsy has declined [1].

The first percutaneous liver biopsy was performed by Paul Ehrlich in Germany in 1883. Its use was popularized in the United States by Baron in the 1930s and then with Menghini and the "one second needle biopsy of the liver" technique in 1958 [2,3]. Liver biopsy techniques have undergone many improvements over time to reduce the risk of complications. To combat the increased risk of bleeding via the percutaneous biopsy in high-risk patients with acquired coagulopathy, the transvenous approach was introduced in 1967 [4]. In an effort to improve sensitivity and reduce the possibility of missing liver cirrhosis, diagnostic laparoscopic liver biopsy became accepted in some practices and has proven to be safe and valuable in the evaluation of patients with chronic liver disease [5]. More recently, endoscopic ultrasound-guided transgastric liver biopsy has emerged as a potential method with promising tissue yields and overall safety profile and may be a viable option in patients already undergoing upper endoscopy with need for concurrent liver biopsy [6].

Notwithstanding the advances in technique which have improved the safety and accuracy of liver biopsy, there remain significant limitations. It is an invasive test that is not acceptable to all patients because of the risk of complications. It samples only a tiny piece of the liver (1/50 000), which is prone to both intra- and interobserver error. Lastly, it is impractical to suggest that all patients worldwide with chronic viral hepatitis be subjected to liver biopsy as a prerequisite to treatment. So while liver biopsy remains the gold standard in diagnosis of liver disease, as

Clinical Dilemmas in Viral Liver Disease, Second Edition. Edited by Graham R. Foster and K. Rajender Reddy.
© 2020 John Wiley & Sons Ltd. Published 2020 by John Wiley & Sons Ltd.

predicted by the American Association for the Study of Liver Disease (AASLD) guideline published in 2009, non-invasive imaging and serum makers are replacing liver biopsy for the evaluation of liver fibrosis [1]. These noninvasive tests and diagnostic modalities can provide us with enough information to assess liver fibrosis and advise patients on the prognosis of their disease, especially in chronic viral hepatitis.

Serologic markers

Panels of serum markers that have been studied and validated include AST to platelet Ratio Index (APRI), FibroTest®/FibroSure®, Hepascore®, FibroSpect II®, and European Liver Fibrosis Study Group panel (ELF). These can be divided into "indirect" serologic markers, which reflect alterations in hepatic function, and "direct" markers that reflect extracellular matrix turnover, which occurs in ongoing liver fibrosis. APRI, FibroTest, and Hepascore can be used to accurately differentiate between significant fibrosis (METAVIR stage F2–F4) and nonsignificant fibrosis (METAVIR F0–F1) [7]. The APRI score, a panel of indirect markers of hepatic fibrosis, is calculated by dividing the AST elevation by the platelet count per millimeter cubed and multiplying that number by 100. Primarily evaluated in patients with hepatitis C virus (HCV) and HIV/HCV coinfection, with a cut-off score of 0.7, it has a sensitivity of 77% and specificity of 72%percent for predicting significant fibrosis [8]. FibroTest and FibroSure, identical tests marketed under different names regionally, have primarily been studied in patients with chronic viral hepatitis B and hepatitis C including levels of alpha-2-macroglobulin, haptoglobin, gammaglobulin, apolipoprotein A1, gamma-glutamyl transferase (GGT), and total bilirubin, as well as demographic factors of age and sex [9]. This assay has a sensitivity of 60–75% and a specificity of 80–90% for detecting significant fibrosis [10–14]. Hepascore has also been validated in patients with hepatitis C with a sensitivity of 82% and specificity of 65% for detecting significant fibrosis when using a cut-off score of ≥0.55 [15].

Of the "direct" markers of liver fibrosis, FibroSpect II and ELF have been shown to be the most accurate. FibroSpect is a combination of serum hyaluronic acid, tissue inhibitor of metalloproteinase-1, and alpha-2-macroglobulin. In chronic hepatitis C patients, FibroSpect can reliably differentiate

between no or mild fibrosis and moderate to severe fibrosis with a sensitivity of 77% and a specificity of 73% [16–18]. ELF which incorporates hyaluronic acid, amino-terminal propeptide of type III collagen level, and tissue inhibitor of metalloproteinase-1, performs well in detecting moderate to severe fibrosis with a sensitivity of 87–90% and a specificity of 41–51% in all liver diseases [19].

Overall, the limitations of serum markers include the inability to differentiate between the individual stages of fibrosis, the fact that they are surrogates, they are affected by clearance rates of the individual patients, none are liver specific therefore they can be affected by other sites of inflammation, the availability of testing is institutionally dependent, and indeterminate results are common.

Imaging alternatives to liver biopsy

Elastography and conventional cross-sectional imaging have also made advancements in providing reliable assessments of fibrosis in chronic viral hepatitis and therefore limiting the role of liver biopsy today. Elastography estimates liver stiffness by applying mechanical waves and measuring their propagation speed through tissue using imaging. Associated imaging modalities include ultrasound (transient elastography [TE], acoustic radiation force impulse imaging [ARFI], two-dimensional shear wave elastography), and magnetic resonance imaging (magnetic resonance elastography [MRE]).

Transient elastography has been validated in large populations and has become widely available. TE uses shear wave imaging to estimate liver stiffness. The procedure involves a mechanical vibrating probe that is applied to the skin overlying the liver; shear waves created by excitation from the probe are measured by an ultrasound detector. In chronic viral hepatitis, TE can be used to accurately diagnosis cirrhosis as well as differentiate reliably between advanced or minimal to no fibrosis. Estimates for the diagnosis of liver cirrhosis are influenced by the etiology of liver disease and the cut-off level for cirrhosis. TE has a high area under the curve receiver operating characteristic (AUROC) for both HCV (fibrosis stage ≥F2: 0.89; fibrosis stage ≥F3: 0.92; fibrosis stage =F4: 0.92) and for HBV (fibrosis stage ≥F2: 0.73; fibrosis stage ≥F3: 0.83; fibrosis stage =F4: 0.90) in large multicenter studies [20,21]. FibroScan®, a compact and transportable TE apparatus, is a readily available point-of-care assessment in Europe and the United States and can be performed at the bedside by trained personnel during a patient's clinic appointment with a result, available in minutes, ready to interpret by the primary provider before the patient leaves the office.

Acoustic radiation force impulse imaging is a form of tissue elastography that uses strain imaging rather than shear wave imaging to estimate liver fibrosis. It is incorporated into some conventional diagnostic ultrasound machines, giving the advantage of obtaining conventional two-dimensional ultrasound images for structural abnormalities and assessing liver fibrosis during the same evaluation. A short-duration, high-intensity acoustic pulse is applied and tissue displacement is measured in the same direction as the stress. One single-center study of 321 patients with chronic liver disease, including those with viral hepatitis, demonstrated comparable detection for early- and late-stage liver fibrosis between ARFI and TE but ARFI performed better for detection of stage F4 fibrosis in nonobese patients [22]. Metanalysis of studies comparing ARFI to liver biopsy has demonstrated good diagnostic accuracy of ARFI for fibrosis stage ≥F2 (AUROC =87%), ≥F3 (AUROC =91%) and =F4 (AUROC =93%) [23].

Unlike ultrasound-based elastography, MRE provides a very robust method to evaluate liver stiffness and thus liver fibrosis as it can evaluate the entire liver and is not limited to a defined volume based on the device. It can be performed as part of conventional MRI with additional hardware and software to conduct elastography in the same instance. A metaanalysis of 12 studies on MRE revealed that when using an optimal cut-off of 3.45 kPa, it has a sensitivity of 73% and specificity of 79% for detecting any fibrosis stage F1 or higher. For detecting significant fibrosis F2 or higher, using a cut-off of 3.66 kPa gives a sensitivity of 79% and specificity of 81%. Advanced fibrosis stage F3 or above can be detected with a sensitivity and specificity of 85% when using a cut-off of 4.11 kPa. Cirrhosis can be detected with a sensitivity of 91% and specificity of 81% when using a cut-off of 4.71 kPa [24]. In comparison with TE, studies have demonstrated that MRE has a higher technical success rate and better diagnostic accuracy [25–27].

Finally, a combination approach with multiple serologic tests or serum testing and imaging improves our ability to assess liver fibrosis. The "SAFE" approach, or sequential algorithm for fibrosis evaluation, which combines APRI and FibroTest/FibroSure in a stepwise fashion, had good overall accuracy for detecting significant fibrosis and reduced the need for liver biopsy in patients with chronic HCV [28]. Furthermore, a combination of FibroTest and TE conducted in chronic HCV patients demonstrated an AUROC of 0.88 for ≥F2, 0.95 for ≥F3, and 0.95 for =F4 [20]. When the TE and FibroTest results were concordant, liver biopsy examination confirmed the stage in 84% of cases for ≥F2 fibrosis, 95% for ≥F3 fibrosis, and 94% for =F4 fibrosis.

A combined approach with serologic testing and imaging can provide reliable and accurate assessments of fibrosis in chronic viral hepatitis, avoiding the need for a liver biopsy. The specific tests chosen will ultimately be determined by institutional availability.

Guidelines

The AASLD guidelines on liver biopsy were last updated in 2009 and stated that liver biopsy is not needed for the diagnosis of HBV or HCV but that biopsy played an important part in staging both diseases, offered some help in assessing prognosis, and was more helpful in the management of HCV-related liver disease than HBV [1]. These statements were very true in the era of interferon therapy for HCV, when a decision to treat patients with a partially successful therapy depended on the degree of disease progression. The guidance document does note that "the role of histological analysis of the liver in the management of patients with liver disease is likely to evolve over time, particularly as noninvasive modalities for assessment of fibrosis … are more positioned in the mainstream." Additionally, given that virtually all patients with HCV infection can achieve a virologic cure with well-tolerated potent direct-acting antiviral therapy, liver biopsy staging is no longer needed as a triage aid. Thus, the current AASLD/Infectious Disease Society of America (IDSA) guideline on recommendations for testing, managing, and treating HCV infection makes no mention of the use of liver biopsy for the evaluation of liver fibrosis [29]. Additionally, the European Association for Study of the Liver (EASL) recommendations on treatment of HCV go further and recommend that noninvasive methods should be used instead of liver biopsy to assess liver disease severity prior to therapy [30].

While noninvasive methods for liver fibrosis assessment may suffice for chronic hepatitis C treatment decisions, these methods tell us little about the degree of liver inflammation, an important parameter in the treatment decision process for patients with chronic HBV infection. Liver biopsy offers the only means of assessing both fibrosis and inflammation and, in the setting of HBV infection, will provide important information for treatment based on the degree of inflammatory activity. The current AASLD treatment guideline for HBV recommends that liver biopsy be considered in HBeAg-positive patients with serum HBV DNA >20 000 U/L or HBeAg-negative patients with HBV DNA >2000 U/L with persistent borderline normal or slightly elevated alanine aminotransferase (ALT) levels, particularly those over 40 years of age who have been infected from a young age, to assess for moderate to severe inflammation with or without fibrosis as a determination for treatment [31].

Importantly, the Asian-Pacific Association for the Study of the Liver (APASL) and the AASLD guidelines on liver biopsy recommend that when counseling the patient on the need for liver biopsy, alternatives such as noninvasive methods for assessing liver fibrosis be discussed [1,32].

What is the trend?

There are few data published on the trend in the use of liver biopsy in the evaluation of patients with viral hepatitis. In one single-center, retrospective study of the pathology database from 1992 to 2007 at a large urban hospital system by Lipp et al, the vast majority of liver biopsies were performed for the management of chronic viral hepatitis [33]. Liver biopsies for chronic hepatitis C increased annually from 1997 to a peak in 2003. The increase in liver biopsies for HCV from 1997 likely followed the National Institutes of Health (NIH) consensus conference in 1997 that included the recommendation for liver biopsy in the management of HCV infection. The reasons for the decline in liver biopsy requests in cases of HCV were multifactorial. The revised 2002 NIH recommendation that liver biopsy was not always necessary in patients with genotype 2 and 3 and the AASLD practice guideline of 2004 that patients with genotype 2 and 3 be treated regardless of liver disease severity might have contributed to the decline in the number of liver biopsies for HCV in the years after 2003.

For HBV, the number of liver biopsies remained stable during the period between 1992 to 2003. This was attributed to the proposed management algorithm by Keeffe et al. and guidelines published by the AASLD suggesting a baseline liver biopsy as part of the initial work-up in

management of chronic HBV [34,35]. A rise thereafter was attributed to the location of this particular medical center amongst a large Chinese immigrant population in an urban setting in addition to bolstering of the hepatology staff around this time, the combination of which supported a rise in percutaneous liver biopsies ordered.

Obviously, these observations are based on the database of a single center in an urban setting. With that being said, they likely reflect the true trend of the current market as the experience at our center is comparable, though the decline in liver biopsy at our center is related to the early adoption of noninvasive measures of liver fibrosis with serum markers and TE.

Is biopsy needed for the complications of chronic viral hepatitis?

The role of liver biopsy in the diagnosis of hepatocellular carcinoma (HCC) has changed over time. The diagnostic pathway for HCC is now based on the radiologic characteristics of the tumor on contrast-enhanced cross-sectional imaging relegating liver biopsy to the controversial cases. The American College of Radiology, through its Liver Imaging Reporting and Data System (LI-RADS) as well as the Organ Procurement and Transplant Network (OPTN), has developed stringent imaging criteria with high specificity for lesions that are >10 mm including enhancement, in combination with washout and/or a capsule. Lesions not meeting these criteria or smaller than 10 mm could be considered in select cases after careful consideration of the risks and benefits. The EASL has similar criteria but also includes a second radiologic confirmation with a different modality and encourages consideration of biopsy only if the second modality fails to demonstrate the typical vascular pattern of HCC [36]. Additional reasons to consider targeted liver biopsy include diagnostic uncertainty, such as hypovascular lesions that could represent HCC, or for the diagnosis of cholangiocarcinoma (CCA) or mixed CCA/HCC variants.

Is there still life in it?

The role of liver biopsy in chronic viral hepatitis has diminished greatly with the widespread availability and accuracy of noninvasive markers of liver fibrosis. Serum markers of liver fibrosis and imaging modalities of liver stiffness can provide us with enough information to treat viral hepatitis appropriately. There may still be a role for liver biopsy in the assessment of liver inflammation in chronic HBV infection. The most efficient approach to fibrosis assessment in these patients is a combination of direct bio-markers coupled with imaging modalities of liver stiffness measurement [37].

However, liver biopsy may still prove useful in objective assessment of inflammation, in detecting coexisting steato-sis secondary to alternative causes of liver injury such as alcohol, and in assessing hepatic iron distribution in cases of elevated serum ferritin. Additionally, while liver biopsy is a useful tool in the diagnosis of HCC complicating viral hepatitis, targeted liver biopsy is only a valid diagnostic choice when imaging fails to diagnose HCC.

Liver biopsy should also be considered for any patient who has discordant results between serologic or liver stiff-ness measurement that could affect clinical decision mak-ing in terms of long-term surveillance for liver cancer and portal hypertension.

References

1. Rockey DC, Caldwell S, Goodman Z et al. Liver biopsy. *Hepatology* 2009;49(3):1017–1044.
2. Baron E. Aspiration for removal of biopsy material from the liver: report of thirty-five cases. *Archives of Internal Medicine* 1939;63(2):276–289.
3. Menghini G. One-second needle biopsy of the liver. *Gastroenterology* 1958;35(2):190–199.
4. Hanafee W, Weiner M. Transjugular percutaneous cholangi-ography. *Radiology* 1967;88(1):35–39.
5. Vargas C, Jeffers L, Bernstein D et al. Diagnostic laparoscopy: a 5-year experience in a hepatology training program. *American Journal of Gastroenterology* 1995;90(8):1258–1262.
6. Diehl DL, Johal A, Khara H et al. Endoscopic ultrasound-guided liver biopsy: a multicenter experience. *Endoscopy International Open* 2015;3(3):E210–215.
7. Chou R, Wasson N. Blood tests to diagnose fibrosis or cir-rhosis in patients with chronic hepatitis C virus infection: a systematic review. *Annals of Internal Medicine* 2013;158(11): 807–820.
8. Lin ZH, Xin Y, Dong Q et al. Performance of the aspartate ami-notransferase-to-platelet ratio index for the staging of hepatitis C-related fibrosis: an updated meta-analysis. *Hepatology* 2011; 53(3):726–736.
9. Imbert-Bismut F, Ratziu V, Pieroni L et al. Biochemical markers of liver fibrosis in patients with hepatitis C virus

infection: a prospective study. *Lancet* 2001;357(9262): 1069–1075.
10. Myers RP, de Torres M, Imbert-Bismut F et al. Biochemical markers of fibrosis in patients with chronic hepatitis C: a comparison with prothrombin time, platelet count, and age-platelet index. *Digestive Diseases and Sciences* 2003;48(1): 146–153.
11. Myers RP, Benhamou Y, Imbert-Bismut F et al. Serum biochemical markers accurately predict liver fibrosis in HIV and hepatitis C virus co-infected patients. *AIDS* 2003; 17(5):721–725.
12. Rossi E, Adams L, Prins A et al. Validation of the FibroTest biochemical markers score in assessing liver fibrosis in hepatitis C patients. *Clinical Chemistry* 2003;49(3):450–454.
13. Halfon P, Bourliere M, Deydier R et al. Independent prospec-tive multicenter validation of biochemical markers (fibrotest-actitest) for the prediction of liver fibrosis and activity in patients with chronic hepatitis C: the fibropaca study. *American Journal of Gastroenterology* 2006;101(3):547–555.
14. Salkic NN, Jovanovic P, Hauser G et al. FibroTest/Fibrosure for significant liver fibrosis and cirrhosis in chronic hepatitis B: a meta-analysis. *American Journal of Gastroenterology* 2014;109(6):796–809.
15. Becker L, Salameh W, Sferruzza A et al. Validation of hepas-core, compared with simple indices of fibrosis, in patients with chronic hepatitis C virus infection in United States. *Clinical Gastroenterology and Hepatology* 2009;7(6):696–701.
16. Mehta P, Ploutz-Snyder R, Nandi J et al. Diagnostic accuracy of serum hyaluronic acid, FIBROSpect II, and YKL-40 for discriminating fibrosis stages in chronic hepatitis C. *American Journal of Gastroenterology* 2008;103(4):928–936.
17. Patel K, Gordon S, Jacobson I et al. Evaluation of a panel of non-invasive serum markers to differentiate mild from moderate-to-advanced liver fibrosis in chronic hepatitis C patients. *Journal of Hepatology* 2004;41(6):935–942.
18. Patel K, Nelson D, Rockey D et al. Correlation of FIBROSpect II with histologic and morphometric evaluation of liver fibrosis in chronic hepatitis C. *Clinical Gastroenterology and Hepatology* 2008;6(2):242–247.
19. Rosenberg WM, Voelker M, Thiel R et al. Serum markers detect the presence of liver fibrosis: a cohort study. *Gastroenterology* 2004;127(6):1704–1713.
20. Castera L, Vergniol J, Foucher J et al. Prospective comparison of transient elastography, Fibrotest, APRI, and liver biopsy for the assessment of fibrosis in chronic hepatitis C. *Gastroenterology* 2005;128(2):343–350.
21. Ziol M, Handra-Luca A, Kettaneh A et al. Noninvasive assessment of liver fibrosis by measurement of stiffness in patients with chronic hepatitis C. *Hepatology* 2005;41(1): 48–54.

22. Cassinotto C, Lapuyade B, Ait Ali A et al. Liver fibrosis: noninvasive assessment with acoustic radiation force impulse elastography – comparison with FibroScan M and XL probes and FibroTest in patients with chronic liver disease. *Radiology* 2013;269(1):283–292.

23. Friedrich-Rust M, Buggisch P, de Knegt R et al. Acoustic radiation force impulse imaging for non-invasive assessment of liver fibrosis in chronic hepatitis B. *Journal of Viral Hepatology* 2013;20(4):240–247.

24. Singh S, Venkatesh S, Wang Z et al. Diagnostic performance of magnetic resonance elastography in staging liver fibrosis: a systematic review and meta-analysis of individual participant data. *Clinical Gastroenterology and Hepatology* 2015;13(3): 440–451.e6.

25. Yin M, Talwalkar J, Glaser K et al. Assessment of hepatic fibrosis with magnetic resonance elastography. *Clinical Gastroenterology and Hepatology* 2007;5(10):1207–1213.e2.

26. Huwart L, Sempoux C, Vicaut E et al. Magnetic resonance elastography for the noninvasive staging of liver fibrosis. *Gastroenterology* 2008;135(1):32–40.

27. Imajo K, Kessoku T, Honda Y et al. Magnetic resonance imaging more accurately classifies steatosis and fibrosis in patients with nonalcoholic fatty liver disease than transient elastography. *Gastroenterology* 2016;150(3):626–637.e7.

28. Sebastiani G, Halfon P, Castera L et al. SAFE biopsy: a validated method for large-scale staging of liver fibrosis in chronic hepatitis C. *Hepatology* 2009;49(6):1821–1827.

29. AASLD-IDSA HCV Guidance Panel. Hepatitis C Guidance 2018 Update: AASLD-IDSA recommendations for testing, managing and treating hepatitis C virus infection. *Clinical Infectious Diseases* 2018;67:1477–1492.

30. EASL, Recommendation on treatment of hepatitis C 2018. *Journal of Hepatology* 2018;69(2):461–511.

31. Terrault NA, Lok A, McMahon B et al. Update on prevention, diagnosis, and treatment of chronic hepatitis B: AASLD 2018 hepatitis B guidance. *Hepatology* 2018;67(4): 1560–1599.

32. Shiha G, Ibrahim A, Helmy A et al. Asian-Pacific Association for the Study of the Liver (APASL) consensus guidelines on invasive and non-invasive assessment of hepatic fibrosis: a 2016 update. *Hepatology International* 2017;11(1):1–30.

33. Lipp MJ, d'Souza L, Clain D et al. Trends in the indication and method of liver biopsy for hepatitis B and C. *Digestive Diseases and Sciences* 2010;55(10):2971–2976.

34. Keeffe EB, Dieterich D, Han S et al. A treatment algorithm for the management of chronic hepatitis B virus infection in the United States. *Clinical Gastroenterology and Hepatology* 2004;2(2):87–106.

35. Lok AS, McMahon BJ. Chronic hepatitis B. *Hepatology* 2001;34(6):1225–1241.

36. Russo FP, Imondi A, Lynch E et al. When and how should we perform a biopsy for HCC in patients with liver cirrhosis in 2018? A review. *Digestive and Liver Disease* 2018;50(7): 640–646.

37. Boursier J, de Ledinghen V, Zarski J et al. Comparison of eight diagnostic algorithms for liver fibrosis in hepatitis C: new algorithms are more precise and entirely noninvasive. *Hepatology* 2012;55(1):58–67.

3 Screening for hepatocellular carcinoma in viral liver disease: any new biomarkers on the horizon?

Saroja Bangaru, Jorge A. Marrero, and Amit G. Singal

Division of Digestive and Liver Diseases, UT Southwestern Medical Center, Dallas, TX, USA

LEARNING POINTS

- The best currently available surveillance strategy for HCC is ultrasound and AFP, although it only has a sensitivity of 63% for early-stage detection.

- Although ultrasound has recognized limitations, including operator dependency, which result in variable sensitivity for early HCC detection, other imaging studies such as CT or MRI have potential concerns, including radiation, gadolinium accumulation, cost, and radiologic capacity, that limit their widespread use for HCC surveillance.

- Several serologic biomarkers have shown promising results in phase 2 (case–control) studies but still require validation in phase 3 (retrospective cohort) studies. Maturation of large cohort studies with stored serum and plasma samples should facilitate evaluation of many serologic biomarkers in the near future.

- Intratumor and intertumor heterogeneity may preclude a single biomarker from achieving sufficient sensitivity for early HCC detection, highlighting the potential value of biomarker panels for HCC surveillance.

Introduction

Hepatocellular carcinoma (HCC) is one of the leading causes of cancer-related death worldwide and has a rapidly rising mortality rate in the United States [1,2]. Chronic hepatitis B (HBV) infection remains the most common cause of HCC globally, whereas most cases in the Western world are related to hepatitis C (HCV)-related cirrhosis [3].

Although direct acting anti-viral (DAA) therapy may reduce HCV-related HCC incidence in the future, patients with HCV-related cirrhosis who achieve sustained virologic response (SVR) remain at risk of HCC [4]. Therefore, HCC incidence may continue to rise over the next several years.

Prognosis for patients with HCC is driven by tumor stage at diagnosis, with curative treatments only available for those with early-stage tumors. Surgical resection and liver transplantation can afford five-year survival rates exceeding 60–70%, whereas patients with advanced HCC are only eligible for palliative therapies and have a median survival of 1–2 years [5]. Therefore, current professional society guidelines, including those of the American Association for the Study of Liver Diseases (AASLD), European Association for the Study of the Liver (EASL), and Asian-Pacific Association for the Study of the Liver (APASL), all recommend HCC surveillance in at-risk patients every six months [5,6].

Historically, the cornerstone of HCC surveillance has been abdominal ultrasound. Ultrasound has many advantages including being readily available, minimally invasive, safe, and inexpensive. However, increasing data have shown that ultrasound is operator dependent, with a wide variation in sensitivity between centers [7]. A systematic review found that the sensitivity of ultrasound for early HCC detection ranged from 21% to 89%, with a pooled sensitivity for early HCC detection of only 47% (95% confidence interval [CI] 33–61%) [8]. Although some providers have started to use alternative imaging such as computed tomography (CT) or magnetic resonance

Clinical Dilemmas in Viral Liver Disease, Second Edition. Edited by Graham R. Foster and K. Rajender Reddy.
© 2020 John Wiley & Sons Ltd. Published 2020 by John Wiley & Sons Ltd.

imaging (MRI), due to frustration with ultrasound's poor accuracy, this strategy is supported by limited data [8]. The only trial comparing CT and ultrasound was a small randomized trial in a single Veterans Affairs (VA) center; however, the authors failed to find a difference in sensitivity for early HCC detection [9]. Further, CT is limited by adverse effects such as radiation and contrast exposure. Although the PRIUS study suggested MRI has higher sensitivity for early HCC detection than ultrasound, this study was conducted in an HBV-infected cohort and these results still require external validation in Western populations [10]. Further, MRI as a routine surveillance test for all patients with cirrhosis may still be limited by issues such as cost, radiologic capacity, and recent concerns about gadolinium accumulation. Early data suggest an abbreviated MRI protocol may be able to address some of these issues while retaining high sensitivity for early detection, but evaluation in large cohort studies is still needed [11,12].

There has been increasing interest in serologic biomarkers for HCC surveillance. For a biomarker to be fully tested, there are five phases of validation (Table 3.1) [13]. Phase 1 biomarker studies are preclinical exploratory pilot studies, whereas phase 2 studies use a case–control design to fully develop assays. The next step, phase 3, typically employs a prospective specimen collection, retrospective blinded evaluation (PRoBE) design to determine if the biomarker can detect preclinical disease. Phase 4 is a prospective study in which the biomarker is used to trigger diagnostic evaluation and can accurately define a biomarker's true-positive and false-positive rates. Finally, phase 5 is a randomized controlled trial in which the biomarker's impact on cancer control is characterized.

To date, alpha-fetoprotein (AFP) is the best-studied serologic test for early HCC detection, having completed all five phases of biomarker validation. Although AFP has insufficient sensitivity to be used alone, it appears to be of significant benefit when combined with ultrasound. A metaanalysis of HCC surveillance studies found a significant increase in sensitivity for early HCC detection when AFP was used in combination with ultrasound (63%, 95% CI 48–75%) compared to ultrasound alone (45%, 95% CI 30–62%) [8]. Although this was associated with a small decrease in specificity, the diagnostic odds ratio for two tests in combination was higher than that of ultrasound alone. Further, provider interpretation of AFP levels appears to mitigate screening-related harms related to false-positive AFP levels in clinical practice [14]. These data informed the most recent AASLD guidelines, which now recommend ultrasound with or without AFP for HCC surveillance [5].

Several other tumor biomarkers (Table 3.2) have demonstrated promising results in phase 2 biomarker studies but have yet to undergo phase 3 evaluation and therefore have insufficient evidence for routine use in clinical practice [15]. There has been growing interest in cell-free DNA for surveillance and/or diagnosis, particularly given promising phase 2 data for mSEPT9 [16], as these data could facilitate personalized treatment decisions; however, these biomarkers still require evaluation in large patient cohorts. The maturation of the Early Detection Research Network (EDRN) Hepatocellular cancer Early Detection Study (HEDS) and initiation of the Cancer Prevention Research Institute of Texas (CPRIT) Texas HCC Consortium (THCCC) cohorts, with stored serum and plasma samples

Table 3.1 Phases of biomarker development for early detection of cancer

Phases of development	Description	Objective
Phase 1	Preclinical exploration pilot study	Identify and prioritize leads for potentially useful biomarkers
Phase 2	Clinical assay and validation (case–control study)	Estimate receiver operating characteristic curve and optimize performance procedures for assay
Phase 3	Retrospective longitudinal cohort study	Evaluate biomarker's capability to detect preclinical disease
Phase 4	Prospective screening cohort study	Determine operating characteristics: detection rate and false referral rate
Phase 5	Cancer control, randomized controlled trial	Assess reductions in cancer mortality afforded by biomarker assay

Table 3.2 Biomarkers undergoing evaluation for hepatocellular carcinoma surveillance

Biomarker	Type of marker	Phase of development
Alpha-fetoprotein (AFP)	Plasma protein	Phase 5
AFP-L3%	Plasma protein	Phase 3
DCP	Abnormal prothrombin	Phase 3
Osteopontin	Extracellular protein in angiogenesis	Phase 2
Dickkopf-1	Wnt signaling pathway inhibitor	Phase 1
Golgi protein-73	Golgi complex transmembrane protein	Phase 2
Glypican 3	Cell surface proteoglycan	Phase 1
Squamous cell carcinoma antigen	Serine protease inhibitor	Phase 2
Annexin A2	Cell surface, phospholipid binding protein	Phase 2
Midkine	Growth factor	Phase 2
Cytokeratin 19	Cytoskeletal protein	Phase 2
miRNA (e.g., miR 21)	Circulating microRNA	Phase 2
Cell-free DNA	Circulating DNA	Phase 2
mSEPT9	Cell-free DNA	Phase 2

from over 4000 combined patients, should facilitate phase 3 validation of biomarkers in the near future.

Intratumor and intertumor heterogeneity may preclude a single biomarker from achieving sufficient sensitivity, and a panel of biomarkers may instead be required. GALAD, which includes gender, age, AFP-L3%, AFP, and DCP, is one of the best studied biomarker panels to date. In a large multinational phase 2 study with 6834 patients (2430 HCC and 4404 chronic liver disease), GALAD achieved sensitivities ranging from 60% to 80% for early HCC detection [17]. Another panel including AFP, fucosylated kininogen, age, gender, alkaline phosphatase, and alanine aminotransferase (ALT) demonstrated a c-statistic of 0.97 (95% CI 0.95–0.99) for early HCC detection, with a true-positive rate of 86% and a 5% false-positive rate in a phase 2 biomarker study with 162 patients (69 early HCC, 93 cirrhosis) [18]. Finally, a phase 2 study with 146 patients (95 HCC and 51 cirrhosis) found a panel including several methylated DNA markers had a c-statistic of 0.96 (95% CI 0.93–0.99), with sensitivity for early HCC detection exceeding 90% [19].

Biomarkers are also being evaluated for risk stratification, classifying patients as high, intermediate, or low risk for incident HCC. Currently, surveillance is recommended in all patients with cirrhosis despite large variations in HCC risk, ranging from ~1% up to >5% per year. For example, a tissue transcriptome signature has been shown to be highly predictive of HCC development in several cohorts of patients with cirrhosis from diverse etiologies. The signature accurately classified patients in a cohort of

216 Child A cirrhosis patients, with annual HCC incidences of 5.8%, 2.2%, and 1.5% for poor-, intermediate-, and good-prognosis signatures, respectively [20]. The investigators recently developed a serum assay surrogating the tissue signature; however, this requires evaluation in a large cohort of cirrhosis patients. By better understanding individual HCC risk, paired with biomarker performance for HCC surveillance, it may be possible to tailor HCC surveillance strategies to patients.

Currently, AFP is the only biomarker to have undergone sufficient validation for HCC surveillance, and we recommend combining ultrasound with AFP to maximize early HCC detection. Other imaging tests, such as contrast-enhanced CT and MRI, have not been adequately evaluated as surveillance tests and should not be used at this time given other potential concerns including radiation, gadolinium accumulation, cost, and radiologic capacity. Several serologic biomarkers, including a couple of multibiomarker panels, have demonstrated promising results in phase 2 studies, with some demonstrating sensitivity for early-stage HCC exceeding that of imaging-based surveillance tests. The availability of at least two large prospective cohorts with stored, clinically annotated serum and plasma samples should facilitate phase 3 validation in the near future – a critical step to these biomarkers being available for routine use in clinical practice.

Therefore, the horizon for the development of new and highly sensitive biomarkers to detect early HCC is promising, which will enhance our care and outcomes in those with this malignancy.

Financial support

This work was conducted with support from NCI RO1 CA212008 and Cancer Prevention Research Institute of Texas (CPRIT) RP150587. The content is solely the responsibility of the authors and does not necessarily represent the official views of the National Institutes of Health.

Conflicts of interest

Amit G. Singal has served as a consultant for Exact Sciences, Glycotest, and Roche. He has also served as a consultant or been on advisory boards for Bayer, Eisai, BMS, Exelixis, and Gilead. He has received research support from Gilead and Abbvie. Jorge Marrero serves as consultant for Glycotest and has been on advisory boards for Exact Sciences.

References

1. Bray F, Ferlay J, Soerjomataram I et al. Global cancer statistics 2018: GLOBOCAN estimates of incidence and mortality worldwide for 36 cancers in 185 countries. *CA: A Cancer Journal for Clinicians* 2018;68:394–424.

2. Cronin KA, Lake AJ, Scott S et al. Annual Report to the Nation on the Status of Cancer, part I: National cancer statistics. *Cancer* 2018;124:2785–2800.

3. El-Serag HB, Kanwal F. Epidemiology of hepatocellular carcinoma in the United States: where are we? Where do we go? *Hepatology* 2014;60:1767–1775.

4. Kanwal F, Kramer J, Asch SM et al. Risk of hepatocellular cancer in HCV patients treated with direct-acting antiviral agents. *Gastroenterology* 2017;153:996–1005.e1.

5. Marrero JA, Kulik LM, Sirlin CB et al. Diagnosis, staging, and management of hepatocellular carcinoma: 2018 practice guidance by the American Association for the Study of Liver Diseases. *Hepatology* 2018;68(2):723–750.

6. Galle PR, Forner A, Llovet JM et al. EASL clinical practice guidelines: management of hepatocellular carcinoma. *Journal of Hepatology* 2018;69(1):182–236.

7. Singal AG, Nehra M, Adams-Huet B et al. Detection of hepatocellular carcinoma at advanced stages among patients in the HALT-C trial: where did surveillance fail? *American Journal of Gastroenterology* 2013;108(3):425–432.

8. Tzartzeva K, Obi J, Rich NE et al. Surveillance Imaging and alpha fetoprotein for early detection of hepatocellular carcinoma in patients with cirrhosis: a meta-analysis. *Gastroenterology* 2018;154(6):1706–1718.e1701.

9. Pocha C, Dieperink E, McMaken KA et al. Surveillance for hepatocellular cancer with ultrasonography vs. computed tomography – a randomised study. *Alimentary Pharmacology and Therapeutics* 2013;38(3):303–312.

10. Kim SY, An J, Lim YS et al. MRI with liver-specific contrast for surveillance of patients with cirrhosis at high risk of hepatocellular carcinoma. *JAMA Oncology* 2017;3(4):456–463.

11. Besa C, Lewis S, Pandharipande PV et al. Hepatocellular carcinoma detection: diagnostic performance of a simulated abbreviated MRI protocol combining diffusion-weighted and T1-weighted imaging at the delayed post gadoxetic acid. *Abdominal Radiology* 2017;42(1):179–190.

12. Goosens N, Singal AG, King L et al. Cost-effectiveness of risk score-stratified hepatocellular carcinoma screening in patients with cirrhosis. *Clinical Translational Gastroenterology* 2017;8(6):e101.

13. Pepe MS, Etzioni R, Feng Z et al. Phases of biomarker development for early detection of cancer. *Journal of the National Cancer Institute* 2001;93:1054–1061.

14. Atiq O, Tiro J, Yopp AC et al. An assessment of benefits and harms of hepatocellular carcinoma surveillance in patients with cirrhosis. *Hepatology* 2017;65(4):1196–1205.

15. Lou J, Zhang L, Lv S et al. Biomarkers for hepatocellular carcinoma. *Biomarkers in Cancer* 2017;9:1–9.

16. Oussalah A, Rischer S, Bensenane M et al. Plasma mSEPT9: a novel circulating cell-free DNA-based epigenetic biomarker to diagnose hepatocellular carcinoma. *EBioMedicine* 2018;30:138–147.

17. Berhane S, Toyoda H, Tada T et al. Role of the GALAD and BALAD-2 serologic models in diagnosis of hepatocellular carcinoma and prediction of survival in patients. *Clinical Gastroenterology and Hepatology* 2016;14(6):875–886.e876.

18. Wang M, Sanda M, Comunale MA et al. Changes in the glycosylation of kininogen and the development of a kininogen-based algorithm for the early detection of HCC. *Cancer Epidemiology, Biomarkers and Prevention* 2017; 26(5):795–803.

19. Kisel JB, Allawi HT, Giakoumopoulos M et al. Hepatocellular carcinoma detection by plasma assay of methylated DNA markers: phase II clinical validation. *Gastroenterology* 2018;154(6S1):S1113.

20. Hoshida Y, Villanueva A, Sangiovanni A et al. Prognostic gene expression signature for patients with hepatitis c-related early-stage cirrhosis. *Gastroenterology* 2013;144(5):1024–1030.

4 Realistic estimates of hepatitis C virus and hepatitis B virus disease burden

Homie Razavi

Center for Disease Analysis Foundation (CDAF), Lafayette, CO, USA

LEARNING POINTS

- Estimates of the disease burden from viral hepatitis rely upon careful evaluation of appropriate local studies.
- Representative studies that take account of the difference in prevalence in different age groups, particularly children, need to be considered.
- For chronic HBV infection, an estimated 292 million people are infected.
- For chronic HCV infection, an estimated 71 million people are infected.

Introduction

The 69th World Health Assembly endorsed the Global Health Sector Strategy for Viral Hepatitis, including a goal to eliminate hepatitis infection as a public health threat by 2030 [1,2], and the World Health Organization (WHO) introduced global targets for the care and management of hepatitis [2]. However, to track progress against these targets, a realistic estimate of hepatitis C virus (HCV) and hepatitis B virus (HBV) infection disease burden is required.

At first glance, there appear to be different estimates of hepatitis disease burden, but that variance narrows once the numbers are critically reviewed. The variance stems from applying adult prevalence estimates to total populations, using nonrepresentative studies, and from the methodologies used to calculate prevalence. Children now account for 30% of the total population in some low-income and middle-income countries (LMIC). Applying the adult figures to this population results in overestimation of the disease burden, since the pediatric population has a lower prevalence due to vaccination (HBV) and fewer risk factors (injection drug use, blood transfusion, medical injections for HCV). The use of nonrepresentative studies can also result in unrealistic estimates. A commonly used data source is blood donors due to the large sample size and availability. However, in most countries blood donors are required to answer a questionnaire to screen out high-risk donors and those found to be infected are not permitted to donate again. Thus, hepatitis prevalence in this population is an underestimate. Studies that used first-generation hepatitis tests overestimated prevalence due to false-positive cases as do studies in high-risk populations. Thus, selection of the study to be used as the basis of a national estimate is critical.

Once the proper study is selected, the methodology used to calculate prevalence is important. The study population rarely matches the general population distribution so the use of the study's prevalence is almost never appropriate. Instead, reported age-specific prevalence should be used to estimate the country's prevalence using the country's population age pyramid. In addition, hepatitis prevalence is rarely constant over time and any reported hepatitis disease burden estimate should be followed by the year of estimate. Hepatitis B prevalence has been declining due to vaccination while hepatitis C prevalence has been declining due to screening of donated blood and the more recent increase in treatment with direct-acting antivirals (DAAs).

Clinical Dilemmas in Viral Liver Disease, Second Edition. Edited by Graham R. Foster and K. Rajender Reddy.
© 2020 John Wiley & Sons Ltd. Published 2020 by John Wiley & Sons Ltd.

On the other hand, the number of individuals with advanced liver disease has been increasing for both infections as the population ages, with the exception of countries with a very high HCV treatment rate.

The lack of published data is another key barrier. This can be overcome by interviewing local experts. It is becoming increasingly difficult to publish single-country manuscripts, but unpublished national and regional data are available that can be used to develop estimates. The lack of data becomes a problem with hepatitis sequalae (cirrhosis or liver-related deaths). Recent studies have shown that even hepatocellular carcinoma burden in high-income countries can be an underestimate by as much as 50% [3,4]. For now, we have to rely on best available data through international organizations (e.g., International Agency for Research on Cancer [IARC]) that use a combination of empirical data and modeling to estimate global hepatitis burden as well as country-level modeling.

Few countries assess the hepatitis prevalence in the national population at regular intervals (e.g., US and France). The most pragmatic approach to estimating hepatitis burden over time is to use mathematical models that take into account prophylaxis measures and treatment for HBV, and treatment and harm reduction for HCV. The models can systematically take into account new infections as well as impact of treatment and mortality. Although the quality of outputs is highly dependent on the inputs used, this approach can provide comparable estimates across countries and regions. Finally, not all countries report hepatitis prevalence. Regional averages can be used to estimate hepatitis prevalence for missing countries. However, nonrepresentative countries need to be removed from the regional average. For example, HCV prevalence in Egypt is high, but unique to that country due to the strategies implemented to manage schistosomiasis. Estimations of HCV prevalence in North Africa have to exclude Egypt since the same risk factor is not applicable to the other countries, with missing data, in the region.

If the above factors are taken into account, the most reliable published estimate for HCV puts the global viremic infection at 71.1 million (95% confidence interval of 62.5–79.4) corresponding to a prevalence of 1.0% (0.8–1.1%) in 2015 [5]. This estimate was adopted by the World Health Organization in 2017 [6]. Modeling the change in prevalence over time would result in an estimated 67.4 million infections (prevalence of 0.9%) at the start of 2018 with a global distribution shown in Figure 4.1 [7]. The drop in prevalence was due to treated cases and mortality outweighing new infections. The burden of HCV in LMIC is 89% of the global estimate. The number of treated HCV patients has increased over time as shown in Figure 4.2 [7]. However, most of this growth came from middle-income countries as the number of treated patients in high-income countries has been decreasing due to the pool of diagnosed and under-care patients being depleted. This highlights the importance of screening strategies to support national hepatitis programs. Without screening programs, the number of treated patients in middle-income countries will decline as well.

The most recent published estimate for HBV puts total HBV infections, defined as those who test positive to HBV surface antigen (HBsAg), at 292 million (252–341) infections, corresponding to a prevalence of 3.9% (3.4–4.6%) in 2016 [8]. The global distribution of this population is shown in Figure 4.3. LMIC account for 99% of all HBV infections. Comparison of Figures 4.1 and 4.3 shows that HBV is much more common than HCV in Africa and Asia where the majority of the world's population lives. Access to treatment remains low despite the introduction of generic antivirals. Globally, 5% of all eligible HBV patients are in treatment, corresponding to 1.5% of all HBV infections. Under current guidelines, only those with a high viral load or cirrhosis are eligible for treatment. The treatment rate in high-income countries, which account for 1% of all infections, is 24% of the eligible population while in LMIC, which account for 99% of HBV infections, it is 4% [8].

Hepatitis B vaccination has resulted in a significant reduction in HBV infection rates among younger age cohorts, with most of the impact in high-income countries and countries with a high vaccination rate (e.g., China, Taiwan, Latin America, and Central Asia) [8]. In 2016, in high-income countries, an estimated 62% of all infants received HBV birth dose and 80% received three doses of HBV vaccine. The coverage of vaccination in these countries is over 95% among mothers who are HBV positive. Vaccination coverage in LMIC is 44% birth dose and 87% for three doses of HBV vaccine [8]. Unfortunately, the estimated prevalence among 5 year olds is 1.8 million (1.6–2.2), due to low prophylaxis rates in LMIC [8].

The estimates of the global burden of HBV and HCV are summarized in Figure 4.4. The mortality rates attributed to

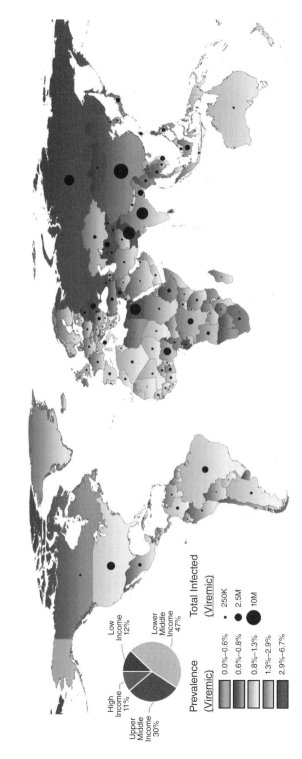

Figure 4.1 Global distribution of HCV infection in 2017.

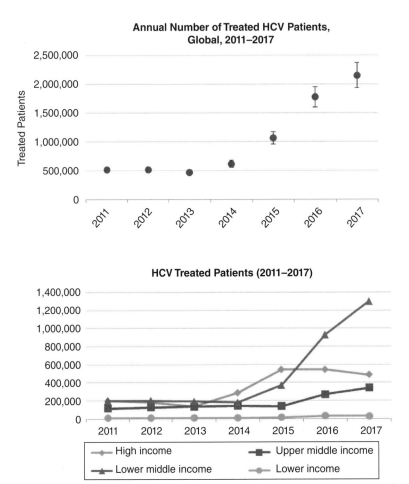

Figure 4.2 Total number of treated HCV patients.

HBV and HCV shown here are higher than those reported previously [9] but those estimates were for 2013, and the same study showed an increase in hepatitis-related mortality that was incorporated in the figures below. The distribution of liver-related deaths attributed to HCV and HBV is also different, mainly due to using an older estimate of HCV prevalence in that study. The key insight from these figures is the massive burden that HBV and HCV represent. Every 20 seconds, someone dies of hepatitis. This figure excludes deaths from nonhepatitis-related causes. The tools needed to tackle both infections and minimize the sequelae and mortality exist today. HBV vaccines have been available for nearly three decades. Antivirals to treat HBV have been available for nearly two decades. Even

though they are not curative, they have been shown to reduce viral load and slow disease progression. The new therapies for HCV provide a sustained viral response in over 95% of patients in 12 weeks or less.

The title of this chapter uses the word *realistic* rather than *accurate*. As scientists, we have a strong desire to collect more data before recommending a path forward and aiming for accuracy will require substantial time and cost. However, the cost of delaying the decision to act is very high for hepatitis, and it is paid for by lives lost. This is especially a problem in low- and middle-income countries. An alternative to the traditional approach is to collect data and improve understanding of hepatitis disease burden while national plans are being implemented. With generic

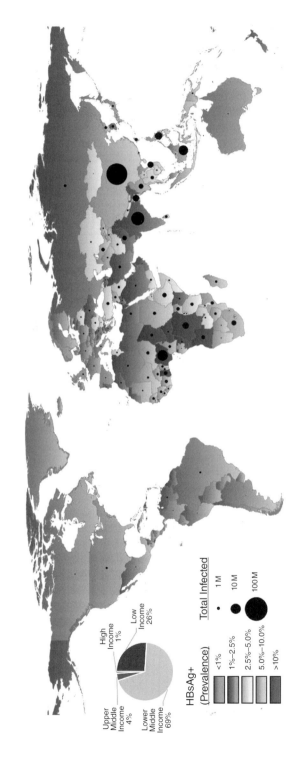

Figure 4.3 Global distribution of HBV infection in 2016.

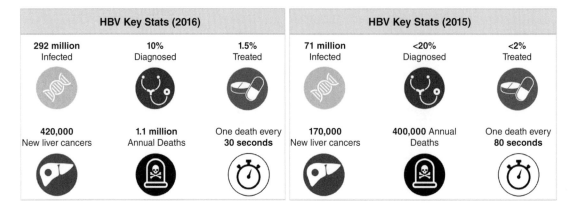

Figure 4.4 HBV and HCV global burden.

HCV therapy and low-cost HBV vaccines and treatment, the economic case for taking action in LMIC is sound. Otherwise, looking back 10–20 years from now, history may not be kind to us.

References

1. World Health Assembly. Draft Global Health Sector Strategies Viral Hepatitis 2016–2021. Geneva: World Health Organization, 2016.

2. World Health Organization. Combating Hepatitis B and C to Reach Elimination by 2030. Geneva: World Health Organization, 2016.

3. Hong TP, Gow P, Fink M et al. Novel population-based study finding higher than reported hepatocellular carcinoma incidence suggests an updated approach is needed. *Hepatology* 2016;63(4):1205–1212.

4. Torner A, Stokkeland K, Svensson A et al. The underreporting of hepatocellular carcinoma to the cancer register and a log-linear model to estimate a more correct incidence. *Hepatology* 2017;65(3):885–892.

5. Blach S, Zeuzem S, Manns M et al. Global prevalence and genotype distribution of hepatitis C virus infection in 2015: a modelling study. *Lancet Gastroenterology and Hepatology* 2017;2(3):161–176.

6. World Health Organization. Global Hepatitis Report 2017. Geneva: Global Hepatitis Programme, Department of HIV/ AIDS, World Health Organization, 2017.

7. Polaris Observatory: CDA Foundation, 2017. http://cdafound. org/polaris/.

8. Razavi-Shearer D, Gamkrelidze I, Nguyen MH et al. Global prevalence, treatment, and prevention of hepatitis B virus infection in 2016: a modelling study. *Lancet Gastroenterology and Hepatology* 2018;3(6):383–403.

9. Stanaway JD, Flaxman AD, Naghavi M et al. The global burden of viral hepatitis from 1990 to 2013: findings from the Global Burden of Disease Study 2013. *Lancet* 2016; 388(10049):1081–1088.

PART II
Today's Therapies

Section 1: HCV

5 Acute hepatitis C: treat immediately or give a chance to spontaneously clear?

David E. Kaplan

Division of Gastroenterology, Department of Medicine, Perelman School of Medicine, University of Pennsylvania, Philadelphia, PA, USA
Corporal Michael J. Crescenz Veterans Affairs Medical Center, Philadelphia, PA, USA

LEARNING POINTS

- A significant proportion of patients with acute hepatitis C spontaneously resolve, largely due to gene polymorphisms associated with innate immune reactivity.

- Success rates with interferon (IFN)-based antiviral therapy were significantly greater with treatment of acute hepatitis C virus (HCV) before the establishment of long-term chronic infection.

- In the postinterferon era, treatment success rates are nearly identical in acute and chronic hepatitis C, mitigating the need to treat hepatitis C early to prevent chronic infection.

- Treating acute hepatitis C, however, has become critical for efforts to eradicate HCV by reducing transmission in the at-risk population.

Introduction

Transmission of hepatitis C most commonly occurs in persons who inject drugs (PWID) and/or individuals who partake in high-risk sexual practices [1–3]. A small fraction of cases come to clinical attention, of which a minority will result in spontaneous resolution but the majority will progress to chronic infection. Predictors of chronicity versus spontaneous clearance are imperfect. Whether or not treatment should be immediately offered, or delayed until the natural history of the individual infection is known, remains a subject of debate. Given the high cost of antiviral therapy, recommendations with regard to treatment in early

acute infection must be based on considerations of efficacy, cost-effectiveness, and distributive justice. In this review, the natural history of acute HCV infection, treatment efficacy, and arguments favoring or opposing early therapy will be discussed.

Defining acute hepatitis C infection

Acute hepatitis C infection, while typically defined temporally as the first six months after initial infection, corresponds to a period of dynamic host–virus interactions that culminates in either spontaneous resolution of the infection or evolution of chronicity [4]. Except in rare settings in which at-risk individuals are undergoing active surveillance, the exact date of infection is often speculative [5]. Except in the 10–36% of patients presenting with symptomatic infection [2,6], characterized by markedly elevated aminotransferase levels (ALT >400 U/L) with or with jaundice and HCV viremia, acute HCV infections are usually established by observation of HCV antibody seroconversion (from prior negative to positive). However, it is infrequent in routine clinical practice for baseline negative HCV antibody testing to be available.

Antibody seroconversion evolves slowly, occurring 7–24 weeks after initial infection [4,6]; by contrast, with current nucleic acid testing, viremia can usually be detected within two weeks [6]. In symptomatic cases, symptoms typically evolve 6–8 weeks after infection [6] but can take significantly longer to evolve based on the size of the viral inoculum [4]. Symptoms most frequently persist for 3–12 weeks and are

Clinical Dilemmas in Viral Liver Disease, Second Edition. Edited by Graham R. Foster and K. Rajender Reddy.
© 2020 John Wiley & Sons Ltd. Published 2020 by John Wiley & Sons Ltd.

typically protean, with flu-like symptoms, myalgias, and fatigue being more common than jaundice [7]. Spontaneous resolution of the infection, in the 5–60% of cases in which it occurs [4,6,8–12], usually happens within six months of infection but can take as long as 12 months [5,13]. Individuals who develop chronic infection typically exhibit slow rates of progressive liver injury, with 20% developing cirrhosis over 20 years; however, individuals older than 50 at the time of acute infection not infrequently progress to cirrhosis within 5–10 years [14].

Risk factors for evolution of chronic infection

Risk factors for progression from acute to chronic infection include age (>15 years old) [15], male gender [2,5,13,16], IFN-lambda 3 polymorphisms (SNP rs12979860; TT > CT > CC) [5,17,18], lack of concomitant chronic hepatitis B [15] or HIV infection [19], HCV genotype (genotype non-1 > genotype 1) [5,20], and higher initial HCV RNA viral load (>400 000 IU/L) [5]. Patients who present with symptomatic acute infection are much more likely to resolve spontaneously; for instance, Gerlach et al. observed in a cohort of 60 acute HCV patients that 52% of symptomatic patients versus 0% of asymptomatic patients cleared infection without treatment [21]. While these variables may be obtainable early in acute infection, no single or combination of variables fully predicts the natural history of an individual infection; therefore, either early treatment or close monitoring must be instituted to ensure that individual patients spontaneously clear infection or receive therapy to prevent chronic infection.

Acute hepatitis C increasing due to opioid epidemic

Until 2010, most literature on acute hepatitis C arose out of focal, small epidemics of acute hepatitis C in human immunodeficiency virus (HIV)-positive and -negative men who have sex with men in urban centers [22–26]. The epidemiology of acute HCV has shifted, with a two-fold increase (from 0.3 to 0.7 cases/100 000, nearly 13 000 new cases/year in the United States) from 2004 to 2014 [27], with significant increases in central Appalachia and other sites in the eastern United States [28]. The largest increase in incidence has been observed in non-Hispanic white and

Hispanic men and women aged 18–39 with injection drug use reported in ≥75% cases.

While this epidemic has been associated with increases in hospital admissions for injection drug use-related complications [27], there is no evidence that this epidemic has yet been associated with increases in liver disease-related hospitalizations or costs due to the rare fulminant nature of acute hepatitis C, the slow natural history of chronic HCV, and competing causes of mortality (e.g., overdose, non-medical mortality) in the PWID population.

Treatment response rates in acute relative to chronic hepatitis C

Treatment of hepatitis C infection prior to *bona fide* establishment of chronicity was supported by multiple retrospective and nonrandomized prospective studies observing significantly greater rates of SVR than observed in contemporary treatments of patients with chronic infection. In 2001, Jaeckel et al. reported a German experience treating 44 patients who were candidates for interferon-based antiviral therapy with a 24-week regimen, resulting in a 98% cure rate [29]. These results were similar to an Italian experience treating inadvertently exposed study volunteers for 20 weeks [30] and American experiences with various regimens [1]. One critique of these studies was that many of the treated patients would have spontaneously resolved, and thus were unnecessarily exposed to interferon.

Several studies attempted to address the questions of how long the treating clinician could wait before triggering antiviral therapy before compromising SVR rates. A follow-up German study demonstrated that waiting 12 weeks for resolution resulted in only modestly reduced SVR rates (80%) [21]. In a metaanalysis of 22 studies and 1075 patients, Corey et al. demonstrated that the overall cure rate for acute hepatitis C using interferon-based, primarily ribavirin-free regimens was 78% compared to a 55.1% spontaneous clearance rate in untreated patients [31]. Earlier treatment before 12 weeks was associated with the highest cure rate (82.5%) although certainly a significant fraction of treated patients would have cleared spontaneously. Cure rates dropped to 66.9% if treatment was delayed to week 12–24 and 62.5% after 24 weeks. The authors argued that the data strongly supported a treatment initiation at week 12 if spontaneous resolutions had yet to occur [31]. Additional studies using modeling based on

IL-28B polymorphisms revealed a reduced likelihood of progression to chronicity with early initiation of antiviral therapy in both C/C and non-C/C individuals independent of symptomatic status [32].

Since the advent of highly effective direct-acting antiviral therapy for chronic hepatitis C, with ≥98% SVR rates in noncirrhotic treatment-naive individuals, treating HCV in the acute setting no longer can be argued based on overall response rates, but efforts have been made to determine if earlier treatment might allow shorter therapy duration and lower treatment cost. To date, such efforts have yielded mixed results. Deterding et al. reported 20/20 cures in genotype 1a or 1b acute HCV monoinfected patients with six weeks of ledipasvir-sofosbuvir [33]. By contrast, a German and British study treating HIV-infected individuals with acute genotype 1 or 4 infection with ledipasvir-sofosbuvir for six weeks yielded a cure rate of only 77% [34]. Similarly, in a study of HIV-positive individuals, SVR12 rate of only 32% was accomplished with a six-week course of ledipasvir-sofosbuvir [35]. Since most of these individuals were noncirrhotic and generally had HCV viral load <6 million IU/mL, the standard therapy would have been eight weeks with SVR rates >95% expected. Thus, expected savings from shorter duration therapy in the acute setting would be relatively modest, particularly as the costs of DAA therapies have markedly declined. Furthermore, any savings were likely offset by the cost of unnecessarily treating the 20–25% of patients who would have cleared spontaneously and the suboptimal efficacy identified in some studies.

Arguments to treat or not to treat in acute hepatitis C (Table 5.1)

In healthcare workers with occupational exposure in whom HCV viremia can be detected within two months following transmission, early treatment has been advocated to minimize the likelihood of chronicity and potential impact on livelihood [32]. Early treatment has also been described in patients with hematologic malignancies with acute HCV for which hepatitis might impede treatment [36].

High treatment success rates, short-duration therapy, and low toxicity associated with DAA therapy in acute HCV have increased interest in using early treatment to reduce transmission, although concerns exist that treatment in potentially low-adherence populations could

Table 5.1 Pros and cons of early antiviral therapy for acute hepatitis C

Pros	Cons
Near certainty of resolution	Cost
Reduced monitoring to determine spontaneous resolution	Unnecessary treatment in up to 28% of individuals
Abrogation of infectivity in active persons who inject drugs	Potential for dissemination during viremic phase
Component of linkage to care for concomitant substance use	Potential for generation of resistance–associated substitutions if poor adherence to therapy
	Most acute infections not clinically observed, not candidates for early therapy

increase circulation of strains with resistance-associated substitutions (RAS) [37].

Few observational data demonstrate that early therapy for acute HCV impacts incidence of new infections, with most data supporting "treatment through prevention" based on modeling studies [38,39]. Some modeling does suggest that treatment as prevention might be cost-effective [40]. Assuming that each acutely infected PWID would transmit infection to 0.2 new individuals, Bethea et al. modeled the clinical and cost-effectiveness of early HCV treatment in PWID, finding cost-effectiveness at a willingness-to-treat threshold <$50 000 per quality-adjusted life-year (QALY) in all scenarios in which the duration of treatment for acute HCV was 2–4 weeks briefer than treatment for chronic infection [40]. In individuals likely to transmit acute HCV, Bethea et al. projected cost savings of nearly $140 000 per QALY by treating acute HCV by preventing downstream infections. Treatment remained cost-effective even if adherence to therapy dropped to 90% and if SVR12 rates fell as low as 44% in high-risk individuals [40].

The primary arguments against treating acute HCV relate to the just allocation of resources. Early treatment prior to potential spontaneous clearance of the 34 000 incident HCV cases each year would cost approximately $300M, of which 28% may be unnecessary expenditure [41]. In the absence of adequate numbers of treating providers and/or healthcare dollars for treatment, individuals with cirrhosis at high short-term risk of liver-related complications and death could be denied access to therapy in lieu of individuals with little to no short-term risk of complications. As treatment costs decline and the pool of individuals with uncured advanced fibrosis/cirrhosis shrinks, concerns regarding the justice of treatment of newly infected individuals should abate. However, to realize the benefits projected by Bethea et al. [40] with universal treatment of acute hepatitis would require a massive investment in infrastructure to identify acute HCV patients, offer comprehensive care for substance abuse, and reduce barriers to access antiviral therapy.

Postexposure prophylaxis (PEP)

In the setting of healthcare worker exposure to chronic hepatitis C-infected blood, the overall rate of transmission of infection has been estimated at approximately <0.1–1.9% [42–45]. Postexposure chemoprophylaxis can be justified for other infections such as HIV and HBV because these infections, unlike HCV, once chronic, cannot be cured. Heller et al. demonstrated that nearly half of healthcare workers with needlestick exposures develop measurable T-cell responses to HCV infection in the absence of antibody seroconversion or viremia [42], suggesting that low-level exposures might boost adaptive T-cell responses that could prevent future infections. In the setting of extremely effective and curative DAA therapy (if needed), highly sensitive assays to detect infection, low likelihood of transmission and high spontaneous clearance rates, routine PEP at this time would be challenging to justify medically and would not be cost-effective [46].

Practical approach to decision making in acute hepatitis C

- Direct testing of hepatitis C virus titers using nucleic acid testing is the preferred diagnostic method in acute hepatitis to detect nascent hepatitis C infection.
- Approximately 1 in 4 acute hepatitis C patients will resolve spontaneously. Individuals presenting with jaundice and low viral loads (<400 000 IU/L) are more likely to resolve and can be given up to 12 weeks to resolve infection. Others should be considered for immediate therapy.
- While six-week direct-acting antiviral regimens may be effective in acute hepatitis C, eight-week regimens used for chronic hepatitis C would be recommended to reduce the risk of relapse.

- Treatment of early hepatitis C infections may prevent spread of virus in high-risk populations, critical to World Health Organization viral hepatitis eradication goals.

References

1. Corey KE, Ross AS, Wurcel A et al. Outcomes and treatment of acute hepatitis C Virus infection in a United States population. *Clinical Gastroenterology and Hepatology* 2006;4:1278–1282.
2. Wang CC, Krantz E, Klarquist J et al. Acute hepatitis C in a contemporary US cohort: modes of acquisition and factors influencing viral clearance. *Journal of Infectious Diseases* 2007;196:1474–1482.
3. Montoya-Ferrer A, Fierer DS, Alvarez-Alvarez B, de Gorgolas M, Fernandez-Guerrero ML. Acute hepatitis C outbreak among HIV-infected men, Madrid, Spain. *Emerging Infectious Diseases* 2011;17:1560–1562.
4. Kaplan DE, Sugimoto K, Newton K et al. Discordant role of CD4 T-cell response relative to neutralizing antibody and CD8 T-cell responses in acute hepatitis C. *Gastroenterology* 2007;132:654–666.
5. Hajarizadeh B, Grady B, Page K et al. Patterns of hepatitis C virus RNA Levels during acute infection: the InC3 Study. *PLoS One* 2015;10:e0122232.
6. Kamal SM. Acute hepatitis C: a systematic review. *American Journal of Gastroenterology* 2008;103:1283–1297; quiz 98.
7. Deterding K, Wiegand J, Gruner N et al. The German Hep-Net acute hepatitis C cohort: impact of viral and host factors on the initial presentation of acute hepatitis C virus infection. *Zeitschrift fur Gastroenterologie* 2009;47:531–540.
8. Lehmann M, Meyer MF, Monazahian M, Tillmann HL, Manns MP, Wedemeyer H. High rate of spontaneous clearance of acute hepatitis C virus genotype 3 infection. *Journal of Medical Virology* 2004;73:387–391.
9. Wawrzynowicz-Syczewska M, Kubicka J, Lewandowski Z, Boron-Kaczmarska A, Radkowski M. Natural history of acute symptomatic hepatitis type C. *Infection* 2004;32:138–143.
10. Maheshwari A, Ray S, Thuluvath PJ. Acute hepatitis C. *Lancet* 2008;372:321–332.
11. Beinhardt S, Payer BA, Datz C et al. A diagnostic score for the prediction of spontaneous resolution of acute hepatitis C virus infection. *Journal of Hepatology* 2013;59:972–977.
12. Bunchorntavakul C, Jones LM, Kikuchi M et al. Distinct features in natural history and outcomes of acute hepatitis C. *Journal of Clinical Gastroenterology* 2015;49:e31–40.
13. Page K, Hahn JA, Evans J et al. Acute hepatitis C virus infection in young adult injection drug users: a prospective study of incident infection, resolution, and reinfection. *Journal of Infectious Diseases* 2009;200:1216–1226.

14. Poynard T, Bedossa P, Opolon P. Natural history of liver fibrosis progression in patients with chronic hepatitis C. *The OBSVIRC, METAVIR, CLINIVIR, and DOSVIRC groups. Lancet* 1997;349:825–832.

15. Zhang M, Rosenberg PS, Brown DL et al. Correlates of spontaneous clearance of hepatitis C virus among people with hemophilia. *Blood* 2006;107:892–897.

16. Micallef JM, Kaldor JM, Dore GJ. Spontaneous viral clearance following acute hepatitis C infection: a systematic review of longitudinal studies. *Journal of Viral Hepatology* 2006;13:34–41.

17. Tillmann HL, Thompson AJ, Patel, et al. A polymorphism near IL28B is associated with spontaneous clearance of acute hepatitis C virus and jaundice. *Gastroenterology* 2010;139: 1586–1592, 92 e1.

18. Hajarizadeh B, Grebely J, Dore GJ. Case definitions for acute hepatitis C virus infection: a systematic review. *Journal of Hepatology* 2012;57:1349–1360.

19. Thomas DL, Astemborski J, Rai RM et al. The natural history of hepatitis C virus infection: host, viral, and environmental factors. *JAMA* 2000;284:450–456.

20. Harris HE, Eldridge KP, Harbour S, Alexander G, Teo CG, Ramsay ME. Does the clinical outcome of hepatitis C infection vary with the infecting hepatitis C virus type? *Journal of Viral Hepatology* 2007;14:213–220.

21. Gerlach JT, Diepolder HM, Zachoval R et al. Acute hepatitis C: high rate of both spontaneous and treatment-induced viral clearance. *Gastroenterology* 2003;125:80–88.

22. Boesecke C, Rockstroh JK. Acute hepatitis C in patients with HIV. *Seminars in Liver Disease* 2012;32:130–137.

23. Urbanus AT, van de Laar TJ, Stolte IG et al. Hepatitis C virus infections among HIV-infected men who have sex with men: an expanding epidemic. *AIDS* 2009;23:F1–7.

24. Brejt N, Gilleece Y, Fisher M. Acute hepatitis C: changing epidemiology and association with HIV infection. *Journal of HIV Therapy* 2007;12:3–6.

25. Gambotti L, Batisse D, Colin-de-Verdiere N et al. Acute hepatitis C infection in HIV positive men who have sex with men in Paris, France, 2001–2004. *Euro Surveillance* 2005;10: 115–117.

26. Gotz HM, van Doornum G, Niesters HG, den Hollander JG, Thio HB, de Zwart O. A cluster of acute hepatitis C virus infection among men who have sex with men – results from contact tracing and public health implications. *AIDS* 2005;19:969–974.

27. Zibbell JE, Asher AK, Patel RC et al. Increases in acute hepatitis C virus infection related to a growing opioid epidemic and associated injection drug use, United States, 2004 to 2014. *American Journal of Public Health* 2018;108:175–181.

28. Viral Hepatitis Surveillance: United States 2014. www.cdc.gov/hepatitis/statistics/2014surveillance/pdfs/2014hepsurveillancerpt.pdf

29. Jaeckel E, Cornberg M, Wedemeyer H et al. Treatment of acute hepatitis C with interferon alfa-2b. *New England Journal of Medicine* 2001;345:1452–1457.

30. Larghi A, Zuin M, Crosignani A et al. Outcome of an outbreak of acute hepatitis C among healthy volunteers participating in pharmacokinetics studies. *Hepatology* 2002;36:993–1000.

31. Corey KE, Mendez-Navarro J, Gorospe EC, Zheng H, Chung RT. Early treatment improves outcomes in acute hepatitis C virus infection: a meta-analysis. *Journal of Viral Hepatology* 2010;17:201–207.

32. Deuffic-Burban S, Castel H, Wiegand J et al. Immediate vs. delayed treatment in patients with acute hepatitis C based on IL28B polymorphism: a model-based analysis. *Journal of Hepatology* 2012;57:260–266.

33. Deterding K, Spinner CD, Schott E et al. Ledipasvir plus sofosbuvir fixed-dose combination for 6 weeks in patients with acute hepatitis C virus genotype 1 monoinfection (HepNet Acute HCV IV): an open-label, single-arm, phase 2 study. *Lancet Infectious Diseases* 2017;17:215–222.

34. Rockstroh JK, Bhagani S, Hyland RH et al. Ledipasvir-sofosbuvir for 6 weeks to treat acute hepatitis C virus genotype 1 or 4 infection in patients with HIV coinfection: an open-label, single-arm trial. *Lancet Gastroenterology and Hepatology* 2017;2:347–353.

35. Martinello M, Gane E, Hellard M et al. Sofosbuvir and ribavirin for 6 weeks is not effective among people with recent hepatitis C virus infection: the DARE-C II study. *Hepatology* 2016;64:1911–1921.

36. Brancaccio G, Sorbo MC, Frigeri F et al. Treatment of acute hepatitis C with ledipasvir and sofosbuvir in patients with hematological malignancies allows early re-start of chemotherapy. *Clinical Gastroenterology and Hepatology* 2018;16:977–978.

37. Gaeta GB, Puoti M, Coppola N et al. Treatment of acute hepatitis C: recommendations from an expert panel of the Italian Society of Infectious and Tropical Diseases. *Infection* 2018;46:183–188.

38. Martin NK, Vickerman P, Grebely J et al. Hepatitis C virus treatment for prevention among people who inject drugs: modeling treatment scale-up in the age of direct-acting antivirals. *Hepatology* 2013;58:1598–1609.

39. Wedemeyer H, Duberg AS, Buti M et al. Strategies to manage hepatitis C virus (HCV) disease burden. *Journal of Viral Hepatology* 2014;21 Suppl 1:60–89.

40. Bethea ED, Chen Q, Hur C, Chung RT, Chhatwal J. Should we treat acute hepatitis C? A decision and cost-effectiveness analysis. *Hepatology* 2018;67:837–846.

41. Congly SE, Lee SS. Treatment of acute hepatitis C virus is cost-effective but at what price? *Hepatology* 2018;67:1640–1641.

42. Heller T, Werner JM, Rahman F et al. Occupational exposure to hepatitis C virus: early T-cell responses in the absence of

seroconversion in a longitudinal cohort study. *Journal of Infectious Diseases* 2013;208:1020–1025.

43. Egro FM, Nwaiwu CA, Smith S, Harper JD, Spiess AM. Seroconversion rates among health care workers exposed to hepatitis C virus-contaminated body fluids: the University of Pittsburgh 13-year experience. *American Journal of Infection Control* 2017;45:1001–1005.

44. Lee JH, Cho J, Kim YJ et al. Occupational blood exposures in health care workers: incidence, characteristics, and transmission of bloodborne pathogens in South Korea. *BMC Public Health* 2017;17:827.

45. Henderson DK. Managing occupational risks for hepatitis C transmission in the health care setting. *Clinical Microbiology Reviews* 2003;16:546–568.

46. Naggie S, Holland DP, Sulkowski MS, Thomas DL. Hepatitis C virus postexposure prophylaxis in the healthcare worker: why direct-acting antivirals don't change a thing. *Clinical Infectious Diseases* 2017;64:92–99.

6 Is ribavirin alive or dead in the current era of HCV therapy?

Vijay Prabhakar[1] and Paul Y. Kwo[2]

[1] Department of Medicine, Stanford University School of Medicine, Stanford, CA, USA
[2] Gastroenterology/Hepatology Division, Stanford University School of Medicine, Stanford, CA, USA

LEARNING POINTS

- The addition of ribavirin to interferon therapy was a major advance in the treatment of hepatitis C.

- In the era of DAA therapy, ribavirin has a limited role.

- The main role of ribavirin is in the treatment of those with decompensated cirrhosis in combination with sofosbuvir and NS5A inhibitors.

- There are limited roles for ribavirin in retreatment strategies and in alternative treatment strategies in the era of pangenotypic DAA options.

- If a third class of DAAs can be developed that is safe in those with decompensated cirrhosis, the role of ribavirin will truly be minimized.

Introduction

The story of hepatitis C is a remarkable one. The rapid path from discovery of the virus in 1989 to clinical use of pangenotypic short-duration therapies in 2019 that successfully treat over 95% of individuals with this chronic infection is a timeline that few chronic diseases and infections have been able to replicate. Moreover, we are beginning to see the fruits of our intensive efforts to identify patients with hepatitis C and to link these individuals to successful therapy worldwide, thus reducing the morbidity and mortality associated with hepatitis C. The treatment of hepatitis C began prior to the identification of the virus, after initial studies in the 1980s demonstrated that a finite course of interferon therapy could normalize alanine aminotransferase (ALT) levels for those with chronic non-A, non-B hepatitis [1]. After the hepatitis C virus was identified and polymerase chain reaction (PCR) testing became available, it was determined that a course of interferon could lead to sustained virologic response (SVR) rates in 10–20% of individuals treated, and interferon therapy for treatment of hepatitis C was officially approved by the FDA in 1991 [2].The course of interferon was not well tolerated by all, and many individuals with medical or psychiatric comorbidities could not be treated with this cytokine-based therapy. Thus, SVR rates remained low in the era of interferon-based therapies.

Ribavirin in the interferon era

Ribavirin was discovered in 1970 and was noted to have antiviral activity against multiple DNA and RNA viruses. Subsequently, it was approved for medical use by the FDA in 1986 for the treatment of respiratory syncytial virus infection in pediatric patients. The exact mechanism of action against hepatitis C remains unclear. Two mechanisms that have been postulated are interference with hepatitis C replication by preventing change elongation through the mechanisms of mutagenesis and inhibition of inosine monophosphate dehydrogenase [3]. Ribavirin was investigated in the early 1990s as a potential monotherapy for hepatitis C. A pilot study demonstrated improvement in ALT levels and a modest reduction in HCV RNA levels though no individual cleared HCV RNA [4]. A subsequent randomized controlled trial confirmed improvement in

Clinical Dilemmas in Viral Liver Disease, Second Edition. Edited by Graham R. Foster and K. Rajender Reddy.
© 2020 John Wiley & Sons Ltd. Published 2020 by John Wiley & Sons Ltd.

ALT levels during treatment, but it did not show improvement in HCV RNA levels [5].

The therapeutic benefit of ribavirin in the treatment of hepatitis C was demonstrated in a seminal study where ribavirin was added to interferon in those who relapsed from a previous course of interferon therapy. In the study, the ribavirin plus interferon arm had a SVR rate of 49% while the interferon monotherapy arm had a SVR rate of 5% [6]. In a treatment-naive hepatitis C population, the addition of ribavirin to interferon improved the SVR rate to 38% compared to an interferon monotherapy treatment SVR rate of 13% [7]. Subsequent studies with PEG-interferon alpha-2b and PEG-interferon alpha-2a demonstrated that the addition of ribavirin to PEG interferon could increase SVR rates in all hepatitis C patients to over 50% and to approximately 40% in those with genotype 1 infection [8]. However, the overall impact of this combination on the global burden of hepatitis C has remained low as the side effects of interferon and ribavirin, such as flu-like symptoms for both and hemolytic anemia in the latter, make the drugs difficult to tolerate. The addition of the first-generation protease inhibitors (telaprevir and boceprevir) to PEG-interferon and ribavirin improved SVR rates considerably in genotype 1-infected individuals though the additional side effects of these protease inhibitors (with exacerbation of anemia) limited the clinical benefit of this higher SVR rate.

Ribavirin in the era of all-oral DAAs

The era of all-oral direct-acting antiviral agents (DAAs) has revolutionized the treatment of hepatitis C, and ribavirin was a key component of the initial reports of successful treatment with DAAs to achieve SVR. The combination of the nucleotide polymerase inhibitor sofosbuvir (NS5B inhibitor) and ribavirin led to a SVR rate of 100% in a pilot study of 10 genotype 2- and 3-infected individuals [9]. This seminal study was followed by additional studies examining whether sofosbuvir monotherapy could achieve similar SVR rates without the side effects and safety monitoring of ribavirin. These studies demonstrated that ribavirin optimized SVR rates by preventing drug resistance-associated substitutions in the viral genome. The combination of sofosbuvir and ribavirin was the first approved all-oral DAA regimen for genotypes 2 and 3 in December 2013. In addition, sofosbuvir and ribavirin was also approved for

genotype 1-infected individuals who were intolerant to interferon. As such, ribavirin remained a key component of hepatitis C therapy as an adjunct to sofosbuvir and made available an all-oral regimen for patients who were unable to tolerate interferon.

Strategies were then explored to create combinations of DAAs to treat hepatitis C that minimized or eliminated the inclusion of ribavirin. The combination of sofosbuvir and ledipasvir (NS5A inhibitor) was investigated with and without ribavirin in durations of eight or 12 weeks in genotype 1-infected individuals with compensated liver disease who were treatment naive or nonresponders to prior therapy in three trials [10–12]. Similar results were found in all three studies with high SVR rates (greater than 95%); importantly, the addition of ribavirin did not incrementally improve the overall SVR in any of the treatment arms though subpopulations did demonstrate benefit (nonresponders to PEG-interferon/ribavirin with cirrhosis). However, the addition of ribavirin was associated with higher rates of constitutional and neuropsychiatric adverse events and increased rates of reduction in hemoglobin (2.5 g/dL) and hyperbilirubinemia, consistent with its known mechanism of action.

A second combination of all-oral DAAs, paritaprevir, ombitasvir, and dasabuvir, was combined with ribavirin to achieve similarly high SVR rates (greater than 95%) in a genotype 1 population [13,14]. Similar to the experience with sofosbuvir and ledipasvir with ribavirin, higher rates of constitutional side effects (nausea, pruritus, insomnia, diarrhea, and asthenia) as well as anemia were noted. The value of ribavirin was demonstrated in a study that compared the combination of paritaprevir, ombitasvir, and dasabuvir with or without ribavirin in genotype 1a- and 1b-infected individuals without cirrhosis [15]. The addition of ribavirin conferred no benefit in genotype 1b-infected individuals, but in genotype 1a-infected individuals, higher rates of virologic failure were noted in the ribavirin-free arm (7.8% versus 2%). Similar to all studies with DAAs combined with ribavirin, higher rates of hemoglobin reduction were seen in those who were randomized to the arms receiving ribavirin.

Another combination of all-oral DAAs, grazoprevir and elbasvir, has been approved for genotype 1 and 4 hepatitis C in those with compensated liver disease. In the United States, the addition of ribavirin and extension of treatment duration from 12 to 16 weeks is required in those with high-level NS5A resistance-associated substitutions and with null response to PEG-interferon though this is no longer a preferred regimen in this patient population [16].

We are now entering the era of pangenotypic DAA regimens that are ribavirin sparing. Both the combinations of sofosbuvir/velpatasvir and glecaprevir/pibrentasvir lead to high SVR rates across all genotypes without ribavirin [17,18]. Moreover, while treatment failure is uncommon in the DAA era, there is now a ribavirin-free salvage regimen of sofosbuvir/velpatasvir/voxilaprevir that has been shown to be highly effective in treating individuals with compensated liver disease that have failed to achieve SVR with DAA therapy [19].

Nevertheless, one group that has consistently been shown to benefit from the addition of ribavirin are individuals with decompensated liver disease, a group that has been historically difficult to treat (Table 6.1). Specifically, patients with Child–Turcotte–Pugh (CTP) class B or C cirrhosis can achieve SVR rates that are somewhat lower than what we see in those with compensated liver disease (approximately 85–90%) and studies to date, while limited, have demonstrated that ribavirin preserves the SVR rate. The benefit of ribavirin was first demonstrated in two seminal studies where the combination of sofosbuvir, ledipasvir, and low-dose ribavirin (600 mg starting dose) was given for 12- or 24-week durations in predominantly genotype 1-infected individuals with decompensated liver disease [20,21] Patients achieved overall SVR rates of 85–90% with no difference noted between 12- and 24-week durations. The combination of sofosbuvir and velpatasvir was also studied with or without ribavirin for 12- and 24-week durations in the ASTRAL-4 trial [22]. The SVR rates were highest in the 12-week ribavirin-containing arm (94%) compared to the 12-week ribavirin-free arm (83%) and 24-week ribavirin-free arm (86%). It should be noted that this study used a higher starting dose of ribavirin (1000/1200 mg) than in earlier studies using sofosbuvir/ledipasvir.

The combination of sofosbuvir and daclatasvir has also been assessed with ribavirin in decompensated individuals with similar findings, and this DAA combination with ribavirin at a starting dose of 600 mg is recommended in those with decompensated liver disease and genotypes 1 and 4 infection(Table 6.1) [23]. Ribavirin is more difficult to tolerate in decompensated cirrhosis and requires either lower doses or careful follow-up of hemoglobin levels to prevent significant anemia. In addition, guidance documents suggest a lower starting dose of ribavirin in CTP class C patients of 600 mg with titration as tolerated. Nonetheless, it appears that SVR rates are optimized in this population when ribavirin can be added to a course of DAAs (sofosbuvir plus NS5A inhibitor).

Postorthotopic liver transplant recurrent hepatitis C infection was for years one of the most problematic challenges faced by transplant hepatologists. The introduction of all-oral DAAs has revolutionized the care of this population, and SVR rates similar to those with compensated liver disease prior to transplant may now be achieved. The first combinations of these DAAs were all studied in combination with ribavirin (paritaprevir/ombitasvir/dasabuvir, ledipasvir/sofosbuvir, daclatasvir/sofosbuvir) and all led to high SVR rates [21,23,24]. The pangenotypic DAA combinations of glecaprevir/pibrentasvir and sofosbuvir/velpatasvir have now been studied post orthotopic liver transplant with high rates of SVR being observed without the use of ribavirin [25,26]. Given that the adverse effects of ribavirin post transplant may be magnified due to preexisting anemia and reduced glomerular filtration rate, ribavirin-free options will likely evolve to be the standard of care with ribavirin being reserved for posttransplant decompensated cirrhosis due to hepatitis C infection, which is becoming uncommon.

Genotype 3-infected individuals have historically been the most difficult to treat successfully in the DAA era. The recent pangenotypic options of glecaprevir/pibrentasvir and sofosbuvir/velpatasvir are highly effective in the treatment of genotype 3 hepatitis C with SVR rates of 95%, with neither combination requiring ribavirin to achieve these high rates. In select cases when high-level resistance-associated substitutions (RAS) are present, ribavirin can be added to sofosbuvir and daclatasvir, and this is now considered an alternative regimen by some guidance documents though in many parts of the world, sofosbuvir/daclatasvir remains an effective low-cost pangenotypic regimen [27]. In those with compensated cirrhosis and genotype 3 infection, ribavirin may be added to sofosbuvir/velpatasvir in those who have failed PEG-interferon and ribavirin as an alternative treatment regimen (Table 6.1).

Historically, ribavirin has been used in most retreatment regimens to salvage those who did not achieve SVR with their first DAA course. However, with the introduction of the pangenotypic NS5A/NS5B polymerase inhibitor and

Table 6.1 Ribavirin-containing regimens: HCV-infected individuals with decompensated cirrhosis or who are post OLT have recommended first-line regimens that contain ribavirin. GT3 DAA treatment failures with compensated cirrhosis also have a recommended ribavirin-containing regimen. All other ribavirin-containing regimens are alternative treatment regimens and have ribavirin-free first-line recommended regimens.

Patient population	Recommended ribavirin-containing regimen	Alternative ribavirin-containing regimen
Child B/C cirrhosis	GT 1, 4, 5, 6 LED/SOF/RBV 600 12 weeks All GT: SOF/VEL/RBV 12 weeks* GT1, 4 SOF/DAC/RBV 600	
DAA failures	GT3: SOF/VEL/VOX/RBV 12 weeks with prior NS5A inhibitor failure and cirrhosis GT 1, 4, 5, 6: LED/SOF/RBV 600 Child B/C SOF only exposure: 24 weeks All GT: SOF/VEL/RBV Child B/C: 24 weeks	GT1: LED/SOF/RBV 12 weeks non-NS5A without cirrhosis/simeprevir exposure
Genotype 1 treatment naive		PrOD/RBV 12 weeks GRZ/ELB/RBV 16 weeks for NS5A RAS
Genotype 4 treatment naive		PrOD/RBV 12 weeks
GT 1 PR failures		LED/SOF/RBV 12 weeks for GT 1 PR failure with cirrhosis GRZ/ELB/RBV 16 weeks for GT 1a with NS5a RAS/or cirrhosis PrOD/RBV 12 weeks GT1a without cirrhosis
Genotype 3 PR failures		SOF/VEL/RBV[2] with Y93H and cirrhosis 12 weeks SOF/DAC/±RBV with cirrhosis 24 weeks
Genotype 4 PR failures		LED/SOF/RBV 12 weeks with cirrhosis GRZ/ELB/RBV 16 weeks without suppression/breakthrough PrOD/RBV 12 weeks
Post-OLT	GT 1, 4, 5, 6 LED/SOF/RBV 600 12 weeks GT 2/3 SOF/VEL/RBV 12 weeks GT 2/3 SOF/DAC/RBV 600 12 weeks	

* Low initial dose of ribavirin (600 mg) is recommended for patients with CTP class C cirrhosis; increase as tolerated.

NS3/4A protease inhibitor DAA combination drug sofosbuvir/velpatasvir/voxilaprevir (SOF/VEL/VOX), the addition of ribavirin is no longer required for the majority of DAA failures. This combination has now become the primary salvage regimen for those who fail to achieve SVR, especially for those with prior NS5A inhibitor exposure. Current guidelines recommend this combination without ribavirin for virtually all patients with compensated liver disease who fail to achieve SVR with sofosbuvir/velpatasvir or glecaprevir/pibrentasvir, with the addition of ribavirin to a combination DAA regimen serving as a retreatment option in selected DAA exposure cases (Table 6.1). As one example, in genotype 3-infected individuals with cirrhosis who have failed previous therapy and have NS5A inhibitor exposure, the addition of ribavirin to SOF/VEL/VOX has been recommended though there are no data yet to justify this recommendation (www.hcvguidelines.org/treatment-experienced/gt3/daa). Additionally, for DAA failures in patients with decompensated liver disease, the approach is similar to those with decompensated liver disease with no prior DAA exposure in that weight-based ribavirin is added to sofosbuvir/velpatasvir or sofosbuvir/ledipasvir. The main treatment difference is extension of the total duration of therapy to 24 weeks [28] (Table 6.1). For genotypes 1, 4, 5, and 6 with decompensated liver disease and DAA failure, 24 weeks of weight-based ribavirin with sofosbuvir/ledipasvir or sofosbuvir/velpatasvir are the preferred regimens. For genotypes 2 and 3 with decompensated liver disease and DAA failure, 24 weeks of sofosbuvir/velpatasvir with weight-based ribavirin is preferred.

Preliminary reports have explored the role of adding ribavirin to glecaprevir and pibrentasvir in those who have failed NS5A inhibitor plus sofosbuvir therapy and those who have failed glecaprevir/pibrentasvir therapy. In a randomized trial of hepatitis C patients with cirrhosis who failed sofosbuvir plus NS5A inhibitor therapy, retreatment with glecaprevir/pibrentasvir and weight-based ribavirin for 12 weeks was compared to 16 weeks of glecaprevir/pibrentasvir. A higher SVR rate was noted in the 16-week glecaprevir/pibrentasvir arm compared to the 12-week ribavirin arm (97% versus 86%), with higher rates of adverse events in the ribavirin-containing arm [29]. A second study examined the efficacy of a 12- or 16-week course of sofosbuvir plus weight-based ribavirin addition to glecaprevir/pibrentasvir for patients who had previous treatment failure with glecaprevir/pibrentasvir. Individuals who had genotypes 1, 2, 4, 5, and 6 without cirrhosis and were not treated with a NS5A inhibitor or protease inhibitor before taking glecaprevir/pibrentasvir the first time were treated for 12 weeks while those with genotype 3, those with cirrhosis, and those who were also previously treated with a NS5A inhibitor or protease inhibitor other than glecaprevir/pibrentasvir were treated for 16 weeks [30]. The overall SVR rates were high at 96% with just one treatment failure (genotype 1a). No ribavirin dose reductions for toxicity were required, with hemoglobin reductions being limited to grades 1–2.

Conclusion

The addition of ribavirin to interferon and all-oral DAA therapies has played a major role in the successful treatment of those with hepatitis C. Indeed, ribavirin has been part of first-line and salvage regimens for decades. However, with the advent of all-oral DAAs, the role of ribavirin is now restricted. Pangenotypic options that are ribavirin free can lead to SVRs of 95% or greater across all genotypes of hepatitis C. The major population that still benefits from the addition of ribavirin to all-oral DAA therapy is the group with decompensated liver disease in whom three classes of DAAs cannot be administered safely due to the unpredictable behavior of the protease inhibitor class in decompensated cirrhosis. DAA treatment failure patients may also benefit in some instances from the addition of ribavirin though the data supporting this recommendation are currently sparse. Nonetheless, when faced with a complicated patient who has failed DAA-based therapies, experienced hepatologists will often include ribavirin as part of a salvage strategy. Postorthotopic liver transplant patients can now be treated with ribavirin-free regimens though the addition of ribavirin remains an option.

In conclusion, ribavirin remains with us in a limited role and will do so for the foreseeable future as long as there are those with decompensated liver disease. If a third class of DAAs can be developed that can be safely administered in decompensated patients, the role of ribavirin will likely be further reduced and given its toxicities, especially in the setting of decompensated liver disease, this would be a welcome advance.

Conflicts of interest

Dr Kwo has the following conflicts of interest. Grant Support: Assembly, BMS, Gilead, Allergan, Abbvie, La Jolla. Advisory Board: Abbvie, BMS, Gilead, Dova, Shionogi, Conatus, Merck, Surrozen, Ferring, Quest, Durect. Shareholder: Durect, DSMB Johnson and Johnson.

References

1. Hoofnagle JH, Mullen KD, Jones DB et al. Treatment of chronic non-A,non-B hepatitis with recombinant human alpha interferon. A preliminary report. *New England Journal of Medicine* 1986;315(25):1575–1578.
2. Davis GL, Balart LA, Schiff ER et al. Treatment of chronic hepatitis C with recombinant alpha-interferon. A multicentre randomized, controlled trial. The Hepatitis Interventional Therapy Group. *Journal of Hepatology* 1990;11 Suppl 1:S31–35.
3. Te,HS, Randall G, Jensen DM. Mechanism of action of ribavirin in the treatment of chronic hepatitis C. *Gastroenterology and Hepatology* 2007;3(3):218–225.
4. di Bisceglie AM, Shindo M, Fong TL et al. A pilot study of ribavirin therapy for chronic hepatitis C. *Hepatology* 1992; 16(3):649–654.
5. Di Bisceglie AM, Conjeevaram HS, Fried MW et al. Ribavirin as therapy for chronic hepatitis C. A randomized, double-blind, placebo-controlled trial. *Annals of Internal Medicine* 1995;123(12):897–903.
6. Davis GL, Esteban-Mur R, Rustgi V et al. Interferon alfa-2b alone or in combination with ribavirin for the treatment of relapse of chronic hepatitis C. International Hepatitis Interventional Therapy Group. *New England Journal of Medicine* 1998;339(21):1493–1499.
7. McHutchison JG, Gordon SC, Schiff ER et al. Interferon alfa-2b alone or in combination with ribavirin as initial treatment for chronic hepatitis C. Hepatitis Interventional Therapy Group. *New England Journal of Medicine* 1998;339(21):1485–1492.

8. McHutchison JG, Lawitz EJ, Shiffman ML et al. Peginterferon alfa-2b or alfa-2a with ribavirin for treatment of hepatitis C infection. *New England Journal of Medicine* 2009;361(6): 580–593.

9. Gane EJ, Stedman CA, Hyland RH et al. Nucleotide polymerase inhibitor sofosbuvir plus ribavirin for hepatitis C. *New England Journal of Medicine* 2013;368(1):34–44.

10. Afdhal N, Reddy KR, Nelson DR et al. Ledipasvir and sofosbuvir for previously treated HCV genotype 1 infection. *New England Journal of Medicine* 2014;370(16):1483–1493.

11. Afdhal N, Zeuzem S, Kwo P et al. Ledipasvir and sofosbuvir for untreated HCV genotype 1 infection. *New England Journal of Medicine* 2014;370(20):1889–1898.

12. Kowdley KV, Gordon SC, Reddy KR et al. Ledipasvir and sofosbuvir for 8 or 12 weeks for chronic HCV without cirrhosis. *New England Journal of Medicine* 2014;370(20):1879–1888.

13. Poordad F, Hezode C, Trinh R et al. ABT-450/r-ombitasvir and dasabuvir with ribavirin for hepatitis C with cirrhosis. *New England Journal of Medicine* 2014;370(21):1973–1982.

14. Feld JJ, Kowdley KV, Coakley E et al. Treatment of HCV with ABT-450/r-ombitasvir and dasabuvir with ribavirin. *New England Journal of Medicine* 2014;370(17):1594–1603.

15. Ferenci P, Bernstein D, Lalezari J et al. ABT-450/r-ombitasvir and dasabuvir with or without ribavirin for HCV. *New England Journal of Medicine* 2014;370(21):1983–1992.

16. Kwo P, Gane EJ, Peng CY et al. Effectiveness of elbasvir and grazoprevir combination, with or without ribavirin, for treatment-experienced patients with chronic hepatitis C infection. *Gastroenterology* 2017;152(1):164–175.e4.

17. Feld JJ, Zeuzem S. Sofosbuvir and velpatasvir for patients with HCV infection. *New England Journal of Medicine* 2016;374(17):1688–1689.

18. Zeuzem S, Foster GR, Wang S et al. Glecaprevir-pibrentasvir for 8 or 12 weeks in HCV genotype 1 or 3 infection. *New England Journal of Medicine* 2018;378(4):354–369.

19. Bourliere M, Gordon SC, Flamm SL et al. Sofosbuvir, velpatasvir, and voxilaprevir for previously treated HCV infection. *New England Journal of Medicine* 2017;376(22):2134–2146.

20. Manns M, Samuel D, Gane EJ et al. Ledipasvir and sofosbuvir plus ribavirin in patients with genotype 1 or 4 hepatitis C virus infection and advanced liver disease: a multicentre, open-label, randomised, phase 2 trial. *Lancet Infectious Diseases* 2016;16:685–697.

21. Charlton M, Everson GT, Flamm SL et al. Ledipasvir and sofosbuvir plus ribavirin for treatment of HCV infection in patients with advanced liver disease. *Gastroenterology* 2015;149(3):649–659.

22. Curry MP, O'Leary JG, Bzowej N et al. Sofosbuvir and velpatasvir for HCV in patients with decompensated cirrhosis. *New England Journal of Medicine* 2015;373(27):2618–2628.

23. Poordad F, Schiff ER, Vierling JM et al. Daclatasvir with sofosbuvir and ribavirin for hepatitis C virus infection with advanced cirrhosis or post-liver transplantation recurrence. *Hepatology* 2016;63(5):1493–1505.

24. Kwo PY, Mantry PS, Coakley E et al. An interferon-free antiviral regimen for HCV after liver transplantation. *New England Journal of Medicine* 2014;371(25):2375–2382.

25. Reau N, Kwo PY, Rhee S et al. Glecaprevir/pibrentasvir treatment in liver or kidney transplant patients with hepatitis C virus infection. *Hepatology* 2018;68(4):1298–1307.

26. Agarwal K, Castells L, Mullhaupt B et al. Sofosbuvir/velpatasvir for 12weeks in genotype 1–4 HCV-infected liver transplant recipients. *Journal of Hepatology* 2018;69(3): 603–607.

27. Nelson DR, Cooper JN, Lalezari JP et al. All-oral 12-week treatment with daclatasvir plus sofosbuvir in patients with hepatitis C virus genotype 3 infection: ALLY-3 phase III study. *Hepatology* 2015;61(4):1127–1135.

28. Gane EJ, Shiffman ML, Etzkorn K et al. Sofosbuvir–velpatasvir with ribavirin for 24 weeks in hepatitis C virus patients previously treated with a direct-acting antiviral regimen. *Hepatology* 2017;66(4):1083–1089.

29. Lok A, Willner I, Reddy R et al. A phase 3b, open-label, randomized, pragmatic study of glecaprevir/pibrentasvir+/− ribavirin (RBV) for HCV genotype 1 subjects who previously failed an NS5A inhibitor+ sofosbuvir (SOF) therapy. *Journal of Hepatology* 2018;68:S104.

30. Wyles D, Weiland O, Yao B et al. Retreatment of patients who failed glecaprevir/pibrentasvir treatment for hepatitis C virus infection. *Journal of Hepatology* 2018;68:S23–S24.

7 Hepatitis C virus genotype and viral testing, and on-treatment monitoring: necessary or overkill?

Sirina Ekpanyapong and K. Rajender Reddy

Department of Medicine, Division of Gastroenterology and Hepatology, University of Pennsylvania, Philadelphia, PA, USA

LEARNING POINTS

- Simplified screening and diagnostic testing, pangenotypic DAA treatment regimens, and simplified monitoring approach are essential steps necessary for wide-scale identification and treatment of chronic HCV, while adherence to therapy can be enhanced – all key elements necessary to achieve HCV global elimination goal by 2030. Current HCV screening and diagnostic strategies are complex and represent an "overkill" for the vast majority of HCV patients encountered globally

- With the advent of highly effective pangenotypic DAA therapy, skipping HCV genotype, for a wider population is a reasonable strategy; certain HCV-infected patients with difficult-to-treat genotype/genotype subtype (e.g., genotype 3 with treatment-experienced; genotype 6 c-l subtype, genotype 4r in Africa have lower responses with first-generation NS5A inhibitor ledipasvir and sofosbuvir) may still need genotype testing before initiating a HCV treatment regimen as they may need a second-generation regimen of velpatasvir/sofosbuvir, glecaprevir/pibrentasvir, a longer duration of HCV therapy and/or combination with ribavirin.

- HCV core antigen and HCV RNA point-of-care testing are new diagnostic and monitoring methods for HCV infection and these require less time to obtain results and have lower cost than current HCV RNA NAAT testing. However, these assays still need to be validated in specific populations (e.g., HBV/HIV coinfection) and evaluated for cost-effectiveness before widespread implementation in a simplified algorithm in real-life practice for ubiquitous use.

- A simplified model of diagnosis and treatment algorithm may not be fit for all global regions, and for special populations, and more studies on cost-effectiveness of a simplified approach are required in different country-specific settings.

Introduction

Hepatitis C virus (HCV) infection is one of the main causes of chronic liver disease worldwide, with approximately 71 million chronically infected individuals [1]. The World Health Organization (WHO) announced a goal of eliminating viral hepatitis as a major public health threat by 2030 [2]. However, in order to achieve the target of HCV global elimination, simplified methods for screening and diagnosis of HCV-infected patients as well as highly effective direct-acting antiviral (DAA) treatment regimens and simplified posttreatment monitoring strategies are important issues.

The American Association for the Study of Liver Diseases and the Infectious Diseases Society of America (AASLD/IDSA) guideline recommended HCV screening in persons with risk behaviors for hepatitis C infection such as injection drug use, intranasal illicit drug use, on long-term hemodialysis, healthcare workers, incarcerated persons, and those who were born between 1945 and 1965, the so-called "baby boomers" [3]. However, HCV screening rates have been low due to the complexity of screening and diagnosis algorithms. The high cost of the required tests has been a major barrier for HCV elimination. Ironically, the high cost and complexity of testing and on-treatment follow-up have been the challenge in an era of highly effective pangenotypic DAA, including generic versions, that have resulted in high cure rates with acceptable safety. This therefore challenges us to implement elimination HCV genotype testing, which while possible for the majority of patients may still leave us with pockets of

Clinical Dilemmas in Viral Liver Disease, Second Edition. Edited by Graham R. Foster and K. Rajender Reddy.
© 2020 John Wiley & Sons Ltd. Published 2020 by John Wiley & Sons Ltd.

challenging populations, such as treatment-experienced genotype 3 HCV-infected patients, particularly those with cirrhosis where genotype and host characteristics might dictate a personalized approach. Additionally, certain genotypes/genotype subtypes (genotype 6 c-l, genotype 4r) may not respond to the first-generation NS5A inhibitor of ledipasvir and sofosbuvir regimen, necessitating genotype testing and use of more robust regimens of velpatasvir/sofosbuvir or glecaprevir/pibrentasvir [4,5].

New simplified methods for diagnosis and monitoring of HCV treatment algorithms are being developed in order to achieve widespread identification of HCV-infected individuals and to treat them effectively. Easy specimen collection and uncomplicated laboratory facilities in decentralized settings are the strengths of these new simplified tools. More data on the clinical performance of these new simplified tests are needed, especially in specific populations such as HBV/HIV coinfection, and the cost-effectiveness analysis should be evaluated in order to implement their usage in a simplified algorithm [6].

Current recommendations on diagnosis and treatment monitoring for HCV infection

The AASLD/IDSA guideline recommendation prior to starting HCV therapy includes HCV genotype, subtype, and quantitative HCV RNA (HCV viral load) apart from other basic laboratory investigations. After four weeks of HCV therapy, quantitative HCV viral load testing is repeated and then followed again at 12 weeks after completion of therapy. If HCV viral load is detectable at week 4 of treatment, repeat quantitative HCV viral load testing is recommended at week 6 of treatment. If quantitative HCV viral load has increased by >10-fold (>1 $\log_{10}$ IU/mL) on repeat testing at week 6 or thereafter, discontinuation of HCV therapy is recommended for lack of efficacy [3].

As per the 2018 European Association for the Study of the Liver (EASL) updated guideline recommendation on hepatitis C treatment, screening for chronic hepatitis C is recommended to be done by anti-HCV antibody testing in serum or plasma by enzyme immunoassay (EIA). Whole blood sampled on dried blood spots can be used as an alternative to serum or plasma obtained by venepuncture for anti-HCV antibody testing, after delivery to a central laboratory where the EIA method is to be performed.

Rapid diagnostic tests (RDTs) using serum, plasma, fingerstick whole blood or salivary fluid can be used instead of classic EIA methods at the patient's care site to improve access. If anti-HCV antibodies are detected, HCV RNA, or alternatively HCV core antigen (if HCV RNA assays are not available), in serum or plasma should be assessed in order to identify patients with active HCV infection. Whole blood sampled on dried blood spots can also be used as an alternative to serum or plasma obtained by venepuncture for HCV RNA testing. Further, anti-HCV antibody screening for HCV infection can be replaced by a point-of-care HCV RNA assay with a lower limit of detection of ≤1000 IU/mL (3.0 $\log_{10}$ IU/mL) or HCV core antigen testing, if the screening strategy proves to be cost-effective. The HCV genotype and genotype 1 subtype (1a or 1b) must be assessed before treatment in order to determine the choice and duration of therapy. However, new pangenotypic DAA regimens can be initiated without genotype testing in areas where the test is not available. Additionally, testing for HCV resistance prior to treatment is not recommended.

The endpoint of therapy can be defined by undetectable HCV RNA in serum or plasma by a sensitive assay (lower limit of detection ≤15 IU/mL) at 12 weeks (SVR12) or 24 weeks (SVR24) after the end of treatment. Alternative approaches can also be used to identify endpoint of therapy, such as undetectable HCV core antigen in serum or plasma at 24 weeks (SVR24) after the end of treatment and/or undetectable HCV RNA using a qualitative HCV RNA assay with a lower limit of detection ≤1000 IU/mL (3.0 $\log_{10}$ IU/mL) in serum or plasma at 24 weeks (SVR24) after the end of treatment [7].

Proposed framework for simplified HCV infection management (Figure 7.1)

Simplified screening for HCV infection

Rapid diagnostic tests (RDTs) have been developed as HCV antibody screening tests with advantages over the traditional EIA techniques. RDTs require less laboratory equipment and maintenance costs, making them more suited for decentralized settings [6]; however, clinical performance of individual tests is still varied depending on the manufacturer and sample type (e.g., fingerstick whole blood, oral fluid, etc.) [8–10]. The WHO has evaluated two new prequalified RDTs which show good sensitivity and

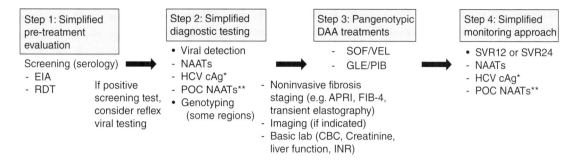

Figure 7.1 Proposed simplified algorithm for HCV management. Source: Modified from [6,7,27].

specificity: OraQuick HCV Rapid Antibody Test Kit and SD Bioline HCV.

Dried blood spot (DBS) sampling is another method for whole-blood specimen collection (by capillary fingerstick or venepuncture). A major advantage of DBS is that multiple spots can be taken at one time on the filter paper, and if the first spot is positive for HCV antibody screening, the second or third spots are used for further reflex HCV RNA testing, which can improve the drop-off rate for HCV RNA confirmatory testing, and the sampling can be done easily by peer workers without special training [6]. The performance of DBS specimens for anti-HCV antibody detection has shown excellent sensitivity and specificity of more than 95% [11]; however, HCV RNA is less reliable, particularly when the viral load is low. Another disadvantage of DBS is that commercial assays have not yet received regulatory approval, and it also needs a centralized laboratory to process the specimen, similar to traditional EIA approaches.

Simplified diagnostic testing

The three possible diagnostic strategies for simplified HCV diagnosis are as follows [6].

HCV core antigen test (HCV cAg)

HCV cAg can be used as a marker of HCV viral replication. This test targets the nucleocapsid peptide 22 (p22) which is released by the infected cells into plasma [12,13]. A systematic review and metaanalysis of HCV cAg testing (44 studies) have shown good sensitivity and specificity, with the Abbott ARCHITECT demonstrating 93.4% sensitivity and 98.8% specificity, and the Ortho ELISA demonstrating 93.2% sensitivity and 99.2% specificity [14].

There were insufficient data on coinfection with hepatitis B or HIV patients, and data on HCV genotype 4–6 infection were scant. HCV cAg assays are less sensitive than HCV RNA assays (lower limit of detection is approximately 500–3000 HCV RNA IU/mL, depending on HCV genotypes) [7,12,15]. Available data on quantitative studies using Abbott ARCHITECT have shown that HCV cAg correlated closely with HCV RNA levels at >3000 IU/mL [14]. The major benefit of HCV cAg is the lower cost of testing compared to HCV RNA [16] and shorter time to obtain the result (<60 minutes). However, this tool still requires centralized laboratory facilities. Other limitations include the false-negative results which can be the case in genotype 3 [17].

New HCV RNA point-of-care (POC) test

This is a new random access qualitative nucleic acid amplification technology (NAAT) which can be used in decentralized settings with the hope of replacing the traditional HCV RNA quantitative NAAT testing, especially in low- and middle-income countries (LMICs). An example of a POC HCV RNA assay which has received WHO pre-qualification is the Xpert HCV Viral Load assay [7,18]. The result can be achieved within 120 minutes with a lower limit of detection of ≤1000 IU/mL (3.0 $\log_{10}$ IU/mL) and the test can be used to provide broad affordable access to HCV diagnosis [7]. However, cost-effectiveness studies are needed to determine whether this test can be used as a first-line diagnostic assay.

The ideal future algorithm would require only one test for both screening and diagnosis of HCV infection. HCV cAg and/or HCV RNA POC test are techniques which can offer one-step screening algorithm if the assays become more affordable in the future.

Skipping HCV genotype

With the advent of pangenotypic DAAs (e.g., sofosbuvir/velpatasvir [SOF/VEL], glecaprevir/pibrentasvir [GLE/PIB]) which achieve high sustained virologic response (SVR) rates in various patient populations, HCV genotype testing may no longer be required. However, there are some challenges for genotype 3 treatment-experienced patients and those with cirrhosis which may require a longer treatment period and possibly even the addition of ribavirin [7].

An experience from Myanmar evaluated the outcomes with generic and pangenotypic SOF/VEL with and without baseline genotype testing (n = 359) where 201 patients did not have baseline genotype tested. Of the 158 participants in whom genotype was tested, 15.2% had genotype 1, 50.6% had genotype 3, and 34.2% had genotype 6. The overall SVR12 rate was 98.6% which was similar in those with and without baseline genotype testing. This study concluded that generic and pangenotypic SOF/VEL ± ribavirin is highly effective and safe, therefore in order to reduce cost, the requirement for baseline genotype can be eliminated [19].

However, in other regions of the world, there might be situations where different HCV genotypes could affect treatment outcomes. The SHARED study in sub-Saharan Africa, that set out to assess the safety and efficacy of sofosbuvir/ledipasvir for chronic HCV genotype 1 or 4 infection in Rwanda (n = 300), noted overall SVR12 of 87%. On genotyping, 83% participants were reported as having genotype 4, 1% genotype 1, and 16% both genotype 1 and 4. Subsequent viral sequencing of genotype 4 infection noted subtype 4k (45%), subtype 4r (16%), subtype 4q (14%), and subtype 4v (8%). In participants with genotype 4r, SVR12 was observed in only 56% compared to 93% with other subtypes, suggesting the importance of genotype testing and/or further viral sequencing in this specific region, and consideration of the use of newer pangenotypic DAA regimens [5].

Pangenotypic DAA regimens

According to the AASLD/IDSA and EASL guideline recommendation on hepatitis C treatment, the suggested pangenotypic DAA regimens are those summarized in Table 7.1.

Sofosbuvir/velpatasvir (SOF/VEL)

Sofosbuvir 400 mg/velpatasvir 100 mg is a coformulation of an NS5B polymerase inhibitor and NS5A inhibitor which is approved for HCV-infected adult patients with genotypes 1–6. A 12-week course of SOF/VEL in genotype 1,2,4,5,6 HCV-infected patients (n = 624), including those with compensated cirrhosis, treatment-naive status, and previous treatment failure with interferon (IFN)-based therapy, resulted in an overall high SVR12 rate of 99% [20]. The ASTRAL-3 study specifically evaluated a 12-week course of SOF/VEL in genotype 3 HCV-infected patients (n = 277), including those with compensated cirrhosis, treatment-naive

Table 7.1 Suggested pangenotypic DAA regimens

Genotype	Prior treatment experience (pegylated IFN-α)	SOF/VEL (noncirrhosis)	SOF/VEL (compensated cirrhosis)	GLE/PIB (noncirrhosis)	GLE/PIB (compensated cirrhosis)
1a, 1b	Treatment naive	12 weeks	12 weeks	8 weeks	12 weeks
	Treatment experienced	12 weeks	12 weeks	8 weeks	12 weeks
2	Treatment naive	12 weeks	12 weeks	8 weeks	12 weeks
	Treatment experienced	12 weeks	12 weeks	8 weeks	12 weeks
3	Treatment-naive	12 weeks	12 weeks*	8 weeks	12 weeks
	Treatment experienced	12 weeks*	SOF/VEL+RBV 12 weeks or SOF/VEL/VOX 12 weeks	12–16 weeks	16 weeks
4	Treatment naive	12 weeks	12 weeks	8 weeks	12 weeks
	Treatment experienced	12 weeks	12 weeks	8 weeks	12 weeks
5, 6	Treatment-naive	12 weeks	12 weeks	8 weeks	12 weeks
	Treatment-experienced	12 weeks	12 weeks	8 weeks	12 weeks

Source: Modified from [3,7].

* RAS testing for Y93H is recommended. If present, ribavirin should be added or daily fixed-dose combination of 12 weeks sofosbuvir (400 mg)/velpatasvir (100 mg)/voxilaprevir (100 mg) should be considered.

DAA, direct-acting antiviral; GLE, glecaprevir; IFN, interferon; PIB, pibrentasvir; RBV, ribavirin; SOF, sofosbuvir; VEL, velpatasvir; VOX, voxilaprevir.

status, and previous failure with IFN-based therapy, and found an overall SVR12 rate of 95% [21]. Patients with decompensated cirrhosis (genotype 1–6) were evaluated in the ASTRAL-4 study (n = 267), which demonstrated SVR12 rates of 83% with a 12-week course of SOF/VEL, 94% with 12 weeks of SOF/VEL+RBV, and 86% with 24 weeks of SOF/VEL [22], suggesting that in these patients with decompensated liver disease, the SOF/VEL regimen should be either for 12 weeks with ribavirin or 24 weeks of SOF/VEL alone.

Glecaprevir/pibrentasvir (GLE/PIB)

Glecaprevir 100 mg/pibrentasvir 40 mg is a coformulation of an NS3/4A protease inhibitor and NS5A inhibitor which is approved for the treatment of HCV genotype 1–6 infected patients. The eight-week regimen of GLE/PIB in HCV-infected patients without cirrhosis can achieve SVR up to 99% in genotype 1 and 95% in genotype 3, whereas a 12-week regimen in those with compensated cirrhosis achieved an SVR of 99% in genotype 1 and 95% in genotype 3 [23]. Another advantage of this regimen is its safety in patients with renal impairment or end-stage renal disease and without the need for dose adjustment [24]. However, a major limitation of this HCV protease inhibitor-containing regimen is the contraindication in patients with decompensated cirrhosis due to potential hepatotoxicity.

Simplified monitoring approach

High SVR rates are achieved with pangenotypic DAA regimens and thus one could argue in favor of eliminating

HCV viral load monitoring during treatments. HCV RNA testing can be reduced to a single posttreatment step to assess SVR at either 12 or 24 weeks after completion of treatment. There are emerging data on HCV cAg to assess response to DAA therapy, compared to conventional HCV RNA. A study evaluating the clinical performance of the HCV cAg assay to monitor HCV treatment efficacy and HCV viral recurrence (335 samples) found high sensitivity and specificity for detection of pretreatment and post-treatment viremia; thus, confirmation of presence or absence of viremia by HCV cAg during the follow-up period is possible [25]. A study of genotype-1 HCV-infected patients (n = 411) who received DAA treatment found an overall concordance between HCV RNA and HCV cAg of 98.6% while concordance in pretreatment samples was 99.5% and 99.24% in posttreatment week 12 samples. Specificity in anti-HCV-positive HCV RNA-negative samples was 100% [26]. However, further studies are needed in specific patient subgroups such as HIV/HBV coinfected patients.

We propose a simplified algorithm for HCV management as shown in Figure 7.1. Pros and cons of eliminating HCV genotype, viral testing, and on-treatment monitoring are summarized in Table 7.2.

Conclusion

The goal of global elimination of HCV infection may need a newly developed simplified framework for HCV diagnosis and treatment. Simplified screening and diagnostic

Table 7.2 Pros and cons of eliminating HCV genotype, viral testing, and on-treatment monitoring

Pros	Cons
• Shorten steps to HCV therapy and decrease the drop-off rate from a complex investigation process • Decrease unnecessary cost from the current investigation process which is most ideal for low- and middle-income countries • Some of the new simplified diagnostic strategies can be performed in decentralized settings and require less time to obtain a result • Could serve as a pathway to achieve the goal of global expanded HCV cure in the future • Use fewer public health resources in order to implement HCV treatment, and also expand provider pool in primary care setting	• Several new screening and diagnostic tools for HCV infection are still under investigation, and have not yet received regulatory approval • Most of the evolving assays are still expensive; thus, not ready for prime time • Patients who are infected with difficult-to-treat genotype/genotype subtype may need genotype testing before initiating a particular regimen and planned duration of HCV therapy • More data on clinical performance of new simplified diagnosis and monitoring tests in specific populations (e.g., HBV/HIV coinfection, genotype 4–6 HCV infection) are still needed

testing, pangenotypic DAA treatment regimens, and a simplified monitoring approach are the key steps towards improving accessibility and adherence to treatment, resulting in successful outcomes. Current diagnosis algorithms remain complex and expensive where there is a requirement for serologic screening with EIA anti-HCV testing, then using NAAT for HCV RNA confirmatory testing, and HCV genotyping, in order to confirm the diagnosis and initiate HCV treatment. However, with the development of new diagnostic tools, one-step screening using HCV cAg or HCV RNA point-of-care test can be a viable option for both screening and diagnosis, especially in high HCV prevalence areas when these assays are likely to be more cost-effective and affordable. Additionally, with the evolution of pangenotypic DAAs, eliminating HCV genotype may also be possible. In the posttreatment monitoring period, only a single posttreatment HCV RNA test with HCV cAg or HCV RNA point-of-care test can be implemented. However, more data on the clinical performance of these new simplified tests are still needed, especially in specific populations and in areas where unique genotypes/genotype subtypes are encountered.

References

1. Polaris Observatory HCV Collaborators. Global prevalence and genotype distribution of hepatitis C virus infection in 2015: a modelling study. *Lancet Gastroenterology and Hepatology* 2017;2(3):161–176.

2. World Health Organization. Draft Global Health Sector Strategy on Viral Hepatitis, 2016–2021. Geneva: WHO, 2016. http://apps.who.int/gb/ebwha/pdf_files/WHA69/A69_32-en.pdf?ua=1.

3. AASLD/IDSA. HCV Guidance: Recommendations for Testing, Managing, and Treating Hepatitis C. www.hcvguidelines.org/sites/default/files/full-guidance-pdf/HCVGuidance_May_24_2018b.pdf.

4. Hlaing NKT, Mitrani RA, Aung ST et al. Safety and efficacy of sofosbuvir-based direct-acting antiviral regimens for hepatitis C virus genotypes 1-4 and 6 in Myanmar: real-world experience. *Journal of Viral Hepatitis* 2017;24(11):927–935.

5. Gupta N, Mbituyumuremyi A, Kabahizi J et al. Treatment of chronic hepatitis C virus infection in Rwanda with ledipasvir-sofosbuvir (SHARED): a single-arm trial. *Lancet Gastroenterology and Hepatology* 2019;4(2):119–126.

6. Fourati S, Feld JJ, Chevaliez S, Luhmann N. Approaches for simplified HCV diagnostic algorithms. *Journal of the International AIDS Society* 2018;21 Suppl 2:e25058.

7. EASL. Recommendations on treatment of hepatitis C 2018. *Journal of Hepatology* 2018;69(2):461–511.

8. Shivkumar S, Peeling R, Jafari Y, Joseph L, Pant Pai N. Accuracy of rapid and point-of-care screening tests for hepatitis C: a systematic review and meta-analysis. *Annals of Internal Medicine* 2012;157(8):558–566.

9. Khuroo MS, Khuroo NS, Khuroo MS. Diagnostic accuracy of point-of-care tests for hepatitis C virus infection: a systematic review and meta-analysis. *PLoS One* 2015;10(3):e0121450.

10. Greenman J, Roberts T, Cohn J, Messac L. Dried blood spot in the genotyping, quantification and storage of HCV RNA: a systematic literature review. *Journal of Viral Hepatitis* 2015;22(4):353–361.

11. Soulier A, Poiteau L, Rosa I et al. Dried blood spots: a tool to ensure broad access to hepatitis C screening, diagnosis, and treatment monitoring. *Journal of Infectious Diseases* 2016;213(7):1087–1095.

12. Chevaliez S, Soulier A, Poiteau L, Bouvier-Alias M, Pawlotsky JM. Clinical utility of hepatitis C virus core antigen quantification in patients with chronic hepatitis C. *Journal of Clinical Virology* 2014;61(1):145–148.

13. Bouvier-Alias M, Patel K, Dahari H et al. Clinical utility of total HCV core antigen quantification: a new indirect marker of HCV replication. *Hepatology* 2002;36(1):211–218.

14. Freiman JM, Tran TM, Schumacher SG et al. Hepatitis C core antigen testing for diagnosis of hepatitis C virus infection: a systematic review and meta-analysis. *Annals of Internal Medicine* 2016;165(5):345–355.

15. Chevaliez S, Feld J, Cheng K et al. Clinical utility of HCV core antigen detection and quantification in the diagnosis and management of patients with chronic hepatitis C receiving an all-oral, interferon-free regimen. *Antiviral Therapy* 2018;23(3):211–217.

16. Cresswell FV, Fisher M, Hughes DJ, Shaw SG, Homer G, Hassan-Ibrahim MO. Hepatitis C core antigen testing: a reliable, quick, and potentially cost-effective alternative to hepatitis C polymerase chain reaction in diagnosing acute hepatitis C virus infection. *Clinical Infectious Diseases* 2015;60(2):263–266.

17. Nguyen LT, Dunford L, Freitas I et al. Hepatitis C virus core mutations associated with false-negative serological results for genotype 3a core antigen. *Journal of Clinical Microbiology* 2015;53(8):2697–2700.

18. Grebely J, Lamoury FMJ, Hajarizadeh B et al. Evaluation of the Xpert HCV Viral Load point-of-care assay from

venepuncture-collected and finger-stick capillary whole-blood samples: a cohort study. *Lancet Gastroenterology and Hepatology* 2017;2(7):514–520.

19. Bwa AH, Nangia G, Win STS et al. Strategy and efficacy of generic and pan-genotypic sofosbuvir/velpatasvir in chronic hepatitis C virus: a Myanmar experience. *Journal of Clinical and Experimental Hepatology* 2019;9:283–293.

20. Feld JJ, Jacobson IM, Hezode C et al. Sofosbuvir and velpatasvir for HCV genotype 1, 2, 4, 5, and 6 infection. *New England Journal of Medicine* 2015;373(27):2599–2607.

21. Foster GR, Afdhal N, Roberts SK et al. Sofosbuvir and velpatasvir for HCV genotype 2 and 3 infection. *New England Journal of Medicine* 2015;373(27):2608–2617.

22. Curry MP, O'Leary JG, Bzowej N et al. Sofosbuvir and velpatasvir for HCV in patients with decompensated cirrhosis. *New England Journal of Medicine* 2015;373(27):2618–2628.

23. Zeuzem S, Foster GR, Wang S et al. Glecaprevir-pibrentasvir for 8 or 12 weeks in HCV genotype 1 or 3 infection. *New England Journal of Medicine* 2018;378(4):354–369.

24. Gane E, Lawitz E, Pugatch D et al. Glecaprevir and pibrentasvir in patients with HCV and severe renal impairment. *New England Journal of Medicine* 2017;377(15):1448–1455.

25. Lamoury FMJ, Soker A, Martinez D et al. Hepatitis C virus core antigen: a simplified treatment monitoring tool, including for post-treatment relapse. *Journal of Clinical Virology* 2017;92:32–38.

26. Rockstroh JK, Feld JJ, Chevaliez S et al. HCV core antigen as an alternate test to HCV RNA for assessment of virologic responses to all-oral, interferon-free treatment in HCV genotype 1 infected patients. *Journal of Virological Methods* 2017;245:14–18.

27. Kapadia SN, Marks KM. Hepatitis C management simplification from test to cure: a framework for primary care providers. *Clinical Therapeutics* 2018; 40(8):1234–1245.

Treatment of hepatitis C virus in renal disease: can we use all the drugs without additional monitoring?

Stanislas Pol

Université Paris Descartes, Hepatology Department, Cochin Hospital, APHP, Paris, France
INSERM U1223, UMS-20 and Center for Translational Science, Institut Pasteur, Paris, France

LEARNING POINTS

- Patients with chronic kidney disease and HCV infection should be considered for treatment with direct-acting antivirals: current DAA regimens lead to a sustained virologic response in over 95% of patients, including those with severe chronic kidney disease.

- Sustained virologic response decreases the risk of both hepatic and extrahepatic complications.

- Impairment of renal function has been reported with DAAs and sofosbuvir, the backbone of several antiviral combinations which is excreted by the kidney, is not recommended, with eGFR <30 mL/min/1.73m^2.

- Additionnal prospective and comparative studies are needed to clarify the potential risk of renal impairment associated with DAAs and to definitively determine that the renal safety of DAAs is not an issue.

Introduction

Hepatitis C virus (HCV) and chronic kidney disease (CKD) are epidemiologically closely related for two main reasons: firstly, because patients with CKD have been overexposed to the virus [1]: the prevalence of HCV in CKD patients remains at least four times higher than in the general population; secondly, because HCV may be directly responsible for renal disease occurrence [2], mostly from glomerulonephritis with or without cryoglobulinemia but also from chronic inflammation, with a

2–2.5 increased risk of developing cardio-, cerebro-, or renovascular-related events, and a 1.5 increased risk of developing insulin resistance and diabetes 2 diabetes which may impact renal function [3,4].

This is why all HCV-infected patients, and especially those with CKD, should be treated. According to KDIGO recommendations, "All patients with CKD and kidney transplant recipients infected with HCV should be evaluated for antiviral therapy" [5] to reduce the risk of hepatic and extrahepatic manifestations (EHM).

Sustained virologic response (SVR) corresponds to a virologic cure [6] and is usually associated with a reduction of the HCV-related hepatic and extrahepatic manifestations, including diabetes, CKD, and end-stage renal disease (ESRD), cardiac complications and stroke, and ESRD-related mortality (lower in treated than untreated patients) [7] and with a better quality of life [8].

This is why we expected an improvement of renal function after direct-acting antiviral (DAA)-associated SVR. Since studies reported a renal impact of DAA [9], one of the remaining issues in HCV therapy is to confidently answer the following question: can we use all the drugs without additional monitoring?

DAA metabolism and general recommendations

Decompensated cirrhosis contraindicates the use of protease inhibitors which can cause liver damage and

Clinical Dilemmas in Viral Liver Disease, Second Edition. Edited by Graham R. Foster and K. Rajender Reddy.
© 2020 John Wiley & Sons Ltd. Published 2020 by John Wiley & Sons Ltd.

decompensation: thus, a protease inhibitor-free combination (sofosbuvir/velpatasvir) should be used for 12 weeks in combination with ribavirin.

Protease inhibitors or NS5A inhibitors are mainly metabolized by the liver and do not require estimated glomerular filtration rate (eGFR) dose adjustment and are good candidates for the treatment of patients with CKD stage 4 and 5 [5]. No dose adjustment to kidney function was needed with simeprevir and daclatasvir but optimal antiviral potency of these two drugs was only achieved in combination with sofosbuvir, the first-in-class nucleotidic NS5B inhibitor which is the backbone of most antiviral combinations and may be coformulated in a single tablet with the NS5A inhibitor ledipasvir or velpatasvir. The standard dose of sofosbuvir (400 mg/d) is not recommended in patients with a GFR below 30 mL/min; the metabolism of sofosbuvir is mainly renal and renal dysfunction (mainly CKD 4–5) has been associated in pharmacokinetics study with overexposure to sofosbuvir and its metabolite (GS-007). A risk of deterioration of renal function has been reported in around 25% of cases [9]. However, pharmacokinetics are reassuring [10] and sofosbuvir-based regimens can be used off-label in patients with an eGFR <30 in the absence of other therapeutic options [11–13].

International guidelines for CKD patients with a eGFR above 30 mL/min/1.73m^2 are the same as in the HCV-infected general population [5]. In patients having a clearance below 30 mL/min/1.73m^2, therapeutic options available for genotypes 1 and 4 infections were before 2017 a combination of paritaprevir/ritonavir boosted, ombitasvir and dasabuvir or grazoprevir/elbasvir for 12 weeks without ribavirin (updated 2018 KDIGO recommendations) [5]. The nonsofosbuvir DAA combinations, including grazoprevir/elbasvir and paritaprevir/ritonavir/ombitasvir/dasabuvir (NS5B), are largely excreted in the feces and did not show significant safety signals in terms of renal toxicity in postmarketing observational studies [14–17]. Excellent results were obtained in genotype 1-infected patients with severe renal impairment including patients receiving dialysis: 99% SVR in per protocol analysis with the grazoprevir/elbasvir (Zepatier) in the largest randomized controlled C-Surfer study [14]; also, the RUBY-1 and -2 trials (paritaprevir/ritonavir, ombitasvir, dasabuvir) with or without ribavirin reported high SVR rates (100% SVR) [17]. Safety was fair and there was no signal regarding the renal function [16]. Although improvement of renal

function was reported ([17], other studies denied such an improvement.

Since sofosbuvir is not approved in patients with eGFR below 30 mL/min/1.73m^2, there was no approved option for genotypes 2, 3, 5, and 6 even if real-life results report a high SVR rate and a good safety profile of sofosbuvir-based regimens [10–14].

Since 2018, the choice of therapy is mainly between sofosbuvir/ledipasvir (Harvoni®), sofosbuvir/velpatasvir (Epclusa®) and grazoprevir/elbasvir (Zepatier®) for 8–12 weeks according to genotype and subtype and underlying liver disease, or the pangenotypic sofosbuvir/ledipasvir/voxilaprevir (Vosevi®) [18] and glecaprevir/pibrentasvir (Maviret®) for eight weeks in noncirrhotic and 12 weeks in cirrhotic patients [19].Given the polemic around the potential negative impact of the sofosbuvir-containing regime, we need to provide confident conclusions, glecaprevir/pibrentasvir appearing as the primary choice in HCV-infected patients with renal impairment.

Non-sofosbuvir recent results

The pangenotypic combination glecaprevir/pibrentasvir (Maviret) may be used irrespective of CKD stage and genotype [19]. In the EXPEDITION 4 study, glecaprevir/pibrentasvir was given to 104 patients with CKD stage 4 or 5, including a majority of patients receiving dialysis (82%) and 19% of cirrhotic patients. A 12-week treatment allowed a SVR rate of 98% in intent-to-treat (ITT) analysis and 100% in modified ITT analysis (failures being related to one death and one loss of follow-up). Tolerance was satisfactory both clinically and biologically and side effects were not related to treatment [20]. The EXPEDITION 5 study, using an eight (n = 84), 12 (n = 13) or 16 (n = 4) week duration according to the US and/or EU label-approved glecaprevir/pibrentasvir regimen, gave similar results (100% SVR12 in modified ITT analysis) in treatment-naive or pegylated interferon/ribavirin/sofosbuvir-experienced HCV genotype 1–6-infected patients with CKD stage 3b, 4, or 5. No patient experienced an adverse event of worsening renal function or started dialysis during or post treatment.

In the overall glecaprevir/pibrentasvir development program in patients who received eight, 12 or 16 weeks of therapy (2238 treated patients), baseline renal function did not change the therapeutic efficacy (SVR 93–100%), nor the clinical or biological tolerance profile [19]. Interestingly, patients with CKD stage 3 had an improvement in renal function, confirming similar data with the grazoprevir/elbasvir combination [15]. Finally, in a study of 100 transplant recipients, including 20 kidney recipients, a 12-week course of glecaprevir/pibrentasvir had a good efficacy and safety profile [21].

In summary, there is no signal regarding a negative impact of the pangenotypic glecaprevir/pibrentasvir combination.

Sofosbuvir-based regimen and renal safety

Some postmarketing studies with methodologic shortcomings and no renal biopsy data have reported renal impairment including decreased eGFR and acute kidney injury (AKI) with DAA treatment including sofosbuvir [9,22]. These are balanced by a growing number of contradictory studies [11–13]. It is unclear whether these observations are related to sofosbuvir or to confounding factors, including underlying liver disease or a concomitant administration of potentially nephrotoxic treatments such as nonsteroidal antiinflammatory drugs, antiretroviral drugs or nucleotide analogs, antidiabetic and antihypertensive drugs, aging, diabetes, hypertension, HIV infection, etc.

The mechanisms of sofosbuvir-associated putative renal toxicity are not clear and are not similar to other NUC-associated kidney-specific toxicities, including organic anion transporter type 1 (OAT1)- and multidrug-resistant protein type 4 (MRP4)-mediated renal proximal tubule accumulation with subsequent mitochondrial toxicities with tenofovir, adefovir or cidofovir treatment [23]. The evolution of the GFR and neutrophil gelatinase-associated lipocalin (NGAL) has been studied in a retrospective cohort study including 102 patients under DAA. eGFR reduction was observed (from 86.2 mL/min/1.73 m^2 at baseline to 84.4 mL/min/1.73 m^2 at follow-up week 12, p=0.049) and mean NGAL increased in 18 patients (from 121.9 to 204.1 ng/mL, p=0.014). At follow-up week 12, 38.8% of patients had a plasmatic NGAL value higher than normal compared with 11.1% at baseline (p=0.054). Authors conclude that a negligible eGFR decline contrasted with a significant NGAL increase in a small subgroup which "could reflect tubular damage during DAA rather than glomerular injury" [24].

We conducted a longitudinal study to model these eGFR variations and to identify the effect of DAA treatment on eGFR among HCV-infected patients without underlying kidney disease or with an early CKD stage [25]. A total of 749 participants (96.5% had an eGFR ≥60 mL/min/1.73 m^2) had longitudinal measurements over a median of 24 weeks between treatment initiation and final eGFR measurement. The difference in mean eGFR between the first and last measurement was calculated and a linear mixed-effects model of the determinants of eGFR variation during the observation period was used. Nonsofosbuvir-based DAA treatment was associated with an increase in eGFR (+2.96 mL/min/1.73 m^2) in contrast with sofosbuvir-based regimens with a mean decrease of 2.6 mL/min/1.73 m^2.

The postmarketing observations suggesting sofosbuvir-associated renal impairment [9,22,25] are in contrast with the absence of reported renal safety signal in sofosbuvir-based premarketing studies [11–13], including the latest studies [18].

This discrepancy cannot be explained by the usual exclusion of patients with an eGFR <50 mL/min/1.73 m^2 by Cockcroft or by the use of insensitive scales to grade adverse events in all sofosbuvir-based premarketing studies, since published data in kidney recipients after DAAs did not suggest renal impairment [26–28]. An international trial with sofosbuvir and ledipasvir for 12 or 24 weeks in renal transplant recipients with a GFR above 40 mL/min/1.73 m^2 reported a high antiviral efficacy (100% in per protocol analysis with 12 or 24 weeks) and fair safety (no renal deterioration during and after therapy) [29].

In addition, a metaanalysis including 264 CKD 4–5 patients treated with sofosbuvir-including regimen or non-sofosbuvir-based therapies did not indicate any signal regarding efficacy (SVR12 of 89.4% and 94.7%, respectively) or safety (the pooled incidence of severe adverse events was 12.1% and the rate of discontinuation related to adverse events 2.2%) [13]. Reassuring results have also been reported in a retrospective study including 97 patients with eGFR <60 mL/min/1.73 m^2 and some degree of proteinuria (42% stage 1–2 CKD and 58% stage 3 CKD, 49% had diabetes, 38% had cirrhosis and 33% had prior solid organ transplant) who were given sofosbuvir-based therapies; regression models were used to examine changes in eGFR from baseline to follow-up [12]. Average baseline eGFR was equivalent to average on-treatment eGFR but seven patients experienced an increase >1.5 times baseline value under sofosbuvir and all but one recovered; CKD stage 3 patients with SVR experienced a 9.3 mL/min/1.73 m^2 improvement of eGFR during the six-month posttreatment follow-up period [12].

Similar results have been reported in 71 CKD patients (84.5% on maintenance hemodialysis and 23.9% with cirrhosis) who were given full-dose generic sofosbuvir in combination with ribavirin in 26 patients for 12 weeks, ledipasvir in 26 for 12 weeks, and daclatasvir in 19 for 12 weeks; SVR12 was seen in 100% of the patients and at week 24 one patient relapsed in the ledipasvir group and at week 48 one more patient in the ribavirin group relapsed [28]. Interestingly, eGFR up to 12 weeks of stopping therapy was analyzed and only two ribavirin-treated patients had a creatinine increase >0.3 mg/dL at the end of therapy from baseline, one with urinary tract infection and the other without clear precipitating factor for creatinine increase. Overall, there was no significant change in median eGFR.

Finally, an unpublished Italian retrospective analysis of a prospective cohort evaluated the kinetics of eGFR (CKD-EPI) in a cohort of 403 patients who were given a DAA regimen. SVR was achieved in 98%. The median eGFR increased throughout treatment from 84.54 to 88.12 mL/min/1.73 m^2 and the rate of CKD stage 1–2 patients increased from 83.1% at baseline to 87.8% at 12 weeks post treatment (p<0.05). A significant eGFR improvement was observed in patients without diabetes (p<0.01), in cirrhotics (p<0.05), only in those treated with the sofosbuvir-ledipasvir regimen (p<0.01) (and not in those treated with ombitasvir/partitaprevir/ritonavir/dasabuvir regimen) or not receiving ribavirin (p<0.05), only in those with a baseline CKD stage higher than 2 (p<0.01) and in those with SVR (p<0.05). Regardless of the presence of comorbidities and the regimen received, CKD grade 3a–3b and 4–5 patients significantly improved their eGFR while those with CKD grade 1–2 did not have significant changes of eGFR between baseline and 12 weeks post treatment.

This study suggests that sofosbuvir-based HCV eradication improves renal function in patients with baseline renal impairment (Coppola N et al., unpublished data). A lesser decline in the renal function of patients achieving SVR12 has been previously reported in 523 patients, whatever the therapeutic option, compared with patients who did not achieve SVR, evidencing the impact of HCV infection on renal function as an extrahepatic manifestation and the need to achieve HCV eradication [30].

These results are in line with those of the ERCHIVES cohort [31] which reported a worsening of renal function in 3728 patients treated with ombitasvir/partitaprevir/ritonavir and dasabuvir regimens and not in the 12 018 treated by a sofosbuvir-based regimen, in contrast with the pooled results of the SAPPHIRE-1 and -2 and RUBY-1 and -2 trials which did not indicate renal dysfunction after treatment [16].

Finally, given the controversy, "analytic" evaluation of renal function kinetics, especially among patients at risk for renal disease progression whatever the DAA, is mandatory [32]. We need to provide strong prospective answers with analytic kinetic renal evaluation (including blood and urine analysis of phosphorus, protein, urine dipsticks, etc.) under DAA not only to explore if there is any renal signal but also to confirm improvement of renal function suggested in most SVR patients. While waiting for renal kinetics to be evaluated further in randomized controlled trials among CKD patients treated with sofosbuvir-containing and sosbuvir-free regimens [28], we cannot use all the drugs without additional monitoring in daily practice, especially at a time when HCV treatment is shifting from tertiary centers to community-based nonspecialist providers.

Conclusion

In summary, results remain controversial regarding the potential risk of renal impairment associated with DAA: most, but not all, results suggest that nonsofosbuvir-based as well as sofosbuvir-based combinations are well tolerated. The main message is that the risk of renal deterioration is low, if any, and that the renal improvement is modest, if any. By following the guidelines, there is no significant risk to patients and an expected benefit for daily clinical practice.

References

1. Fissell RB, Bragg-Gresham J, Woods J et al. Patterns of hepatitis C prevalence and seroconversion in hemodialysis units from three continents: the DOPPS. *Kidney International* 2004;65:2335–2342.

2. Lee MH, Yang H, Lu S et al. Chronic hepatitis C virus infection increases mortality from hepatic and extrahepatic

diseases: a community-based long-term prospective study. *Journal of Infectious Diseases* 2012;206:469–477.

3. Cacoub P, Desbois AC, Comarmond C, Saadou, D. Impact of sustained virological response on the extrahepatic manifestations of chronic hepatitis C: a meta-analysis. *Gut* 2018;67:2025–2034.

4. Pol S, Parlati L, Jadoul M. Hepatitis C virus and the kidney. *Nature Review Nephrology* 2019;15:73–86.

5. Jadoul M, Berenguer M, Doss W et al. Executive summary of the 2018 KDIGO Hepatitis C in CKD Guideline: welcoming advances in evaluation and management. *Kidney International* 2018;94:663–673.

6. Fontaine H, Chaix ML, Lagneau JL, Brechot C, Pol S. Recovery from chronic hepatitis C in long-term responders to ribavirin plus interferon alfa. *Lancet* 2000;356:41.

7. Hsu YC, Ho H, Huang Y et al. Association between antiviral treatment and extrahepatic outcomes in patients with hepatitis C virus infection. *Gut* 2015;64:495–503.

8. Bruchfeld A, Roth D, Martin P et al. Elbasvir plus grazoprevir in patients with hepatitis C virus infection and stage 4–5 chronic kidney disease: clinical, virological, and health-related quality-of-life outcomes from a phase 3, multicentre, randomised, double-blind, placebo-controlled trial. *Lancet Gastroenterology and Hepatology* 2017;2:585–594.

9. Saxena V, Koraishy F, Sise M et al. Safety and efficacy of sofosbuvir-containing regimens in hepatitis C infected patients with reduced renal function: real-world experience from HCV-target. *Journal of Hepatology* 2015;62:S267.

10. Desnoyer A, Pospai D, Le M et al. Pharmacokinetics, safety and efficacy of a full dose sofosbuvir-based regimen given daily in hemodialysis patients with chronic hepatitis C. *Journal of Hepatology* 2016;65:40–47.

11. Sise ME, Backman E, Ortiz G et al. Effect of sofosbuvir-based hepatitis C virus therapy on kidney function in patients with CKD. *Clinical Journal of the American Society of Nephrology* 2017;12:1615–1623.

12. Li T, Qu Y, Guo Y et al. Efficacy and safety of direct-acting antivirals-based antiviral therapies for hepatitis C virus patients with stage 4–5 chronic kidney disease: a meta-analysis. *Liver International* 2017;37:974–981.

13. Sharma S, Mukherjee D, Nair RK, Datt B, Rao A. Role of direct antiviral agents in treatment of chronic hepatitis C infection in renal transplant recipients. *Journal of Transplantation* 2018;28:7579689.

14. Roth D, Nelson D, Bruchfeld A et al. Grazoprevir plus elbasvir in treatment-naïve and treatment-experienced patients with hepatitis C virus genotype 1 infection and stage 4–5 chronic kidney disease (the C-SURFER study): a combination phase 3 study. *Lancet* 2015;386:1537–1545.

15. Reddy KR, Roth D, Bruchfeld A et al. Elbasvir/grazoprevir does not worsen renal function in patients with hepatitis C

virus infection and pre-existing renal disease. *Hepatology Research* 2017;47:1340–1345.

16. Mehta DA, Cohen E, Charafeddine M et al. Effect of hepatitis C treatment with ombitasvir/paritaprevir/r + dasabuvir on renal, cardiovascular and metabolic extrahepatic manifestations: a post-hoc analysis of phase 3 clinical trials. *Infectious Diseases and Therapy* 2017;6:515–529.

17. Pockros PJ, Reddy K, Mantry P et al. Efficacy of direct-acting antiviral combination for patients with hepatitis C virus genotype 1 infection and severe renal impairment or end-stage renal disease. *Gastroenterology* 2016;150:1590–1598.

18. Bourliere M, Gordon S, Flamm S et al. Sofosbuvir, velpatasvir, and voxilaprevir for previously treated HCV infection. *New England Journal of Medicine* 2017;376:2134–2146.

19. Puoti M, Foster G, Wang S et al. High SVR12 with 8-week and 12-week glecaprevir/pibrentasvir therapy: an integrated analysis of HCV genotype 1–6 patients without cirrhosis. *Journal of Hepatology* 2018;69:293–300.

20. Gane E, Lawitz E, Pugatch D et al. Glecaprevir and pibrentasvir in patients with HCV and severe renal impairment. *New England Journal of Medicine* 2017;377:1448–1455.

21. Reau N, Kwo P, Rhee S et al. Glecaprevir/pibrentasvir treatment in liver or kidney transplant patients with hepatitis C virus infection. *Hepatology* 2018;68:1298–1307.

22. Maan R, Al Marzooqi S, Klair J et al. The frequency of acute kidney injury in patients with chronic hepatitis C virus infection treated with sofosbuvir-based regimens. *Alimentary Pharmacology and Therapeutics* 2017;46:46–55.

23. Kohler JJ, Hosseini S, Green E et al. Tenofovir renal proximal tubular toxicity is regulated by OAT1 and MRP4 transporters. *Laboratory Investigation* 2011;91:852–858.

24. Strazzulla A, Coppolino G, Barreca G et al. Evolution of glomerular filtration rates and neutrophil gelatinase-associated lipocalin during treatment with direct acting antivirals. *Clinical and Molecular Hepatology* 2018;24:151–162.

25. Mallet V, Parlati L, Dorval O et al. Estimated glomerular filtration rate variations and direct acting antivirals treatment for chronic hepatitis C: a retrospective longitudinal study. *Journal of Hepatology* 2018;68:S22.

26. Kamar N, Marion O, Rostaing L et al. Efficacy and safety of sofosbuvir-based antiviral therapy to treat hepatitis c virus infection after kidney transplantation. *American Journal of Transplantation* 2016;16:1474–1479.

27. Fernandez I, Munoz Gomez R, Pascasio J et al. Efficacy and tolerability of interferon-free antiviral therapy in kidney transplant recipients with chronic hepatitis C. *Journal of Hepatology* 2017;66:718–723.

28. Kumar M, Nayak SL, Gupta E, Kataria A, Sarin SK. Generic sofosbuvir based direct-acting antivirals in hepatitis C virus

infected patients with chronic kidney disease. *Liver International* 2018;38:2137–2148.

29. Colombo M, Aghemo A, Liu H et al. Treatment with ledipasvir-sofosbuvir for 12 or 24 weeks in kidney transplant recipients with chronic hepatitis C virus genotype 1 or 4 infection: a randomized trial. *Annals of Internal Medicine* 2017;166:109–117.

30. Aby ES, Dong TS, Kawamoto J et al. Impact of of sustained virologic response on chronic kidney disease progression in hepatitis C. *World Journal of Hepatology* 2017;9:1352–1360.

31. Butt AA, Wang X, Fried LF. HCV infection and the incidence of CKD. *American Journal of Kidney Disease* 2011;57: 396–402.

32. Oppong Y, Chute D, Davis M et al. AKI effects of treatment of hepatitis C virus infection on kidney function (abstract). file:///C:/Users/Owner/Downloads/Oppong_American JournalofKidneyDiseases.pdf

9 Does directly acting antiviral therapy improve quality of life?

Daniel M. Forton

St George's University Hospitals NHS Foundation Trust, London, UK

LEARNING POINTS

- Hepatitis C infection *per se* causes a reduction in quality of life which is likely related to interactions between direct physical effects of the virus and psychosocial consequences of infection.

- Viral clearance, whether through interferon or DAA therapy, improves quality of life in nearly all studies, although studies in patients with multiple comorbidities indicate that the benefits may be reduced by other illnesses.

- A small minority of patients develop persistent fatigue even after HCV clearance.

- The mechanism of the effects of hepatitis C on health-related quality of life is unclear and further work will be required.

Introduction

The impact of directly acting antiviral (DAA) therapy on hepatitis C (HCV) virologic cure has been one of the most important developments in modern medicine, with sustained virologic response (SVR) rates of greater than 95% across all genotypes and in most indications. Despite initial claims, based on a systematic review of clinical trials, that virologic cure does not directly equate to important clinical outcomes [1], there are increasing numbers of published studies which refute this and evidence important reductions in liver-related and nonliver-related morbidity and mortality. In addition to reductions in early mortality after virologic cure of patients with compensated [2] and decompensated cirrhosis [3], there are improvements in other hard endpoints such as listing for liver transplantation [4] and incidence of hepatocellular carcinoma [5]. Surrogate markers of portal hypertension [6] and liver fibrosis improve [7] after DAA therapy and there are reductions in nonliver mortality [2] and improvements in carotid atherosclerosis [8] and in glycemic control in diabetic patients [9].

These assessments of the clinical sequelae of HCV infection have been made by investigators. In order to understand the full impact of HCV infection and its treatment, patient-reported outcomes of health-related quality of life (HRQL) are also needed. This refers to an individual patient's personal assessment or perception of his/her physical, mental and/or social well-being and experience. Just as virologic cure is an important endpoint of DAA therapy, the impact of HCV infection and its treatment on patient-reported outcome (PRO) measures is an important reflection of the patients' lived experience and the perceived benefit of treatment.

Several generic and disease-specific tools have been developed to measure HRQL across a number of domains including physical, emotional, and social functioning (the generic SF-36) [10], fatigue and its impacts (FACIT-F) [11], and liver-specific measures such as energy (CLDQ-HCV) [12]. Attempts have been made to define clinically important differences in HRQL which can be used in group comparisons, such as HCV-infected individuals versus the general population, and in comparisons of disease states, such as before and after SVR.

Clinical Dilemmas in Viral Liver Disease, Second Edition. Edited by Graham R. Foster and K. Rajender Reddy.
© 2020 John Wiley & Sons Ltd. Published 2020 by John Wiley & Sons Ltd.

Health-related quality of life in chronic hepatitis C infection

The results from several large studies challenge the perception that HCV infection is an "asymptomatic" disease, with general agreement that physical and mental HRQL is significantly reduced in HCV-infected patients, compared to published normative data [13][1;6;7;12]. In a systematic review of 15 large cohorts of HCV-infected patients who completed the SF-36 questionnaire and were compared to healthy controls [14], impairments were seen across each of the eight domains with weighted mean reductions of between 7.0 and 15.8; a 3–5-point difference was considered to be clinically important. It was concluded that the impact of HCV on HRQL is moderate to large, with the most important impairments being in social and physical function, general health, and vitality.

A more recent study from Baltimore examined standardized differences from US population means and found impairments in physical health, with a medium to large effect size, but only small differences in the mental health domain [15]. Reductions in HRQL are seen across all stages of liver fibrosis and appear independent of ALT [16], although cirrhosis and decompensated liver disease are associated with more severe impacts [17].

In patients with compensated liver disease, fatigue appears to be an important determinant of the impaired HRQL, with a reported prevalence ranging from 20% to 80% in different cohorts [18]. Fatigue severity does not appear to correlate with the degree of biochemical hepatitis although one study found associations between fatigue scores and the inflammatory profile of 47 immune factors measured in plasma using a multiplex microbead methodology [19], suggesting that peripheral immune activation may potentially contribute to this symptom. However, the relative contribution of a biological mechanism for fatigue in HCV infection remains unclear as multiple, interrelating social, psychologic, and comorbid factors are undoubtedly relevant. The impacts of diagnosis, health-related anxiety, and stigmatization are all thought to be determinants of HRQL [20].

The role of labelling was suggested in a study of subjects who were admitted to hospital in the 1970s with acute hepatitis, a proportion of whom were unaware of their diagnosis of chronic HCV infection. Those who were aware of their serostatus rated significantly worse on seven

of eight SF-36 scales compared to population norms, whereas those who did not know their diagnosis scored significantly worse in only three scales [20]. However, other prospective studies of blood donors have revealed impaired SF-36 scores in HCV-infected individuals prior to knowledge of their diagnosis, compared both to donors who tested HCV negative and those who had a false-positive result [21,22]. The data together suggest an independent effect of HCV infection itself on HRQL, which may be compounded by the impact of diagnosis. Other important adverse factors which have emerged from surveys in different parts of the world include greater age, low income, comorbidities including diabetes mellitus [15,23], intravenous drug (ID) use [24], emotional distress, posttraumatic stress disorder [25], and depression. Depression is a common and clinically important finding in HCV-infected patients, affecting 51% of previous ID users in a cohort of over 6000 patients in the National HCV Research UK Biobank, compared to 27% of non-IDUs [26]. The relationship between HCV and depression is undoubtedly complex. ID use is a key risk factor for both HCV acquisition and depression [27]. Conversely, depression may exist as a secondary phenomenon to HCV infection. This may take the form of a reactive depression, related to the diagnosis and concerns over long-term health, or may be associated with symptoms such as fatigue and cognitive impairment, which may in part have a biological basis [28].

An independent biological basis for impairments in HRQL and symptoms, such as fatigue and mild cognitive impairment, is supported by neuroimaging studies. Cerebral magnetic resonance imaging, spectroscopy, positron emission tomography, and nuclear medicine techniques have revealed brain abnormalities in small cohorts of patients with HCV infection (see [18] for review). In parallel, mild impairments in cognitive performance have been reported, with diminished abilities in the areas of concentration, attention, verbal learning, working memory, executive function, and psychomotor performance, although there have been inconsistent correlations with neuroimaging data. Furthermore, the studies have not consistently controlled for the psychosocial factors described previously. A number of hypotheses have been suggested linking these findings, including neuroinflammatory models as consequence of neuroinvasion and/or a central effect of peripheral immune activation and changes in tryptophan metabolites (see [18] for review). The absence of an animal model to test these hypotheses has limited the conclusions.

The question as to whether there is a direct virologic cause for impaired HRQL in HCV infection has become unnecessarily dichotomized between biological and psychosocial models [24]. In this context, measuring the impact of DAA therapy on HRQL and other functions in properly controlled studies is of great interest, not only in terms of quantifying patient benefit but also to gain insights into the pathogenesis of the symptoms that patients experience.

Direct-acting antiviral therapy and health-related quality of life

The advent of DAA therapy, with its generally excellent adverse effect profile, provides an opportunity to study the impact of viral eradication on HRQL. In the pre-DAA era, improvements in HRQL and reductions in fatigue levels were widely reported in patients after an SVR to treatment with pegylated interferon and ribavirin [13], drugs with associated physical, mental and cognitive effects during and, sometimes, after the end of therapy. The positive impacts were only evident after cessation of treatment. In contrast, clinically significant improvements in PROs have been reported as early as four weeks into ribavirin-free DAA therapy as viremia is suppressed [29].

In a double-blind placebo-controlled randomized clinical trial of sofosbuvir/velpatasvir in 750 patients with hepatitis C, subjects completed questionnaires that assessed 25 PROs at baseline and every four weeks through treatment and to 24 weeks after the end of treatment in those who had an SVR [29]. The patients were unaware of their viral status when completing the assessments in this double-blind trial. Most large DAA studies to date had included ribavirin and/ or were not placebo controlled. This study provided an excellent opportunity to determine the impact of direct virologic suppression on HRQL. By week 4 of treatment, statistically significant improvements were seen in general health, emotional well-being, and fatigue compared to baseline in the patients on active treatment, which were not seen in the placebo group. Most PROs continued to improve in the treatment group, but not the placebo group, to the end of treatment at week 12 and then improved further to the last time point, 24 weeks after the end of treatment. A multivariable analysis was performed, which took into account

baseline levels of the PROs in addition to clinical and demographic factors, and demonstrated that treatment emergent improvements in the PROs, such as fatigue scores, during and then continuing after treatment were independently predicted by receiving antiviral treatment as opposed to placebo. Early virologic clearance was associated with improvements in HRQL but these improvements continued long after complete viral clearance from serum, implying additional mechanisms. The authors postulated an improvement in the inflammatory milieu and its impact on the brain. Similar findings have been reported with other sofosbuvir-containing regimes [30], in cirrhotic [31] and HIV coinfected patients [32] and in different cohorts of patients from the USA, Europe [33], and Asia [34] with different cultural backgrounds and with other DAA regimes [35].

In contrast to these data, derived largely from registration trials, some real-world reports reveal less profound improvements in PROs. In a study of 236 US patients, there was only a small improvement in mental health domains and no improvement in physical health domains after interferon and ribavirin-free DAA therapy [15]. In this cohort, the physical health scores were much lower than both the US population and patients in registration trials and, furthermore, baseline factors such as hypertension, high BMI, pulmonary conditions, number of comorbidities, and public health insurance were the strongest negative predictors of HRQL. This study demonstrates that the health benefits of HCV eradication have to be considered in the context of other comorbidities, which need to be treated separately to improve the health burden on such patients. The authors did recognize that early HCV treatment might prevent metabolic and cardiovascular complications, with impacts on long-term HRQL, but such studies have not been performed to date.

Very few studies to date have examined the impact of DAA therapy on mood, cognitive function, and biological correlates. Two small studies report interesting findings which need to be examined in larger prospective studies. In 20 mono- or HIV coinfected patients, DAA therapy improved fatigue and mental health together with several cognitive domains such visual memory, learning, and processing speed but not attention and working memory [36]. In another recently published study, 24 patients were assessed for fatigue and depression before, during, and after therapy with a variety of DAAs including ribavirin-containing regimes (79% with a sofosbuvir-based protocol)

[37]. In addition, blood was analyzed for levels of the amino acids tryptophan and kynurenine, which are intermediates in the metabolic regulation of serotonin concentrations. Antiviral treatment resulted in significant reduction of depression scores, which was not seen in patient controls. This was accompanied by significant elevations in kynurenine and reductions in tryptophan, findings which are also reported in interferon therapy and have been invoked as a cause for interferon-induced depression. The findings are somewhat counterintuitive but indicate a biological impact of DAAs on serotonin metabolites and require further investigation in larger studies.

Conclusion

The positive impact of an SVR on HRQL was demonstrated previously with interferon-containing regimes but was only evident at SVR24 or later, with substantial on-treatment decrements. In contrast, large datasets from the DAA registration studies show early improvements in HRQL, fatigue, and work productivity on treatment, which continue to increase after the end of therapy. Real-world data are less reported but indicate that the positive impact of DAA therapy on HRQL as a consequence of viral eradication may be abrogated by impairments due to the frequent multiple comorbidities that characterize the aging HCV-infected cohort.

The biological mechanisms that underlie the early, later and sustained improvements in HRQL are incompletely understood but may be related to beneficial changes in the inflammatory milieu and its impact on abnormal cerebral and somatic systems, such as insulin resistance. A small minority of patients remain quite symptomatic after DAA therapy with, for example profound fatigue [38], and this may be related to more permanent impacts of HCV infection or significant unconnected comorbidities. There is therefore still a need to understand the biological mechanisms causing fatigue, depression, and cognitive impairment in HCV infection as well as offering patients strategies to manage important comorbidities.

References

1. Jakobsen JC, Nielsen EE, Feinberg J et al. Direct-acting antivirals for chronic hepatitis C. *Cochrane Database of Systematic Reviews* 2017;9:Cd012143.

2. Backus LI, Belperio PS, Shahoumian TA, Mole LA. Impact of sustained virologic response with direct-acting antiviral treatment on mortality in patients with advanced liver disease. *Hepatology* 2017;10.1002/hep.29408.

3. Cheung MCM, Walker AJ, Hudson BE et al. Outcomes after successful direct-acting antiviral therapy for patients with chronic hepatitis C and decompensated cirrhosis. *Journal of Hepatology* 2016;65(4):741–747.

4. Belli LS, Berenguer M, Cortesi PA et al. Delisting of liver transplant candidates with chronic hepatitis C after viral eradication: a European study. *Journal of Hepatology* 2016;65(3):524–531.

5. Kanwal F, Kramer J, Asch SM, Chayanupatkul M, Cao Y, El-Serag HB. Risk of hepatocellular cancer in HCV patients treated with direct-acting antiviral agents. *Gastroenterology* 2017;153(4):996–1005.e1.

6. Lens S, Alvarado-Tapias E, Marino Z et al. Effects of all-oral antiviral therapy on hvpg and systemic hemodynamics in patients with hepatitis C virus-associated cirrhosis. *Gastroenterology* 2017;153(5):1273–1283.e1.

7. Knop V, Hoppe D, Welzel T et al. Regression of fibrosis and portal hypertension in HCV-associated cirrhosis and sustained virologic response after interferon-free antiviral therapy. *Journal of Viral Hepatology* 2016;23(12):994–1002.

8. Petta S, Adinolfi LE, Fracanzani AL et al. Hepatitis C virus eradication by direct-acting antiviral agents improves carotid atherosclerosis in patients with severe liver fibrosis. *Journal of Hepatology* 2018;69(1):18–24.

9. Hum J, Jou JH, Green PK et al. Improvement in glycemic control of type 2 diabetes after successful treatment of hepatitis C virus. *Diabetes Care* 2017;40(9):1173–1180.

10. Ware JE Jr, Sherbourne CD. The MOS 36-item short-form health survey (SF-36). I. Conceptual framework and item selection. *Medical Care* 1992;30(6):473–483.

11. Webster K, Peterman A, Lent L, Cella D. The Functional Assessment of Chronic Illness Therapy (FACIT) measurement system: validation of version 4 of the core questionnaire. *Quality of Life Research* 1999;8:604.

12. Younossi ZM, Guyatt G, Kiwi M, Boparai N, King D. Development of a disease specific questionnaire to measure health related quality of life in patients with chronic liver disease. *Gut* 1999;45(2):295–300.

13. Bonkovsky HL, Woolley JM. Reduction of health-related quality of life in chronic hepatitis C and improvement with interferon therapy. *The Consensus Interferon Study Group.* *Hepatology* 1999;29(1):264–270.

14. Spiegel BM, Younossi ZM, Hays RD, Revicki D, Robbins S, Kanwal F. Impact of hepatitis C on health related quality of life: a systematic review and quantitative assessment. *Hepatology* 2005;41(4):790–800.

15. Thuluvath PJ, Savva Y. Mental and physical health-related quality of life in patients with hepatitis C is related to baseline comorbidities and improves only marginally with hepatitis C cure. *Clinical and Translational Gastroenterology* 2018;9(4):149.

16. Miller ER, Hiller JE, Shaw DR. Quality of life in HCV-infection: lack of association with ALT levels. *Australian and New Zealand Journal of Public Health* 2001;25(4):355–361.

17. Cordoba J, Flavia M, Jacas C et al. Quality of life and cognitive function in hepatitis C at different stages of liver disease. *Journal of Hepatology* 2003;39(2):231–238.

18. Yarlott L, Heald E, Forton D. Hepatitis C virus infection, and neurological and psychiatric disorders – a review. *Journal of Advanced Research* 2017;8(2):139–148.

19. Huckans M, Fuller BE, Olavarria H et al. Multi-analyte profile analysis of plasma immune proteins: altered expression of peripheral immune factors is associated with neuropsychiatric symptom severity in adults with and without chronic hepatitis C virus infection. *Brain and Behavior* 2014;4(2):123–142.

20. Rodger AJ, Jolley D, Thompson SC, Lanigan A, Crofts N. The impact of diagnosis of hepatitis C virus on quality of life. *Hepatology* 1999;30(5):1299–1301.

21. Strauss E, Porto-Ferreira FA, de Almeida-Neto C, Teixeira MC. Altered quality of life in the early stages of chronic hepatitis C is due to the virus itself. *Clinics and Research in Hepatology and Gastroenterology* 2014;38(1):40–45.

22. Ferreira FA, de Almeida-Neto C, Teixeira MC, Strauss E. Health-related quality of life among blood donors with hepatitis B and hepatitis C: longitudinal study before and after diagnosis. *Revista Brasileira de Hematologia e Hemoterapia* 2015;37(6):381–387.

23. Jang ES, Kim YS, Kim KA et al. Factors associated with health-related quality of life in Korean patients with chronic hepatitis C infection using the SF-36 and EQ-5D. *Gut and Liver* 2018;12(4):440–448.

24. Helbling B, Overbeck K, Gonvers JJ et al. Host- rather than virus-related factors reduce health-related quality of life in hepatitis C virus infection. *Gut* 2008;57(11):1597–1603.

25. Lim JK, Cronkite R, Goldstein MK, Cheung RC. The impact of chronic hepatitis C and comorbid psychiatric illnesses on health-related quality of life. *Journal of Clinical Gastroenterology* 2006;40(6):528–534.

26. Hudson B, Walker AJ, Irving WL. Comorbidities and medications of patients with chronic hepatitis C under specialist care in the UK. *Journal of Medical Virology* 2017;89(12):2158–2164.

27. Johnson ME, Fisher DG, Fenaughty A, Theno SA. Hepatitis C virus and depression in drug users. *American Journal of Gastroenterology* 1998;93(5):785–789.

28. McDonald J, Jayasuriya J, Bindley P, Gonsalvez C, Gluseska S. Fatigue and psychological disorders in chronic hepatitis C. *Journal of Gastroenterology and Hepatology* 2002;17(2):171–176.

29. Younossi ZM, Stepanova M, Feld J et al. Sofosbuvir/velpatasvir improves patient-reported outcomes in HCV patients: results from ASTRAL-1 placebo-controlled trial. *Journal of Hepatology* 2016;65(1):33–39.

30. Younossi ZM, Stepanova M, Henry L, Nader F, Hunt S. An in-depth analysis of patient-reported outcomes in patients with chronic hepatitis C treated with different anti-viral regimens. *American Journal of Gastroenterology* 2016;111(6):808–816.

31. Younossi ZM, Stepanova M, Afdhal N et al. Improvement of health-related quality of life and work productivity in chronic hepatitis C patients with early and advanced fibrosis treated with ledipasvir and sofosbuvir. *Journal of Hepatology* 2015;63(2):337–345.

32. Younossi ZM, Stepanova M, Sulkowski M, Naggie S, Henry L, Hunt S. Sofosbuvir and ledipasvir improve patient-reported outcomes in patients co-infected with hepatitis C and human immunodeficiency virus. *Journal of Viral Hepatology* 2016;23(11):857–865.

33. Cacoub P, Bourliere M, Asselah T et al. French patients with hepatitis C treated with direct-acting antiviral combinations: the effect on patient-reported outcomes. *Value in Health* 2018;21(10):1218–1225.

34. Younossi ZM, Stepanova M, Henry L et al. Sofosbuvir and ledipasvir are associated with high sustained virologic response and improvement of health-related quality of life in East Asian patients with hepatitis C virus infection. *Journal of Viral Hepatology* 2018;25(12):1429–1437.

35. Ng X, Nwankwo C, Arduino JM et al. Patient-reported outcomes in individuals with hepatitis C virus infection treated with elbasvir/grazoprevir. *Patient Preference and Adherence* 2018;12:2631–2638.

36. Kleefeld F, Heller S, Jessen H, Ingiliz P, Kraft A, Hahn K. Effect of interferon-free therapy on cognition in HCV and HCV/HIV infection: a pilot study. *Neurology* 2017;88(7):713–715.

37. Hahn D, Stokes CS, Kaiser R, Meyer MR, Lammert F, Gruenhage F. Antidepressant effects of direct-acting antivirals against hepatitis C virus-Results from a pilot study. *European Journal of Clinical Investigation* 2018;48(12):e13024.

38. Dirks M, Pflugrad H, Haag K et al. Persistent neuropsychiatric impairment in HCV patients despite clearance of the virus?! *Journal of Viral Hepatology* 2017;24(7):541–550.

10 Morbid obesity and hepatitis C: treat as normal or are there additional issues to consider?

María Fernanda Guerra[1], Javier Ampuero[2], and Manuel Romero-Gómez[2]

[1] Digestive Diseases Department, Virgen Macarena University Hospital, Sevilla, Spain
[2] UCM Digestive Diseases and CIBEREHD, Virgen del Rocío University Hospital, Institute of Biomedicine of Seville, University of Seville, Sevilla, Spain

LEARNING POINTS

- Thirty-seven percent of American adults are obese, 8% showed morbid obesity, and 21% of patients with chronic hepatitis C are obese.

- Obesity is an independent risk factor for nonalcoholic fatty liver disease (NAFLD) and nonalcoholic steatohepatitis (NASH) and independently increases the risk of hepatocellular carcinoma.

- Chronic hepatitis C is a cause of insulin resistance, type 2 diabetes, and hepatic steatosis and all these factors are related to fibrosis progression.

- Insulin resistance, obesity, and type 2 diabetes were associated with a reduced sustained virologic response rate using an interferon-based regimen. However, orally administered direct antiviral agent success rate was not affected by these metabolic disorders.

- Eradication of the virus improves fibrosis and HOMA-IR in patients with preexisting insulin resistance and type 2 diabetes but cannot reverse features of metabolic syndrome once they have been established.

- Obese patients should be closely followed after sustained virologic response, because regression of fibrosis and steatosis is scarce and slower.

Obesity as a health problem

Obesity (Body Mass Index [BMI] $\geq 30\,kg/m^2$) is a complex multifactorial disease that today, together with being overweight, affects more than a third of the world's population.

According to CDC data [1], the prevalence of obesity was 39.6% and it affected about 93.3 million American adults in 2015–2016. The prevalence of obesity increased in women and in adults aged 40–59 years. Data from the National Health and Nutrition Survey (NHANES) in the US reported a standardized prevalence by age of severe obesity (BMI $\geq 40\,kg/m^2$) in adults of 7.7% (95% confidence interval [CI] 6.6–8.9%) in 2015–2016 compared to 5.7% (95% CI 4.9–6.7%) in 2007–2008 [2], which shows a clear and alarming increase.

In a recent NHANES study for the period 1999–2012, of patients with chronic hepatitis C (CHC), it was estimated that the demographic-adjusted prevalence of obesity was 20.9% (95% CI 12.4–29.5), and type 2 diabetes mellitus (T2DM) was 17.9% (95% CI 11.2–27.5). Overall, 69.6% of persons with CHC had at least one major cardiometabolic comorbidity (95% CI 62.1–76.2%) [3], increasing the risk of early death.

Obesity-related comorbidities

Obesity has been considered an independent risk factor for NAFLD and NASH and was significantly associated with metabolic disorders (such as insulin resistance [IR], T2DM, and dyslipidemia), tissue inflammation, and liver fibrosis [4]. Obesity is also associated with an increased risk of hepatocellular carcinoma (HCC).

The large amount of visceral adipose tissue in severe obese patient contributes to a high prevalence of NAFLD. The visceral fat secretes adipokines and induces inflammatory

Clinical Dilemmas in Viral Liver Disease, Second Edition. Edited by Graham R. Foster and K. Rajender Reddy.
© 2020 John Wiley & Sons Ltd. Published 2020 by John Wiley & Sons Ltd.

processes that impair insulin sensitivity in tissues such as liver and muscle. Also, the accumulation of visceral fat is a surrogate indicator of ectopic lipid accumulation and lipotoxicity [5].

The prevalence of steatosis in hepatitis C ranges from 40% to 86% [6], which is associated with features of metabolic syndrome and IR in non-3 genotype-infected cases or viral steatosis related to viral load in genotype 3-infected cases [7]. Hepatitis C virus interacts with host lipid metabolism by several mechanisms, such as promotion of lipogenesis, reduction of fatty acid oxidation, and decrease of lipid export, leading to hepatic steatosis and hypolipidemia [8]. In non-3 genotype, genetic backgrounds such as interleukin and patatin-like phospholipase-3 (PNPL3) polymorphism are associated with an increased risk of hepatocyte steatosis.

Assessment of fibrosis in obese patients

The prevalence of severe fibrosis in morbidly obese patients who underwent bariatric surgery was around 12%. The prevalence of NAFLD in this group is estimated to be 84–96% and NASH 5–25% [9,10]. The correct evaluation of fibrosis in these patients remained elusive. Liver biopsy is the gold standard for assessing the degree of fibrosis and steatosis, but this is an invasive method. Noninvasive techniques are gaining interest. Development of the XL probe for transient elastography (TE) increases the success of liver stiffness measurement rates up to 82% in obese patients compared with the standard M probe [11]. Many studies showed the combination of serum (APRI, Forns, FibroTest®) and imaging-based noninvasive (ARFI, 2D-SWE, MR elastography) methods as increasing the accuracy of fibrosis diagnosis and avoiding liver biopsy [12]; however, they had reduced accuracy for distinguishing early fibrosis stages (F1–F2). Other methods not applied in clinical practice (NASHMRI with FibroMRI [13], lipidomic serum test [12]) are showing good results in terms of diagnostic accuracy for steatohepatitis and NAFLD [14] in the obese population.

Obesity and sustained virologic response with interferon therapies

In the era of interferon (INF) therapies, cure of infection was achieved in 45% of genotype 1 [15] and 65% of genotype 3 cases. There were some predictive factors associated with a low response to this therapy including viral load,

polymorphism IL28B, genotype, age, sex, race, fibrosis, and metabolic disorders.

Obesity was associated with lower sustained virologic response (SVR) rates regardless of viral genotype due to the following factors [16].

- Adipose tissue is an active endocrine organ secreting several hormones called adipokines (adiponectin and leptin), which regulate body weight, insulin sensitivity, inflammation, and vascular function. Leptin has proinflammatory properties, upregulating the production of Th1, interleukins, and tumor necrosis factor alpha (TNF-alpha) and decreasing production of the antiinflammatory cytokines (interleukin [IL]-10) [17]. All this translates into a decrease in response to interferon.
- High TNF-alpha levels can interfere with the IFN-alpha receptor and signaling proteins via induction of the suppressor of cytokine signaling (SOCS) family. Studies reported that obese subjects infected with hepatitis C virus (HCV) genotype 1 had increased hepatic expression of SOCS-3 [18].
- Insulin resistance is thought to be due to a combination of host- and virus-mediated pathways. HCV core protein in the hepatocyte upregulates TNF-alpha, which causes the phosphorylation of insulin receptor substrate types 1 and 2 (IRS-1/IRS-2) [19]. Also, HCV core protein upregulates SOCS protein which causes ubiquitination of IRS1/IRS-2, and these both prevent the downstream activation of protein kinase B (AKT). HCV core protein leads to oxidative stress, increasing inflammatory cytokines, which promotes a state of hyperinsulinemia, decreases apolipoprotein B-100, enhances triglyceride accumulation in the liver, and leads to steatosis [20]. In general, SOCS-3 overexpression and hepatic steatosis promote intrahepatic and systemic lipid oxidation, thus leading to peripheral and hepatic insulin resistance [21]. Insulin resistance is associated with steatosis and fibrosis and also impairs responses to combination therapy.
- Decreased bioavailability of IFN-alpha in obese patients due to impaired drug absorption. While the volume of distribution of PEG-interferon alpha 2a (PEG-IFN-alpha 2a) was not affected by body weight, it varied according to body weight with PEG-IFN-alpha 2b. This difference could be explained, at least in part, by a variation in molecular weights of these proteins. Studies in

obese patients with escalating doses of PEG-IFN-α 2a up to 360 µg/week failed to demonstrate better efficacy [22].

Several strategies to improve IR during IFN-based therapy have been assessed (using antidiabetic drugs), but did not demonstrate a clear improvement in SVR [23,24]. Weight loss was a common adverse event in IFN therapies, and they did not show an increase in SVR.

Obesity and SVR in the new direct-acting antivirals

Development of direct-acting antiviral drugs (DAAs) targeting viral proteins has revolutionized the treatment of chronic hepatitis C, reaching response rates close to 100%, and leaving behind the poor response of predictive factors to interferon therapies. Pharmacokinetic dosage adjustments based on age, body weight, and sex were not necessary for these therapies.

Table 10.1 shows the SVR rate according to subgroup stratified by BMI. SVR was similar across all groups.

Obesity as a predictor of fibrosis progression beyond SVR

Liver fibrosis as a consequence of hepatic stellate cell activation remains after SVR, mainly in patients with advanced fibrosis and/or severe comorbidities [25–27] in the era of interferon therapies. Activation of the hepatic stellate cells is induced by cytokines and chemokines in the intrahepatic tissues or through indirect mechanisms mediated by HCV viral proteins. Stellate cells can respond to cytokines and growth factors after the first stimulation, producing an accumulation of extracellular matrix [28] (overproduction of collagen type I). Approximately 10% of HCV patients present a persistent or even progressive fibrosis following SVR due to an underlying liver disease like NAFLD, although this percentage increases in patients with basal advanced fibrosis [29].

Patients who achieved SVR reduced by half the incidence of T2DM and/or impaired fasting glucose during posttreatment follow-up with interferon therapies [30]. With the new DAAs, SVR improved homeostatis model assessment (HOMA)-IR and fasting glucose in patients with existing IR and T2DM, although the values did not return to normal; this persistence of IR was observed in

patients with advanced fibrosis. Data suggested that a reduction of beta-cell distress can prevent or delay the development of T2DM. Eradication of the hepatitis C virus could delay the onset of metabolic syndrome, but this has not been definitely established. Weight loss was a common adverse event in IFN therapies, whereas with the new DAAs, no BMI changes have been reported after the therapies.

It is known that patients with HCV genotype 3 showed more hepatocyte steatosis than other genotypes. Also, after IFN-induced HCV clearance, resolution of hepatocyte steatosis has been commonly seen. However, in non-3 genotype or in patients treated with DAAs with metabolic comorbidities, disappearance of steatosis after SVR is not homogeneous. In non-3 genotype patients treated with DAA, Noureddin et al. reported a prevalence of hepatic steatosis around 47.5% post SVR, despite normal liver enzymes [31]. Changes in lifestyle after SVR, with more relaxed habits in diet and alcohol consumption, could explain this, at least in part.

In a multicenter Spanish study, Ampuero et al. showed the importance of evaluation of basal comorbidities at the time of steroidogenic acute regulatory protein (StAR) DAA in CHC patients [32]. They demonstrated how the combination of Charlson index, age, INR, albumin, and bilirubin (HepCom score) was able to identify a high-risk group of patients who would die or suffer a relevant clinical event within the first two years of DAA therapy. As expected, obesity was not an independent variable associated with outcomes in DAA-treated patients. In this study, the two-year rate of mortality was 5.4%, and 20% of patients developed a relevant clinical event. Only one-third of these events were related to hepatic complications. This emphasizes the importance of monitoring comorbidities like obesity, IR, and T2DM after SVR.

Accuracy of noninvasive tests in staging post-SVR fibrosis has been addressed in several studies. However, guidelines do not recommend their use because they have not been validated. Variables included in these models could change irrespective of virus clearance. Thus, obese patients with hepatitis C after SVR should be closely monitored to prevent liver cancer and development of comorbidities. The current European and American guidelines recommend treating all patients with hepatitis C, suggesting that patients with associated cofactor-related liver disease (history of alcohol drinking, a metabolic syndrome

Table 10.1 SVR rate in obese patients with different genotypes and therapeutic regimens

Authors/study	Treatment	Genotype	BMI	SVR %
Afdhal et al. [33] ION-1 Naive	Ledipasvir + sofosbuvir 12 weeks Ledipasvir + Sofosbuvir 24 weeks	1	≥30	100 100
Afdhal et al. [34] ION-2 Previously treated	Ledipasvir + sofosbuvir 12 weeks Ledipasvir + sofosbuvir 24 weeks	1	≥30	95.3 100
Kowdley et al. [35] ION-3 Naive	Ledipasvir + sofosbuvir 8 weeks Ledipasvir + sofosbuvir 12 weeks	1	≥30	95.3 96.5
Feld et al. [36] SAPPHIRE-I Naive	Paritaprevir/r + ombitasvir + dasabuvir + ribavirin* 12 weeks	1	<30 ≥30	97 91.5
Zeuzem et al. [37] SAPPHIRE-II Previously treated	Paritaprevir/r + ombitasvir + dasabuvir + ribavirin 12 weeks	1	<30 ≥30	97.1 93.2
Zeuzem et al. [38] C-EDGE	Grazoprevir/elbasvir 12 weeks	1, 4 and 6	BMI** mean 26 (DE 5.22)	95
Feld et al. [39] ASTRAL-1	Sofosbuvir + velpatasvir 12 weeks	1 2, 4, 6 5	≥30 ≥30 ≥30	98.6 100 100
Foster et al. [40] ASTRAL 2–3	Sofosbuvir + velpatasvir 12 weeks	2 and 3	≥30	98
Bourlière et al. [41] POLARIS-1 and POLARIS-4	Sofosbuvir + velpatasvir + voxilaprevir 12 weeks Sofosbuvir + velpatasvir 12 weeks	1, 2, 3, 4, 5 and 6	≥30	97 99
Zeuzem et al. [42] ENDURANCE-1	Glecaprevir/pibrentasvir 8 weeks Glecaprevir/pibrentasvir 12 weeks	1	BMI** mean 25 (18–41) 25 (18–54)	99.1 99.7
ENDURANCE-3	Glecaprevir/pibrentasvir 8 weeks Glecaprevir/pibrentasvir 12 weeks	3	26 (18–44) 25 (17–49)	95 95
EXPEDITION-1 [43]	Glecaprevir/pibrentasvir 12 weeks	1,2,4,5, and 6	29.2 (5.8)	99–100

* Ribavirin: 1000 mg daily body weight <75 kg, 1200 mg daily body weight ≥75 kg.
** No subgroup (BMI) analysis.
BMI, Body Mass Index; SVR, sustained virologic response.

possibly associated with obesity and/or T2DM) should be additionally evaluated. HCC surveillance every six months is mandatory and must be continued indefinitely in patients with advanced fibrosis.

Conclusion

In summary, metabolic syndrome coexists in approximately 30% of patients with hepatitis C. Obesity is related to NAFDL, mainly in patients with obesity showing insulin resistance or diabetes. These comorbidities have no impact on SVR rates with new DAAs. However, baseline liver injury such as steatosis, steatohepatitis, and fibrosis could continue to promote fibrosis progression to cirrhosis or liver cancer even after SVR (Figure 10.1). Thus, these patients should be closely followed up to prevent liver-related and extrahepatic complications. The identification of biomarkers able to predict outcomes in obese patients with hepatitis C after SVR and the development of drugs able to reverse hepatic stellate cell activation are two major unmet needs in this field. Further studies addressing both goals are warranted.

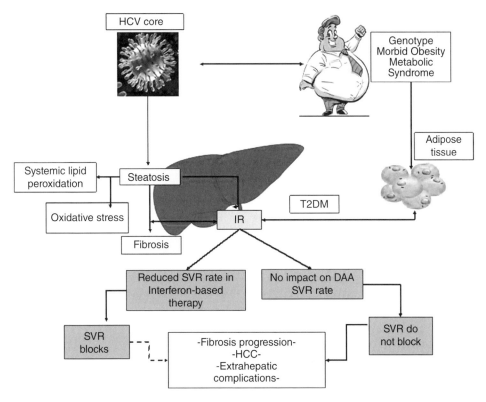

Figure 10.1 Schematic representation of the interaction between obesity, lipid metabolism, insulin resistance, and outcomes of hepatitis C after sustained virologic response. DAA, direct-acting antiviral drug; HCC, hepatocellular carcinoma; IR, insulin resistance; SVR, sustained virologic response; T2DM, type 2 diabetes mellitus.

References

1. Centers for Disease Control and Prevention (CDC). Viral Hepatitis Statistics and Surveillance – United States, 2016. www.cdc.gov/hepatitis/statistics/2016surveillance/index.htm.

2. Hales C, Fryar C, Carroll M et al. Trends in obesity and severe obesity prevalence in US youth and adults by sex and age, 2007–2008 to 2015–2016. *JAMA* 2018;319:1723–1725.

3. Lazo M, Nwankwo C, Daya NR et al. Confluence of epidemics of hepatitis c, diabetes, obesity,and chronic kidney disease in the united states population. *Clinical Gastroenterology and Hepatology* 2017;15:1957–1964.e7

4. Lu FB, Hu ED, Xu LM et al. The relationship between obesity and the severity of non-alcoholic fatty liver disease: systematic review and meta-analysis. *Expert Reviews in Gastroenterology and Hepatology* 2018;12:491–502.

5. Esteve Rafols M. Adipose tissue: cell heterogeneity and functional diversity. *Endocrinologia y Nutricion* 2014;61: 100–112.

6. Lonardo A, Adinolfi LE, Loria P et al. Steatosis and hepatitis C virus: mechanisms and significance for hepatic and extra-hepatic disease. *Gastroenterology* 2004;126:586–597.

7. Castera L. Steatosis, insulin resistance and fibrosis progression in chronic hepatitis C. *Minerva Gastroenterologica e Dietologica* 2006;52:125–134.

8. Romero-Gómez M, Rojas Á. Sofosbuvir modulates the intimate relationship between hepatitis C virus and lipids. *Hepatology* 2015;61:744–747.

9. Carmona I, Cordero P, Ampuero J et al. Role of assessing liver fibrosis in management of chronic hepatitis C virus infection. *Clinical Microbiology and Infection* 2016;22:839–845.

10. Losekann A, Weston A, de Mattos A et al. Non-alcoholic steatohepatitis (NASH): risk factor in morbidly obese patients. *International Journal of Molecular Sciences* 2015;16: 25552–25559.

11. De Lédinghen V, Vergniol J, Foucher J et al. Feasibility of liver transient elastography with FibroScan using a new probe for obese patients. *Liver International* 2010;30:1043–1048.

12. Castera L, Sebastiani G, Le Bail B et al. Prospective comparison of two algorithms combining non-invasive methods for staging liver fibrosis in chronic hepatitis C. *Journal of Hepatology* 2010;52:191–198.

13. Gallego-Durán R, Cerro-Salido P, Gómez-González E et al. Imaging biomarkers for steatohepatitis and fibrosis detection in non-alcoholic fatty liver disease. *Scientific Reports* 2016; 6:31421.

14. Mayo R, Crespo J, Martínez-Arranz I et al. Metabolomic-based noninvasive serum test to diagnose nonalcoholic steatohepatitis: results from discovery and validation cohorts. *Hepatology Communications* 2018;2:807–820.

15. Jacobson IM, Brown RS, Freilich B et al. Peginterferon alfa-2b and weight-based or flat-dose ribavirin in chronic hepatitis C patients. A randomized trial. *Hepatology* 2007;46:971–981.

16. Charlton MR, Pockros PJ, Harrison SA. Impact of obesity on treatment of chronic hepatitis C. *Hepatology* 2006;43: 1177–1186.

17. Coelho M, Oliviera T, Fernandez R. Biochemistry of adipose tissue: an endocrine organ. *Archives of Medical Science* 2013;9:191–200.

18. Walsh MJ, Jonsson JR, Richardson MM et al. Non-response to antiviral therapy is associated with obesity and increased hepatic expression of suppressor of cytokine signaling 3 (SOCS-3) in patients with chronic hepatitis C, viral genotype 1. *Gut* 2006;55:529–535.

19. Banerjee S, Saito K, Ait-Goughoulte M et al. Hepatitis C virus core protein upregulates serine phosphorylation of insulin receptor substrate-1 and impairs the downstream akt/protein kinase B signaling pathway for insulin resistance. *Journal of Virology* 2008;82:2606–2612.

20. Hum J, Jou J. The link between hepatitis C virus and diabetes mellitus: improvement in insulin resistance after eradication of hepatitis C virus. *Clinical Liver Disease* 2018;11:73–76.

21. Vanni E, Abate ML, Gentilcore E et al. Sites and mechanisms of insulin resistance in nonobese, nondiabetic patients with chronic hepatitis C. *Hepatology* 2009;50:697–706.

22. Bressler B, Wang K, Grippo JF et al. Pharmacokinetics and response of obese patients with chronic hepatitis C treated with different doses of PEG-IFN alpha-2a (40KD) (PEGASYS). *British Journal of Clinical Pharmacology* 2009; 67:280–287.

23. Romero-Gómez M, Diago M, Andrade RJ et al. Treatment of insulin resistance with metformin in naïve genotype 1 chronic hepatitis C patients receiving peginterferon alfa-2a plus ribavirin. *Hepatology* 2009;50:1702–1708.

24. Yu JW, Sun LJ, Zhao YH et al. The effect of metformin on the efficacy of antiviral therapy in patients with genotype 1 chronic hepatitis C and insulin resistance. *International Journal of Infectious Diseases* 2012;16:e436–441.

25. Van de Mer AJ, Berenguer M. Reversion of disease manifestations after HCV eradication. *Journal of Hepatology* 2016; 65(1 Suppl):S95–S108.

26. Poynard T, McHutchison J, Manns M et al. Impact of pegylated interferon alfa-2b and ribavirin on liver fibrosus in patients with chronic hepatitis C. *Gastroenterology* 2002;122: 1303–1313.

27. Simmons B, Saleem J, Heath K et al. Long-term treatment outcomes of patients infected with hepatitis C virus: a systematic review and meta-analysis of the survival benefit of achieving a sustained virological response. *Clinical Infectious Diseases* 2015;61:730–740.

28. Morozov V, Sylvie Lagaye S. Hepatitis C virus: morphogenesis, infection and therapy. *World Journal of Hepatology* 2018;10:186–212.

29. Hsu YC, Ho HJ, Huang YT et al. Association between antiviral treatment and extrahepatic outcomes in patients with hepatitis C virus infection. *Gut* 2015;64:495–503.

30. Romero-Gómez M, Fernández-Rodríguez CM, Andrade RJ et al. Effect of sustained virological response to treatment on the incidence of abnormal glucose values in chronic hepatitis C. *Journal of Hepatology* 2008;48:721–727.

31. Noureddin M, Wong M, Todo T et al. Fatty liver in hepatitis C patients post-sustained virological response with direct-acting antivirals. *World Journal of Gastroenterology* 2018;24: 1269–1277.

32. Ampuero J, Jimeno C, Quiles R et al. Impact of comorbidities on patient outcomes after interferon free therapy-induced viral eradication in hepatitis C. *Journal of Hepatology* 2018;68: 940–948.

33. Afdhal N, Zeuzem S, Kwo P et al., ION-1 Investigators. Ledipasvir and sofosbuvir for untreated HCV genotype 1 infection. *New England Journal of Medicine* 2014;370: 1889–1898.

34. Afdhal N, Reddy KR, Nelson DRIO et al., ION-2 Investigators. Ledipasvir and sofosbuvir for previously treated HCV genotype 1 infection. *New England Journal of Medicine* 2014;370:1483–1493.

35. Kowdley KV, Gordon SC, Reddy KR et al., ION-3 Investigators. Ledipasvir and sofosbuvir for 8 or 12 weeks for chronic HCV without cirrhosis. *New England Journal of Medicine* 2014;370:1879–1888.

36. Feld JJ, Kowdley KV, Coakley E et al. Treatment of HCV with ABT-450/r-ombitasvir and dasabuvir with ribavirin. *N Engl J Med* 2014;370:1594–603.

37. Zeuzem S, Jacobson IM, Baykal T et al. Retreatment of HCV with ABT-450/r-ombitasvir and dasabuvir with ribavirin. *New England Journal of Medicine* 2014;370:1604–1614.

38. Zeuzem S, Ghalib R, Reddy KR et al. Grazoprevir-elbasvir combination therapy for treatment-naive cirrhotic and

noncirrhotic patients with chronic hepatitis C virus genotype 1, 4, or 6 infection: a randomized trial. *Annals of Internal Medicine* 2015;163:1–13.

39. Feld JJ, Jacobson IM, Hézode C et al., ASTRAL-1 Investigators. Sofosbuvir and velpatasvir for HCV genotype 1, 2, 4, 5, and 6 infection. *New England Journal of Medicine* 2015;373:2599–2607.

40. Foster GR, Afdhal N, Roberts SK et al., ASTRAL-2 Investigators, ASTRAL-3 Investigators. Sofosbuvir and velpatasvir for HCV genotype 2 and 3 Infection. *New England Journal of Medicine* 2015;373:2608–2617.

41. Bourlière M, Gordon SC, Flamm SL et al., POLARIS-1 and POLARIS-4 Investigators. Sofosbuvir, velpatasvir, and voxilaprevir for previously treated HCV infection. *New England Journal of Medicine* 2017;376:2134–2146.

42. Zeuzem S, Foster GR, Wang S et al. Glecaprevir-pibrentasvir for 8 or 12 weeks in HCV genotype 1 or 3 infection. *New England Journal of Medicine* 2018;378:354–369.

43. Forns X, Lee SS, Valdes J et al. Glecaprevir plus pibrentasvir for chronic hepatitis C virus genotype 1, 2, 4, 5, or 6 infection in adults with compensated cirrhosis (EXPEDITION-1): a single-arm, open-label, multicentre phase 3 trial. *Lancet Infectious Diseases* 2017;17:1062–1068.

11 Generic direct-acting antiviral agents: do they work well?

Omar Salim Al Siyabi[1] and Seng-Gee Lim[2,3]

[1] Division of Gastroenterology and Hepatology, Department of Medicine, Royal Hospital, Oman
[2] Division of Gastroenterology and Hepatology, Department of Medicine, National University Health System, Singapore
[3] Faculty of Medicine, Yong Loo Lin School of Medicine, National University of Singapore, Singapore

LEARNING POINTS

- Access to HCV therapy is essential if WHO targets for the elimination of HCV are to be met by 2030; approximately 60% of HCV-infected individuals reside in low- to middle-income countries.

- There are various mechanisms by which generic medications can be accessed by low- to middle-income countries such as voluntary licensing, compulsory licensing, absence of patent law or buyers' club.

- HCV therapy, in over 100 countries, can be procured as generic medicine and at much reduced prices from licensees.

- Bioequivalence studies of generics have shown comparable pharmacokinetics to the original DAA and there is clinical evidence of efficacy, similar to clinical trials, of generics from multiple real-world studies.

Introduction

In May 2016, the World Health Assembly endorsed the Global Health Sector Strategy (GHSS) for 2016–2021 on viral hepatitis (HBV and HCV infection), which aims that by 2030, viral hepatitis as a public health danger should be eliminated. Elimination is defined as a 90% reduction in new chronic infections and a 65% reduction in mortality compared with the 2015 baseline [1]. In 2015, the World Health Organization (WHO) estimated HCV infection rates of around 71 million persons. However, only 20% of them were diagnosed, 7% (1.1 million) had been started on treatment, and 1.75 million new infections occurred, leaving a gap of 73% to reach the WHO goal of HCV elimination by 2030 [2]. There are several reasons proposed for such a gap including deficiencies in screening and diagnosis, access to specialty care, high cost of direct-acting antiviral agents (DAA), new infections, reinfection, and lack of a vaccine [3].

The American Association for the Study of Liver Diseases (AASLD) and the Infectious Diseases Society of America (IDSA) [4], European Association for the Study of the Liver (EASL) [5], and WHO guidelines [6] recommend treatment for all individuals diagnosed with HCV infection above the age of 12 years, irrespective of disease stage, except those with an estimated life expectancy <1 year. With the availability of pangenotype DAA regimens with a high cure rate of >95%, the treatment of chronic HCV is much easier and requires less personal and laboratory input.

One of the major steps towards achieving the WHO vision of elimination by 2030 is to make the highly effective DAAs available at affordable cost, which has been generally achieved by increasing competition, especially from generic manufacturers. In 2017, 62% of those infected with HCV lived in countries where generic medicines could be procured, and this is an enabler for HCV eradication programs by lowering the costs of therapy. However, there are still some doubts over the efficacy of generic medications. The aim of this chapter is to review the available data on the effectiveness and safety of generic drugs worldwide.

Clinical Dilemmas in Viral Liver Disease, Second Edition. Edited by Graham R. Foster and K. Rajender Reddy.
© 2020 John Wiley & Sons Ltd. Published 2020 by John Wiley & Sons Ltd.

Access to generic DAAs

There are several ways to access generic DAAs (Table 11.1): voluntary license, compulsory license, buyers' club, clinical trials, or unavailable patent law. The originator companies Gilead and Bristol-Myers Squibb (BMS) have signed voluntary license agreements that enable other producers to manufacture and/or sell generic versions of sofosbuvir, ledipasvir, velpatasvir (Gilead), and daclatasvir (BMS) in countries listed in the agreements. All countries included in the list (105 from Gilead and 112 from BMS) can procure generic medicine at affordable prices from licensees. As of November 2017, several mostly upper middle-income countries, including Brazil, China, Colombia, Mexico, Kazakhstan, and Turkey, which together are home to an estimated 14 million people living with HCV, were not included in the license agreements [7]. On November 12, 2018, Abbvie signed a license agreement with the Medicines Patent Pool to provide royalty-free glecaprevir/pibrentasvir to 99 low- and middle-income countries, ensuring that two of the most important pangenotypic regimens will now be accessible to patients in these countries [8].

Countries not included in voluntary licensing can still access generic DAA by other means. For instance, Pakistan did not sign relevant patents, while Malaysia obtained generic DAA under the provisions of the World Trade Organization (WTO) Trade Related Aspects of Intellectual Property Rights (TRIPS) agreement by compulsory license. Buyers' clubs are internet facilitators for individual DAA purchases from generic companies. Although such methods of importation are not encouraged in many countries, some (including Australia, Italy, Switzerland, and the United Kingdom) do allow individuals to import a treatment course for personal use.

While competition from generic manufacturers has driven down the price of DAAs, most generic suppliers do not yet offer prequalified products or products approved by a stringent regulatory authority.

Bioequivalent pharmacokinetics for generic and originator DAAs

As of February 2018, the WHO had prequalified three generic sofosbuvir medications, as well as the daclatasvir tablets of the originator company [7,9]. The WHO has also prequalified the Active Pharmaceutical Ingredient (API) for sofosbuvir. The majority of generic DAAs, however, are neither WHO prequalified (largely because the producers have not applied for prequalification) nor authorized by any other stringent regulatory authority. So far, only sofosbuvir from Mylan Laboratories, Cipla Ltd, and Hetero Labs Ltd has been granted WHO prequalification [9]. Consequently, it is important to ascertain if generic DAAs are as effective as the original DAAs.

Bioequivalence is an important investigation to establish that generic versions of the same drugs have similar pharmokinetics since formulations may be different. A study was performed to determine whether generic forms of sofosbuvir and daclatasvir had bioequivalent pharmacokinetics to the originator versions. Seven generic companies (European Egyptian Pharmaceutical Industries [Egypt], Beker [Algeria], Hetero, Natco, Mylan, and Virchow [India]) provided sofosbuvir and daclatasvir to conduct bioequivalence studies and compared it to the original sofosbuvir (Gilead) and daclatasvir (BMS) [10]. These were randomized, open-label, variable-period pharmacokinetic studies in groups of 22–54 healthy volunteers. The pharmacokinetics of generic sofosbuvir and daclatasvir were bioequivalent to the originator versions for all seven generic companies [10]. This crucial step not only secured prequalification of the manufacture of these drugs from these companies but also demonstrated that the quality of the generic medications was indeed of a high standard.

Table 11.1 Ways to access generic DAAs

Methods of access	Definition
Voluntary license	License to produce generic product given by the original company for specific manufacturer who can produce and export to all countries (usually low–middle-income countries) listed in the agreement. This covers around 62% of HCV-infected people
Compulsory license	An individual or company seeking to use another's intellectual property can do so without seeking the rights holder's consent and pays the rights holder a set fee for the license
Medicine is not patented	Some countries have no patent law for some medicine and can get supplies of generic medicine from both compulsory and voluntary licensees
Buyers' club	Websites that act as middlemen by providing details of trusted online pharmacies and drug manufacturers
WHO prequalified products	WHO makes available technical advice and technical assistance to help companies understand how to meet prequalification requirements, and, in the case of specific deficiencies, how to overcome them

Results of generic DAAs by country

The Center for Disease Analysis estimates that China has the largest HCV epidemic (almost 10 million people living with HCV in 2015), followed by Pakistan (7.2 million), India (6.2 million), and Egypt (5.6 million) [2]. These four countries account for almost 40% of all people living with HCV. Table 11.2 shows studies that have used generic versions of DAAs and their 12-week sustained virologic response (SVR12).

Table 11.2 Studies of real-world generic DAA regimen efficacy in various countries, their genotypes and cirrhosis status.

	Study size	Cirrhosis %	GT1 regimen (SVR)	GT3 regimen (SVR)	Other GT regimen (SVR)
Asia Lim et al. [11]	2171	41.8%	SR12–24w (88%) SD±R 12–24w (100%) SL±R 12–24w (92%)	SR12–24w (96%) SD±R 12–24w (98%)	GT 2 SR12–24w (100%) SD±R12–24w (100%) SL±R12–24w (100%) GT6 SR12 (100%) SD±R12 (100%) SL12 (74%) SLR12 (89%)
China Li et al. [13]	HIV/HCV155	19.9%	SVR12 (96%) SD±R12w SL±R12w	SVR12 (100%) SD±R12w SL±R12w	GT6 SVR12 (100%) SD12w SL12w
China Zeng et al. [14]	192	32.8%	SR12w (96.8%) SLR8w (96.9%) SL8w(96.9%)		
India Gupta et al. [15]	490	30%	SL12w (90.3%) SR12w (94.7%)	SD12w (97.5%)	
Taiwan Liu et al. [16]	519	36%	SL12w (93.5%)	SD12w (96.0%)	GT2 SR12w (85.3%) GT1–6 SV12w (97.7%) Mixed SD12w (96.0%)
Taiwan Liu et al [18]	HCV159 HIV/HCV69	22.8%	SV12w (97.1% HCV) (98.1% HCV/HIV)	SV12w (100%)	Decompensated cirrhosis GT1,2,6 SVR12w (93%)
Argentina Marciano et al. [19]	184	91%	SD±R12–24w (91%)		GT2 (95–96%) SD±R12w SR12–24w GT3 (79–81%) SD±R24w
Egypt Omar et al. [20]	18378	49.9%			GT4 Noncirrhosis/naive SD12w 95.1% Cirrhosis/treatment experienced SDR12w 94.7%
Buyers' club Freeman et al. [22]	448	28%	SL12w (91%)	SD±R12w (100%)	GT2,4,6 SL12w or SD±R12w (100%)
Buyers' club Hill et al. [23]	250	11%	SL±R12–24w (99%)	SD±R12–24w (98%)	GT2,4,6 SL/SD±R12–24w (100%)

D, daclatasvir; GT, genotype; HCV, hepatitis C virus; HIV, human immunodeficiency virus; L, ledipasvir; R, ribavirin; S, sofosbuvir; SVR, sustained virologic response; V, velpatasvir; w, weeks.

Asia

The largest real-world dataset in Asia was reported by Lim et al. [11] but not all countries used generic DAAs. The countries where generics were used included India (n = 977), Myanmar (n = 552), and Pakistan (n = 406) out of a total of 2171 patients, with 42% having cirrhosis. The overall SVR was 89.5%, and by genotype (GT) based on those who completed treatment was 92% for GT1, 100% GT2, 97% GT3, 95% GT4, and 87% GT6. Patients with cirrhosis had a lower SVR of 85% versus noncirrhosis patients at 93%. Patients with GT1 and GT3 treated with sofosbuvir/ribavirin had 88% and 89% SVR12 respectively but those with GT6 treated with sofosbuvir/ledipasvir had only 77.6% SVR12.

China

Although China has the highest prevalence of chronic HCV, it has yet to gain access to generic DAAs. In August 2018, China's State Intellectual Property Office (SIPO) cancelled key patent claims that had been previously granted to Gilead Sciences for the oral hepatitis C drug sofosbuvir [12]. China will now be in a position to either import or produce its own generics of sofosbuvir. Li et al. studied generic sofosbuvir with daclatasvir or ledipasvir with or without ribavirin produced by Indian companies in 155 patients with HCV/HIV coinfection [13]. The majority of patients were male, infected with GT1 or 3 (78.7%), and 19.9% had cirrhosis (see Table 11.2). They found that SVR12 was 96% for GT1 and 100% for GT3 and GT6 using either sofosbuvir/ledipasvir or sofosbuvir/daclatasvir with or without ribavirin for 12–24 weeks, and side effects were no different from those of original DAAs.

Zeng et al. also studied generic sofosbuvir with ledipasvir with or without ribavirin, also from Indian companies, in 192 patients with GT1b (32.8% cirrhotic) and the response rate was >96% [14]. Reported side effects included fatigue 17.8%, diarrhea 10.9%, and headache 9.9%. No patient stopped medications because of side effects.

India

Gupta et al. reviewed 490 patients, mainly GT3 (75%), treatment naive (88%); the SVR12 was >95% with generic sofosbuvir, ledipasvir and ribavirin produced by local companies, and no major side effect was reported, except anemia in 10% of patients who were on ribavirin [15].

Taiwan

In Taiwan, Liu et al. conducted a study across all genotypes with 519 patients, some of whom had HIV coinfection [16]. They also used generic sofosbuvir/velpatasvir from Beacon Pharmaceutical, Bangladesh, a company which has no license agreement with Gilead to produce the drug [17]. Again, the SVR12 was >95% with good safety profile.

In another study, 288 chronic HCV patients (159 HCV monoinfection, 69 HCV-HIV coinfection) with varying genotypes were treated with sofosbuvir/velpatasvir (Beacon Pharmaceuticals) for 12 weeks with 97–98% SVR12 regardless of HIV coinfection [18]. Decompensated cirrhotics were treated with sofosbuvir/velpatasvir + ribavirin for 12 weeks with 93% SVR12 (genotypes 1, 2, and 6).

Argentina

Marciano et al. reported no difference in response to treatment or adverse effects in 321 patients with chronic HCV (91% cirrhotic) when using original sofosbuvir (Sovaldi®, Gilead Sciences, n = 135) or generic sofosbuvir (Probirase®, Laboratorios RICHMOND, n = 184) in combination with original daclatasvir ± ribavarin, with SVR12 of 91% in those receiving original sofosbuvir compared to 89% receiving generic sofosbuvir [19].

Egypt

Omar et al. reported the largest studied population on generic DAAs from Egypt where 18 373 patients with chronic HCV GT4 were treated with locally produced sofosbuvir and daclatasvir with SVR12 of 95.1% [20]. The response rate was also high (SVR12 94.7%) in difficult-to-treat patients who have cirrhosis or treatment-experienced patients where ribavirin was added. In a study of 971 chronic HCV patients comparing generic to original sofosbuvir in a regimen of sofosbuvir/ledipasvir or sofosbuvir/daclatasvir (ribavirin added for those treatment experienced or with cirrhosis), SVR12 was 98.2% in those with original sofosbuvir compared to 98.1% in those taking generic sofosbuvir [21].

Buyers' club global access programs

Countries that lack access to generic DAAs are almost exclusively in the upper middle-income and high-income categories, which are typically not included in voluntary license agreements and represent about 38% of people living with HCV globally. They include, for example, Brazil, China, Colombia, Kazakhstan, Mexico, and Turkey. For patients in these countries, access to generic DAAs is made possible by a third party through internet buyers' clubs, where patient can buy generic DAAs even if they have no prescription.

At the International Liver Congress 2017, Freeman et al. presented preliminary results on a cohort of 448/1087 patients from REDMPTION-1 where patients globally could purchase prescriptions of DAAs for their individual use through the fixhepc.com website [22]. The cohort included a high proportion of treatment-experienced patients (42%), of which 28% had cirrhosis. The genotype distribution was 1 (67%), 2 (6%), and 3 (23%). The overall SVR12 was 90% with no new or unexpected adverse effects reported.

Hill et al. gathered results of 616 patients: 199 from an Australian buyers' club, 205 from a South-East Asian buyers' clubs, and 212 from an Eastern European buyers' club representing 38 different countries [23]. The generic DAAs were marketed by 24 different companies and achieved a SVR12 of 99% where reported (only 41% reported SVR) with no adverse events.

Results of generic DAA by genotype, cirrhosis and treatment regimen – comparison with clinical trial data

Rates of SVR12 from studies of generic therapy are usually real-world data and should be evaluated by regimen, genotype, duration of therapy, presence of cirrhosis, and use of ribavirin. This is largely due to the early first-generation all-oral DAA which was not pangenotypic such as sofosbuvir and ribavirin and sofosbuvir and ledipasvir. These treatments also required longer therapy in cirrrhotics and treatment-experienced patients. For use of sofosbuvir and ribavirin in GT1, SVR12 rates were 88–96.8%, keeping in mind that the largest study had 42% cirrhotics (see Table 11.2), and compares very favorably with clinical trial data showing SVR12 of 68.5% (Table 11.3).

The metaanalysis of GT1 therapy with sofosbuvir and ribavirin was conducted in Caucasians [24,25] but a clinical trial in India with original sofosbvuvir showed SVR12 of 90–96% [26], suggesting that Asians may respond differently from Caucasians to DAA therapy (see Table 11.3). Sofosbuvir/ledipasvir ± ribavirin was one of the most common regimens for GT1 and SVR ranged from 90.3% to 99%, while sofosbuvir/daclatasvir ± ribavirin had SVR12 of 100% (see Table 11.2), and also compares favorably to clinical trial data showing SVR ≥95% [24,25] (see Table 11.3).

Table 11.3 Clinical trial summary of SVR12 from metaanalyses of different DAA regimens in various genotypes based on presence or absence of cirrhosis. Where there is absence of metaanalysis, clinical trial data were used

Genotype	Cirrhosis status	SR 12–24w	SL±R 12w	SD±R 12–24w	SV 12w
GT1	No cirrhosis	68.5%	≥95%	95–100%	>98%
	Cirrhosis	(90–96%*)	97% (+R)		
GT2	No cirrhosis	92%		92–100%	99–100%
	Cirrhosis				
GT3	No cirrhosis	76%		94–97%	95%
	Cirrhosis	(93–100%*)		83–89% (+R)	
GT4	No cirrhosis	82%	93–95%	97%**	100%
	Cirrhosis				
GT5	No cirrhosis		95%		97%
	Cirrhosis				
GT6	No cirrhosis		96%		100%
	Cirrhosis				

Sources: Ferrerira et al. [24], Falade-Nwulia et al. [25].

* Study conducted in India by Shah et al. [26].

** Study conducted in Egypt by Yakoot et al. [28].

D, daclatasvir; GT, genotype; L, ledipasvir; R, ribavirin; S, sofosbuvir; V, velpatasvir; w, weeks.

For the more difficult to treat GT3, sofosbuvir/daclatasvir 12 weeks led to SVR12 of 96–100% with cirrhosis present in about 30% (see Table 11.2) and is comparable to clinical trial data showing SVR12 of 94–97% [24,25]. Sofosbuvir/daclatasvir ± ribavirin for 12–24 weeks had a consistently high rate of SVR12 of 98%, a regimen usually given to cirrhotics and/or treatment-experienced patients and again shows better results than clinical trials of 83–89% [24,25] (see Table 11.3). For other genotypes (see Table 11.2), SVR12 rates were >90% except for GT2 using sofosbuvir/ribavirin for 12 weeks (SVR12 85.4%) which is not a usual therapy for this genotype, and also GT6 where sofosbuvir/ledipasvir had a SVR12 of 74% but sofosbuvir/ledipasvir + ribavirin had SVR12 of 89% [24,25]. The poor response of GT6 with sofosbuvir/ledipasvir is largely from Myanmar and has been reported in other studies [27]. It is not clear if this is due to subgenotype response as this is a distinct variation from the high SVR12 rates reported in clinical trials [24,25] (see Table 11.3).

Finally genotype 4 data come mainly from Egypt and the SVR12 is 95% using sofosbuvir/daclatasvir ± ribavirin (see Table 11.2) consistent with clinical trial data of 97% [28] (see Table 11.3).

There is only one report of generic sofosbuvir/velpastasvir since this regimen has only recently been approved but the report from Taiwan showed a high SVR12 whether in HCV monoinfection or coinfection with HIV. Even patients with decompensated cirrhosis had SVR12 of 92% with addition of ribavirin (see Table 11.2). These findings are again consistent with clinical trial data [25,29,30] (see Tables 11.3 and 11.4a, 11.4b).

Conclusion

Generic DAAs are accessible to over 60% of patients in HCV-infected countries but there has been some concern about their efficacy and safety. The access to generics may be through different mechanisms in low- and middle-income countries but buyers' clubs provide individuals in high-income countries with access as well. Reassurance that generics are efficacious comes from bioequivalence testing showing that the pharmacokinetics of generics are comparable to those of the original compounds but, more importantly, that generics show comparable SVR12 rates to those of the original regimens. In some instances, the results differ; for example, sofosbuvir/ribavirin for GT1 showed surprisingly better results than clinical trials but a clinical

Table 11.4a Clinical trial summary of SVR12 of DAA therapy in decompensated cirrhosis of different genotypes

Genotype	SOF-LDV+R	SOF-DCV+R	SOF-VEL+R
GT1	85–87%	82%	94%
GT2		80%	100%
GT3			85%
GT4	87–89%		100%
GT5			
GT6			100%

Sources: Falade-Nwulia et al. [25], Charlton et al. [29].
DCV, daclatasvir; GT, genotype; LDV, ledipasvir; R, ribavarin; SOF, sofosbuvir; VEL, velpatasvir.

Table 11.4b Real-world summary of SVR12 of DAA therapy in decompensated cirrhosis of different genotypes

Genotype	SOF-LDV+R	SOF-DCV+R	SOF-VEL+R
GT1	92%	85%	
GT2			
GT3	61%	73%	
GT4			
GT5			
GT6			

Source: Foster et al. [30].
DCV, daclatasvir; GT, genotype; LDV, ledipasvir; R, ribavarin; SOF, sofosbuvir; VEL, velpatasvir.

trial in India showed better SVR12 rates than Caucasians, suggesting that in certain settings Asians may respond better to DAA therapy. For GT6, the SVR12 rates with sofosbuvir/ledipasvir are suboptimal compared to clinical trial data and further data are required from countries with more GT6 patients, such as Thailand and Vietnam.

Overall, data from generic DAA studies are generally not from the latest pangenotypic regimens such as sofosbuvir/velpatasvir which are superior to the older regimens of soforbuvir/ribavirin, sofosbuvir/daclatasvir, and sofosbuvir/ledipasvir but the results to date are certainly comparable to clinical trial data. Based on the current available data, there is no reason to suspect generic DAAs are inferior to the original compounds, and should not be a barrier to purchase of HCV therapy.

The goal of HCV elimination cannot be achieved without widespread acceptance and use of generic DAAs, and future reviews should examine the efficacy of the more recent pangenotypic therapies in this context.

Conflicts of interest

Seng Gee Lim: Advisory Board – Gilead Sciences, Merck Sharpe and Dohme, Abbvie, Abbott. Speakers Bureau – Gilead Sciences, Abbott, Merck Sharpe and Dohme, Roche. Educational/research funding: Abbott, Merck Sharpe and Dohme, Gilead Sciences.

Omar Salim Al Siyabi: No disclosures to report.

References

1. World Health Organization. Global Health Sector Strategy On Viral Hepatitis 2016–2021. www.who.int/hepatitis/strategy2016-2021/ghss-hep/en/

2. Polaris Observatory HCV Collaborators. Global prevalence and genotype distribution of hepatitis C virus infection in 2015: a modelling study. *Lancet Gastroenterology and Hepatology* 2017;2:161–176.

3. Konerman MA, Lok AS. Hepatitis C treatment and barriers to eradication. *Clinical and Translational Gastroenterology* 2016;7:e193.

4. AASLD-IDSA HCV Guidance Panel. Hepatitis C Guidance 2018 Update: AASLD-IDSA Recommendations for Testing, Managing, and Treating Hepatitis C Virus Infection. *Clinical Infectious Diseases* 2018;67:1477–1492.

5. European Association for the Study of the Liver. Recommendations on treatment of hepatitis C 2018. *Journal of Hepatology* 2018;69:461–511.

6. World Health Organization. Guidelines for the Care and Treatment of Persons Diagnosed with Chronic Hepatitis C Virus Infection. www.ncbi.nlm.nih.gov/pubmed/30307724.

7. World Health Organization. Progress Report on Access to Hepatitis C Treatment: Focus on Overcoming Barriers in Low- and Middle-Income Countries. www.who.int/hepatitis/publications/hep-c-access-report-2018/en/

8. Medicines Patent Pool. The Medicines Patent Pool signs licence with AbbVie to expand access to key hepatitis C treatment, glecaprevir/pibrentasvir. https://medicinespatentpool.org/mpp-media-post/the-medicines-patent-pool-signs-licence-with-abbvie-to-expand-access-to-key-hepatitis-c-treatment-glecaprevirpibrentasvir/

9. World Health Organization. WHO prequalifies first generic active ingredient for hepatitis C medicines. www.who.int/medicines/news/2017/1st_generic-hepCprequalified_active_ingredient/en/

10. Hill A, Tahat L, Mohammed MK et al. Bioequivalent pharmacokinetics for generic and originator hepatitis C direct-acting antivirals. *Journal of Virus Eradication* 2018;4:128–131.

11. Lim SG, Phyo WW, Shah SR et al. Findings from a large Asian chronic hepatitis C real-life study. *Journal of Viral Hepatitis* 2018;25:1533–1542.

12. Médecins Sans Frontières. Gilead loses monopoly control of its blockbuster hepatitis C medicine in China. https://msfaccess.org/gilead-loses-monopoly-control-its-blockbuster-hepatitis-c-medicine-china

13. Li Y, Li L et al. Tolerable and curable treatment in HIV/HCV co-infected patients using anti-HCV direct antiviral agents: a real-world observation in China. *Hepatology International* 2018;12:465–473.

14. Zeng QL, Xu GH, Zhang JY et al. Generic ledipasvir-sofosbuvir for patients with chronic hepatitis C: a real-life observational study. *Journal of Hepatology* 2017;66:1123–1129.

15. Gupta S, Rout G, Patel AH et al. Efficacy of generic oral directly acting agents in patients with hepatitis C virus infection. *Journal of Viral Hepatitis* 2018;25:771–778.

16. Liu CH, Huang YJ, Yang SS et al. Generic sofosbuvir-based interferon-free direct acting antiviral agents for patients with chronic hepatitis C virus infection: a real-world multicenter observational study. *Scientific Reports* 2018;8:13699.

17. Rajagopal D. US' Gilead faces competition from Bangladesh's Beacon pharma. Economic Times 2016. https://economictimes.indiatimes.com/industry/healthcare/biotech/pharmaceuticals/us-gilead-faces-competition-from-bangladeshs-beacon-pharma/articleshow/53407488.cms

18. Liu CH, Sun HY, Liu CJ et al. Generic velpatasvir plus sofosbuvir for hepatitis C virus infection in patients with or without human immunodeficiency virus coinfection. *Alimentary Pharmacology and Therapeutics* 2018;47:1690–1698.

19. Marciano S, Haddad L, Reggiardo MV et al. Effectiveness and safety of original and generic sofosbuvir for the treatment of chronic hepatitis C: a real world study. *Journal of Medical Virology* 2018;90:951–958.

20. Omar H, El Akel W, Elbaz T et al. Generic daclatasvir plus sofosbuvir, with or without ribavirin, in treatment of chronic hepatitis C: real-world results from 18 378 patients in Egypt. *Alimentary Pharmacology and Therapeutics* 2018;47:421–431.

21. Abozeid M, Alsebaey A, Abdelsameea E et al. High efficacy of generic and brand direct acting antivirals in treatment of chronic hepatitis C. *International Journal of Infectious Diseases* 2018;75:109–114.

22. Freeman J, Khwairakpam G, Dragunova J et al. Sustained virological response for 94% of people treated with low-cost, legally imported generic direct acting antivirals for hepatitis C: analysis of 1087 patients in 4 treatment programmes. *Journal of Hepatology* 2017;66:S55–56.

23. Hill A, Khwairakpam G, Wang J et al. High sustained virological response rates using imported generic direct acting antiviral treatment for hepatitis C. *Journal of Virus Eradication* 2017;3:200–203.

24. Ferreira VL, Tonin FS, Assis Jarek NA, Ramires Y, Pontarolo R. Efficacy of interferon-free therapies for chronic hepatitis C: a systematic review of all randomized clinical trials. *Clinical Drug Investigation* 2017;37:635–646.

25. Falade-Nwulia O, Suarez-Cuervo C, Nelson DR, Fried MW, Segal JB, Sulkowski MS. Oral direct-acting agent therapy for hepatitis C virus infection: a systematic review. *Annals of Internal Medicine* 2017;166:637–648.

26. Shah SR, Chowdhury A, Mehta R et al. Sofosbuvir plus riba-virin in treatment-naive patients with chronic hepatitis C virus genotype 1 or 3 infection in India. *Journal of Viral Hepatitis* 2017;24:371–379.

27. Hlaing NKT, Mitrani RA, Aung ST et al. Safety and efficacy of sofosbuvir-based direct-acting antiviral regimens for hepatitis C virus genotypes 1–4 and 6 in Myanmar: real-world experi-ence. *Journal of Viral Hepatitis* 2017;24:927–935.

28. Yakoot M, Abdo AM, Abdel-Rehim S, Helmy S. Response tailored protocol versus the fixed 12 weeks course of dual sofosbuvir/daclatasvir treatment in Egyptian patients with chronic hepatitis C genotype-4 infection: a randomized, open-label, non-inferiority trial. *EBioMedicine* 2017;21: 182–187.

29. Charlton M, Everson GT, Flamm SL et al. Ledipasvir and sofosbuvir plus ribavirin for treatment of HCV infection in patients with advanced liver disease. *Gastroenterology* 2015;149:649–659.

30. Foster GR, Irving WL, Cheung MC et al. Impact of direct acting antiviral therapy in patients with chronic hepatitis C and decompensated cirrhosis. *Journal of Hepatology* 2016;64:1224–1231.

12 Impact and management of patients with multiple hepatitis C virus genotypes

Peter Ferenci

Department of Internal Medicine III, Division of Gastroenterology and Hepatology, Medical University of Vienna, Vienna, Austria

LEARNING POINTS

- Hepatitis C virus (HCV) may be divided into at least seven major genotypes and 67 subtypes according to the phylogenetics of available HCV sequences.

- Approximately 5–10% of patients may have an infection with multiple genotypes/genotype subtypes. This may vary in high-risk individuals such as in persons who inject drugs where superinfection of concurrent coinfection may occur.

- There are challenges with identifying these multiple infections with routinely available genotyping assays.

- In the current era of potent and safe pangenotypic DAA regimens, successful treatment of multiple genotype/multiple genotype subtypes is not challenging.

Introduction

Hepatitis C virus may be divided into at least seven major genotypes and 67 subtypes according to the phylogenetics of available HCV sequences [1]. Moreover, even in patients infected with a single HCV subtype, HCV circulates as a group of variants with up to 10% nucleotide sequence difference, termed *quasi-species*. Perhaps due to the lack of protective immunity, superinfection by different HCV isolates in patients with chronic HCV is clinically observed, particularly in individuals at very high risk for infection, such as injection drug users, HIV-infected patients, patients on hemodialysis, and those who received multiple blood transfusions in the era before HCV screening of blood donors was introduced. Multiple infections by different HCV genotypes may still impact the response to interferon-free direct-acting antivirals (DAA) in some patients.

One attractive explanation for the persistence of multiple different genotypes of HCV is that the different genotypes may persist in different viral reservoirs. Extensive distribution of HCV genomes throughout nonhepatic reservoirs has been described, and some evidence supports the hypothesis that different HCV variants may acquire specific tropism for hepatic versus nonhepatic reservoirs. However, the issue remains controversial, and one of the major limitations in reaching consensus about this aspect of HCV virology is that there are many technical approaches described for assessing HCV genotype [2].

Extent of the problem

The extent of infection with multiple different subtypes/genotypes of HCV simultaneously in a given individual is controversial. Basically, there are two different scenarios that may result in the presence of more than one genotype: superinfection by another genotype of a patient already infected with a single genotype [3] or coinfection with multiple genotypes. Using serologic methods, it has been shown that patients infected with a single genotype of HCV may experience transient or occult superinfection with different genotypes of HCV [4].

By the most commonly used genotyping testing, the line probe assay, multiple HCV genotypes were detected in 10.8% of HCV monoinfected patients [5] and in 5% of

Clinical Dilemmas in Viral Liver Disease, Second Edition. Edited by Graham R. Foster and K. Rajender Reddy.
© 2020 John Wiley & Sons Ltd. Published 2020 by John Wiley & Sons Ltd.

HCV/HIV coinfected patients [6]. Other studies demonstrate that 0–39% of high-risk, HCV-infected individuals harbor mixed genotypes; however, standardized, sensitive methods of detection are lacking. In 1159 Polish patients, the dominant genotype was genotype 1b. A mixed genotype infection was detected in 26 patients (2.2%) [7]. The most common mixed genotype was 1a+1b detected in 17/26 patients (65%). Antiviral therapy with DAA led to complete elimination of both genotypes in 50% of patients with 1b+3a infection and in 33% of patients with 1b+4a infection.

In a large study from Spain, subtype distribution showed a higher level of heterogeneity than was expected, particularly for genotype 2 [8]. Prevalence of mixed infections was around 1%.

In 506 UK patients infected with genotypes 1a or 3a, the overall prevalence rate of mixed infection was 3.8% [9]; however, this rate was unevenly distributed, with 6.7% of individuals diagnosed with genotype 3 (as dominant strain) harboring genotype 1a strains and only 0.8% of samples from genotype 1a patients harboring genotype 3 (p<0.05). Analysis of a subset of the cohort by Illumina PCR next-generation sequencing resulted in a much greater incidence rate than obtained by PCR.

By next-generation sequencing (NGS) in three of 76 Polish seronegative, HCV-RNA-positive blood donors [10], mixed-genotype HCV were detected. One (1.3%) mixed-genotype (1b+3a) infection was found in a sample diagnosed as genotype 3a only by routine testing. Two samples were identified with different genotypes, compared to routine testing. NGS is a sensitive method for HCV genotyping. These few cases represent acute infections in the incubation period, but the prevalence of mixed-genotype HCV infections in blood donors is low.

A recent study compared PCR amplicon [11], random primer (RP), and probe enrichment (PE)-based deep sequencing methods coupled with a custom sequence analysis pipeline to detect multiple HCV genotypes in two clinical trials of HCV treatment in high-risk individuals (ACTIVATE [12], DARE-C II [13]) and a cohort of HIV/HCV coinfected individuals (Canadian Coinfection Cohort [CCC] [14]). Sequencing of ACTIVATE and DARE-C II demonstrated, on average, 2% and 1% of HCV reads mapping to a second genotype using RP and PE, respectively; however, none passed the mixed infection

cut-off criteria and phylogenetics confirmed no mixed infections. From CCC, one mixed infection was confirmed while the other was determined to be a recombinant genotype. This study underlines the risk for false identification of mixed HCV infections and stresses the need for standardized methods to improve prevalence estimates and to understand the impact of mixed infections for management and elimination of HCV.

Chimeric hepatitis C virus

Genetic recombination is considered as an alternate mechanism to create divergent HCV genomes. The intergenotypic recombinant HCV strain RF_2k/1b was first described in 2002 [15]. HCV genotype 2k/1b chimeras are typically described as HCV genotype 2 by the commercially used hybridization genotyping assays. Detection of the chimeric virus requires Sanger-based sequencing. Most patients with 2k/1b chimeras (88%) were originally from eight different areas of the former Soviet Union [16]. Treatment with sofosbuvir plus ribavirin is insufficient, but genotype 1-based regimens seem to be effective [17]. Other recombinant HCV strains (2b/1a, 2b/1b, 2k/5a, 2i/6p, and 2b/6w) were described sporadically

Clinical implications of infection with multiple genotypes

The results of studies about frequency and clinical implications of coinfections are conflicting, possibly due to problems associated with testing for HCV genotype and subtypes. Hepatitis C virus mixed genotype infections can affect treatment outcomes and may have implications for vaccine design and disease progression. In mixed infections, more drug-resistant genotypes such as genotype 3 could lead to treatment failure as a result of emerging dominance during treatment [9]. NGS methodologies that routinely captured these data would therefore represent an important advance. In a small group of 84 Spanish patients, six (7%) were infected with more than one subtype, and two of them failed DAA-based triple therapy [18]. The clinical implications of infection with multiple HCV genotypes have become of minor interest since the availability of pangenotypic antiviral treatments.

The setting of liver transplantation where both recipient and donor are infected with different HCV strains provides an interesting scenario for studying host–virus and virus–virus interactions, although the immunosuppression used to prevent rejection of the transplanted liver may modify the nature of the interactions. In six HCV-positive liver donor–recipient pairs, serial serum samples were collected at multiple time points. Detailed genetic analyses showed that only one strain of HCV could be identified at each time point in all six cases. Recipient HCV strains took over in three cases, whereas donor HCV strains dominated after liver transplantation in the remaining patients. Similarly, a genotype conversion was observed after transplantation in four HCV-infected recipients receiving HCV-infected donor organs [19].

In all six cases studied, no genetic recombination was detected among HCV quasi-species or between donor and recipient HCV strains [20]. Similar observations have been made by others [21] and suggest that in multiply infected patients, one viral sequence will dominate.

Conclusion

Infections with multiple HCV genotypes may occur in some patients, but technical issues regarding optimal test procedures have to be resolved before the clinical implications of this condition can safely be assessed. Some studies indicate that the presence of multiple genotypes has important implications for choosing therapeutic regimens but this has not been universally accepted. In clinical practice, the dominance of one viral genotype will usually ensure that only one viral strain is detected but it is prudent to ensure that a recent genotyping result is used to determine treatment duration as reinfection (or reactivation) of other strains may lead to a change in the dominant genotype over time. In patients who relapse following therapy, many clinicians repeat the viral genotyping assessment to ensure that activation is with the dominant pretreatment strain.

References

1. Smith DB, Bukh J, Kuiken C et al. Expanded classification of hepatitis C virus into 7 genotypes and 67 subtypes: updated criteria and genotype assignment web resource. *Hepatology* 2014;59:318–327.
2. Li H, Thomassen LV, Majid A et al. Investigation of putative multisubtype hepatitis C virus infections in vivo by heteroduplex mobility analysis of core/envelope subgenomes. *Journal of Virology* 2008;82:7524–7532.
3. Aberle JH, Formann E, Steindl-Munda P et al. Prospective study of viral clearance and CD4(+) T-cell response in acute hepatitis C primary infection and reinfection. *Journal of Clinical Virology* 2006;36:24–31.
4. Toyoda H, Fukuda Y, Hayakawa T et al. Presence of multiple genotype-specific antibodies in patients with persistent infection with hepatitis C virus (HCV) of a single genotype: evidence for transient or occult superinfection with HCV of different genotypes. *American Journal of Gastroenterology* 1999;94:2230–2236.
5. Giannini C, Giannelli F, Monti M et al. Prevalence of mixed infection by different hepatitis C virus genotypes in patients with hepatitis C virus-related chronic liver disease. *Journal of Laboratory and Clinical Medicine* 1999;134:68–73.
6. van Asten L, Prins M. Infection with concurrent multiple hepatitis C virus genotypes is associated with faster HIV disease progression. *AIDS* 2004;18:2319–2324.
7. Gowin E, Bereszyńska I, Adamek A et al. The prevalence of mixed genotype infections in Polish patients with hepatitis C. *International Journal of Infectious Diseases* 2016;43:13–16.
8. Rodriguez-Frias F, Nieto-Aponte L, Gregori J et al. High HCV subtype heterogeneity in a chronically infected general population revealed by high-resolution hepatitis C virus subtyping. *Clinical Microbiology and Infection* 2017;23:775.e1–775.e6.
9. McNaughton AL, Sreenu VB, Wilkie G, Gunson R, Templeton K, Leitch ECM. Prevalence of mixed genotype hepatitis C virus infections in the UK as determined by genotype-specific PCR and deep sequencing. *Journal of Viral Hepatology* 2018;25:524–534.
10. Janiak M, Caraballo Cortés K, Perlejewski K et al. Next-generation sequencing of hepatitis C virus (HCV) mixed-genotype infections in anti-HCV-negative blood donors. *Advances in Experimental Medicine and Biology* 2018;1096:65–71.
11. Olmstead AD, Montoya V, Chui CK et al. A systematic, deep sequencing-based methodology for identification of mixed-genotype hepatitis C virus infections. *Infection, Genetics and Evolution* 2019;69:76–84.
12. Midgard H, Hajarizadeh B, Cunningham EB et al. Changes in risk behaviours during and following treatment for hepatitis C virus infection among people who inject drugs: the ACTIVATE study. *International Journal of Drug Policy* 2017;47:230–238.
13. Martinello M, Gane E, Hellard M et al. Sofosbuvir and ribavirin for 6 weeks is not effective among people with recent hepatitis C virus infection: the DARE-C II study. *Hepatology* 2016;64:1911–1921.
14. Klein MB, Saeed S, Yang H et al. Cohort profile: the Canadian HIV-hepatitis C co-infection cohort study. *International Journal of Epidemiology* 2010;39:1162–1169.

15. Kalinina O, Norder H, Mukomolov S, Magnius LO. A natural intergenotypic recombinant of hepatitis C virus identified in St. Petersburg. *Journal of Virology* 2002;76:4034–4043.

16. Susser S, Dietz J, Schlevogt B et al. Origin, prevalence and response to therapy of hepatitis C virus genotype 2k/1b chimeras. *Journal of Hepatologgy* 2017;67:680–686.

17. Hedskog C, Doehle B, Chodavarapu K et al. Characterization of hepatitis C virus intergenotypic recombinant strains and associated virological response to sofosbuvir/ribavirin. *Hepatology* 2015;61:471–480.

18. Del Campo JA, Parra-Sánchez M, Figueruela B et al. Hepatitis C virus deep sequencing for sub-genotype identification in mixed infections: a real-life experience. *International Journal of Infectious Diseases* 2018;67:114–117.

19. Adekunle R, Jonchhe S, Ravichandran B, Wilson E, Husson J. Hepatitis C genotype change after transplantation utilizing hepatitis C positive donor organs. *Transplant Infectious Disease* 2018;20:e12925.

20. Fan X, Lang DM, Xu Y et al. Liver transplantation with hepatitis C virus-infected graft: interaction between donor and recipient viral strains. *Hepatology* 2003;38:25–33.

21. Vargas HE, Laskus T, Wang L et al. Outcome of liver transplantation in hepatitis C virus-infected patients who received hepatitis C virus-infected grafts. *Gastroenterology* 1999;117:149–153.

Hepatitis C virus and injecting drug use: what are the challenges?

Olav Dalgard

Akershus University Hospital, Oslo, Norway
University of Oslo, Oslo, Norway

LEARNING POINTS

- Liver disease is an important cause of death among HCV-infected people who inject drugs (PWID) older than 50 years.

- Adherence to treatment and SVR rates after treatment with DAAs have been very good among PWID and comparable to those seen in non-PWID populations.

- Reinfection must be expected and surveillance for new infection should be offered to all successfully treated PWID every 6–12 months.

- To engage PWID in HCV care, new models of care must be developed and scaled up.

Introduction

The consensus among experts involved in hepatitis C virus (HCV) elimination programs is that management and treatment of people who inject drugs (PWID) will be key to any successful elimination initiative. However, there are a number of challenges in such programmes.

Challenge 1: Identification of those with cirrhosis

The most immediate challenge will be to identify those who have developed advanced liver fibrosis or cirrhosis and who are at risk of developing liver failure, hepatocellular carcinoma, and death.

The importance of liver disease as a cause of death among PWID was demonstrated in a cohort of HCV-infected PWID retrospectively identified to have had HCV disease during the late 19702 [1]. In this cohort, it was found that liver disease was the most important cause of death among those who died older than 50 years. This is in line with the findings of a Scottish study that through linkage showed the importance of liver disease among older HCV-infected PWID, especially among those with harmful alcohol consumption [2]. Scaling up testing for HCV among PWID followed by assessment of liver disease stage in those with chronic HCV infection is therefore urgently needed. Noninvasive testing for liver fibrosis with liver stiffness measurement or serum markers of fibrosis are effective methods that are acceptable to patients [3,4].

Challenge 2: Halting the spread of HCV

Halting the transmission of HCV among PWID is another challenge that needs to be addressed. The size of the problem is difficult to estimate as most transmissions occur in low- and middle-income countries with very limited surveillance of the HCV epidemic. For example, in Russia it is feared that 1 million PWID are living with HCV infection without good surveillance data being available [5].

In the United States, the recent increase in injecting opiate use has translated into a new increase in the incidence of HCV and in Stockholm, the incidence of new HCV infection among PWID was recently found to be 22/100 year [6]. The main driver of the high incidence of HCV among

Clinical Dilemmas in Viral Liver Disease, Second Edition. Edited by Graham R. Foster and K. Rajender Reddy.
© 2020 John Wiley & Sons Ltd. Published 2020 by John Wiley & Sons Ltd.

PWID is new recruitment to injecting drug use. Adding to the problem is the poor access to harm reduction in most countries [7]. Needle and syringe programs (NSP) combined with opiate agonist therapy (OAT) have been shown to reduce the incidence of HCV by 75% [8]. Despite this, there is poor access to NSP and OAT in many countries, including the United States and Russia [7]. In Western Europe, access to harm reduction has been good for many years but despite this, the prevalence of chronic HCV infection among PWID is still 40% in this region [5]. The high prevalence despite availability of harm reduction may be explained by the fact that most infections occur in the first few years after injecting drug use has been initiated and before good access to harm reduction has been established.

Challenge 3: Providing treatment as prevention

Mathematical modeling suggests that elimination of HCV among PWID can best be achieved by providing harm reduction in combination with treatment as prevention [9]. Incidence is dependent on prevalence. Thus, in theory, treatment may work as prevention. The modeling suggests, for instance, that elimination can be achieved in several European countries provided there is good coverage of NSP, high uptake of OAT, and HCV treatment is administered to at least 50 per 1000 PWID (uninfected and infected) per year until 2026 [9]. A PWID in this analysis is defined as a person who has recently injected drugs, is receiving OAT or both.

It has been shown that as soon as a PWID is engaged in HCV care, treatment results are excellent and comparable to those achieved among people not injecting drugs. For instance, a *post hoc* analysis of phase 2 and phase 3 trials of DAA therapy demonstrated similar sustained virologic response (SVR) rates in patients receiving, as in those not receiving, OAT [10–15]. Furthermore, in the phase 3 C-EDGE CO-STAR trial, patients on OAT and with HCV genotype 1 or 4 infection who were treated with DAAs had a SVR of 92%, similar to that observed in other phase 3 trials. Importantly, ongoing drug use (47% noncannabinoids) did not affect SVR. Neither did drug use have an impact on adherence. This is in line with the Simplify study in which only persons who reported recent injecting drug use were included and treated with DAAs. In this study, adherence was 94% and SVR12 was obtained in 94% (97/103) of cases.

Drug use within the month preceding the start of therapy was reported by 74% of patients. SVR12 in this subgroup was 96% and did not differ from that in patients who did not report drug use in the preceding month (94%).

Among PWID treated outside strict clinical trials in real-world studies, high rates of treatment completion (93–100%), as well as high SVR rates (80–96%) have been confirmed.

Challenge 4: Poor linkage to care

In most countries, PWID are not engaged in HCV care. In Norway, we found that only 15% of people on OAT notified with HCV infection had received treatment in the interferon era prior to 2014 [16]. The number receiving treatment has increased tremendously since 2014 when interferon-free treatment became available but it is uncertain to what extent the increase has included PWID. In Norway, at a large treatment center we found that less than 5% of those who received DAAs between 2014 and 2018 reported recent injecting drug use (data on file). In comparison, recent drug use is thought to be present in 35% of those living with HCV infection in Norway [17]. In Australia, an apparently higher treatment uptake has been reported among PWID as 38% of users of a NSP eligible for HCV treatment had been administered treatment within 2017 [18].

Challenge 5: Reinfection

After successful treatment of HCV in PWID, the risk of reinfection remains a problem. However, the size of the problem is not known. A metaanalysis of several small studies showed that during the interferon era, reinfection appeared in 5% per year among those with recent drug use successfully treated for HCV [19,20]. This reinfection rate is lower than the incidence of new HCV infection among PWID that in a European metaanalysis has been reported to be 13% per year [20]. The relatively low reinfection rates after treatment reported to date suggest that only a selected group of PWID who rarely take part in risk behavior were administered interferon-based treatment.

It has been speculated that DAA treatment that is much more acceptable to patients than interferon may engage more marginalized PWID in HCV care and, as a consequence, more reinfections will occur, with rates approaching the incidence of new infections. So far, there are no data confirming this. A pooled analysis of two HCV treatment trials of DAAs that included PWID showed a reinfection rate of 5% per year among those who recently injected [21]. This is encouraging, but it should be kept in mind that within only seven years, one in three will be reinfected, given a 5% reinfection rate [22].

Models suggesting that elimination may be achieved through treatment suggest that it is important to reach patients among whom risk behavior is most prevalent. This is based on the assumption that those with high risk of HCV reinfection are also those with the highest risk of transmitting the virus to others. The relatively low reinfection rate observed to date may therefore paradoxically be an unfortunate sign that those most important to treat are not being reached.

Challenge 6: Standard models of care are not suited for PWID

With all-oral, effective HCV treatment with few side effects, HCV tests with excellent test performance and noninvasive methods to identify those with advanced HCV disease, we do have most of the tools to help us succeed in elimination of HCV among PWID. The main challenge in the future will be engaging PWID in HCV care. To achieve this, we need to develop and scale up models of care capable of reaching this population.

The most successful models of HCV care adapted for PWID populations have been built upon already existing infrastructures of health services for PWID. As such, these integrated models have covered diagnostics and treatment under the same roof with concurrent access to harm reduction services and other relevant health services for PWID. Multidisciplinary models typically include clinician and nursing staff, drug and alcohol support services, psychiatric services, social work, peer support, and options for directly observed therapy. Utilizing these principles, HCV treatment for PWID has been successfully delivered in various clinical settings such as OAT clinics, community-based low-threshold services, and general practice, as well as in secondary/tertiary hepatology units [23].

Conclusion

The availability of DAAs has opened up a new era in HCV care. In high- and middle-income countries, the majority of HCV patients have injected drugs. To successfully diminish HCV as a health problem among PWID will require that new models of care are developed to address the special needs of this population.

References

1. Kielland KB, Skaug K, Amundsen EJ, Dalgard O. All-cause and liver-related mortality in hepatitis C infected drug users followed for 33 years: a controlled study. *Journal of Hepatology* 2013;58:31–37.
2. Innes HA, Hutchinson SJ, Barclay S et al. Quantifying the fraction of cirrhosis attributable to alcohol among chronic hepatitis C virus patients: implications for treatment cost-effectiveness. *Hepatology* 2013;57:451–460.
3. Wai CT, Greenson JK, Fontana RJ et al. A simple noninvasive index can predict both significant fibrosis and cirrhosis in patients with chronic hepatitis C. *Hepatology* 2003;38:518–526.
4. Castera L, Vergniol J, Foucher J et al. Prospective comparison of transient elastography, Fibrotest, APRI, and liver biopsy for the assessment of fibrosis in chronic hepatitis C. *Gastroenterology* 2005;128:343–350.
5. Grebely J, Larney S, Peacock A et al. Global, regional, and country-level estimates of hepatitis C infection among people who have recently injected drugs. *Addiction* 2019;114:150–166.
6. Zibbell JE, Asher AK, Patel RC et al. Increases in acute hepatitis C virus infection related to a growing opioid epidemic and associated injection drug use, United States, 2004 to 2014. *American Journal of Public Health* 2018;108:175–181.
7. Larney S, Peacock A, Leung J et al. Global, regional, and country-level coverage of interventions to prevent and manage HIV and hepatitis C among people who inject drugs: a systematic review. *Lancet Global Health* 2017;5:e1208–e1220.
8. Platt L, Minozzi S, Reed J et al. Needle syringe programmes and opioid substitution therapy for preventing hepatitis C transmission in people who inject drugs. *Cochrane Database of Systematic Reviews* 2017;9:CD012021.
9. Fraser H, Martin NK, Brummer-Korvenkontio H et al. Model projections on the impact of HCV treatment in the prevention of HCV transmission among people who inject drugs in Europe. *Journal of Hepatology* 2018;68:402–411.
10. Grebely J, Dore GJ, Zeuzem S et al. Efficacy and safety of sofosbuvir/velpatasvir in patients with chronic hepatitis C virus infection receiving opioid substitution therapy: analysis of Phase 3 ASTRAL trials. *Clinical Infectious Diseases* 2016;63:1479–1481.
11. Grebely J, Jacobson IM, Kayali Z et al. SOF/VEL/VOX for 8 or 12 weeks is well tolerated and results in high SVR12 rates

in patients receiving opioid substitution therapy. *Journal of Hepatology* 2017;66:S513.

12. Grebely J, Mauss S, Brown A et al. Efficacy and safety of ledipasvir/sofosbuvir with and without ribavirin in patients with chronic HCV genotype 1 infection receiving opioid substitution therapy: analysis of Phase 3 ION trials. *Clinical Infectious Diseases* 2016;63:1405–1411.

13. Grebely J, Puoti M, Wedemeyer H et al. Safety and efficacy of ombitasvir, paritaprevir/ritonavir and dasabuvir with or without ribavirin in chronic hepatitis C patients receiving opioid substitution therapy: a pooled analysis across 12 clinical trials. *Journal of Hepatology* 2017;66:S514.

14. Lalezari J, Sullivan JG, Varunok P et al. Ombitasvir/paritaprevir/r and dasabuvir plus ribavirin in HCV genotype 1-infected patients on methadone or buprenorphine. *Journal of Hepatology* 2015;63:364–369.

15. Grebely J, Feld JJ, Wyles D et al. Sofosbuvir-based direct-acting antiviral therapies for HCV in people receiving opioid substitution therapy: an analysis of Phase 3 studies. *Open Forum Infectious Diseases* 2018;5:ofy001.

16. Midgard H, Bramness JG, Skurtveit S, Haukeland JW, Dalgard O. Hepatitis C treatment uptake among patients who have received opioid substitution treatment: a population-based study. *PLoS One* 2016;11:e0166451.

17. Midgard H. Management of hepatitis C virus infection among people who inject drugs. Treatment uptake, reinfection and risk behaviours. Thesis. Faculty of Medicine, University of Oslo, 2017.

18. Iversen J, Dore GJ, Catlett B, Cunningham P, Grebely J, Maher L. Association between rapid utilisation of direct hepatitis C antivirals and decline in the prevalence of viremia among people who inject drugs in Australia. *Journal of Hepatology* 2019;70:33–39.

19. Aspinall EJ, Corson S, Doyle JS et al. Treatment of hepatitis C virus infection among people who are actively injecting drugs: a systematic review and meta-analysis. *Clinical Infectious Diseases* 2013;57 Suppl 2:S80–89.

20. Wiessing L, Ferri M, Grady B et al. Hepatitis C virus infection epidemiology among people who inject drugs in Europe: a systematic review of data for scaling up treatment and prevention. *PLoS One* 2014;9:e103345.

21. Cunningham E, Grebely J, Dalgard O, Hajarizadeh B, Conway B, Powis J. Reinfection following successful HCV DAA therapy among people with recent injecting drug use: the SIMPLIFY and D3FEAT studies. https://az659834.vo.msecnd.net/eventsairaueprod/production-ashm-public/b8181b9f24f64ac78ed5fc68b1f7e44d

22. Midgard H, Bjoro B, Maeland A et al. Hepatitis C reinfection following sustained virological response – seven-year follow-up of patients infected through injecting drug use. *Journal of Hepatology* 2016;64:1020–1026.

23. Bruggmann P, Litwin AH. Models of care for the management of hepatitis C virus among people who inject drugs: one size does not fit all. *Clinical Infectious Diseases* 2013;57 Suppl 2:S56–61.

14 Hepatitis B virus reactivation while on hepatitis C virus direct-acting antiviral therapy: is that a real concern and when is it a concern?

Marina Serper

Division of Gastroenterology and Hepatology, Perelman School of Medicine, University of Pennsylvania, Philadelphia, PA, USA

LEARNING POINTS

- In 2016, the United States Food and Drug Administration issued a warning recommending screening of all HCV-infected patients for current or previous HBV infection. This warning was initially based on 29 reports of HBV reactivation, which were submitted to the adverse report database.

- Due to these emerging data, the American Association for the Study of Liver Diseases (AASLD) and Infectious Disease Society of America (IDSA) recommended HBV vaccination for all susceptible individuals, testing of HBV DNA (in those HBsAg positive) before HCV DAA therapy in anyone at risk for active viral replication, and regular monitoring of patients with HBV DNA.

- In a pooled analysis of 242 patients, the risk of HBV reactivation was 24% among those with HBsAg+ and 9% when using the AASLD definition. This risk was similar whether or not HBV DNA was quantifiable at baseline.

- Several studies have investigated HBV reactivation among patients with resolved HBV (HBsAg-/HBcAb+). The pooled HBV reactivation rate was < 1%. VA studies showed a less than 1% reactivation rate. Hepatitis B surface antibody status was not protective against HBV reactivation.

- This risk of reactivation in chronic HBV is high enough to warrant preemptive HBV antiviral therapy at the time of DAA initiation in most cases. However, it is reasonable to have a risk-benefit discussion of preemptive HBV antivirals versus careful monitoring among those with chronic HBV and an undetectable HBV DNA at baseline. Patients with resolved HBV (HBsAg-/HBcAb+) have a very low risk of reactivation and monitoring with serial ALT is generally sufficient.

Introduction

The advent of all-oral direct-acting antivirals (DAAs) has revolutionized treatment for chronic hepatitis C virus (HCV) and has broadly expanded HCV therapy criteria to be nearly universal. Commonly, patients with HCV are affected by chronic hepatitis B virus (HBV) coinfection (hepatitis B surface antigen positive [HBsAg+]) or have evidence of resolved HBV (HBsAg-, hepatitis B core antibody+ [HBcAb+]) due to residing in endemic areas or high-risk behaviors for parenteral transmission. In general, HCV replication is suppressed in the presence of HBV, but reactivation can occur following HCV eradication [1]. In the previous era of HCV therapy, cases of HBV reactivation (HBVr) had been reported with pegylated interferon and ribavirin and recent data have emerged regarding reactivation with DAAs [2].

In 2016, the United States Food and Drug Administration (FDA) issued a warning recommending screening of all HCV-infected patients for current or previous HBV infection. As HBsAg+ patients were specifically excluded from HCV DAA registration trials, this warning was initially based on 29 reports of HBVr, which were submitted to the adverse report database [3]. Of the cases reported, one patient had severe enough HBVr to require liver transplantation and two patients died [3]. Of concern, HBVr was reported in HCV DAA-treated patients with both chronic (HBsAg+) and resolved (HBsAg-/HBcAb+) infection. Unfortunately, due to the nature of the reporting system,

Clinical Dilemmas in Viral Liver Disease, Second Edition. Edited by Graham R. Foster and K. Rajender Reddy.
© 2020 John Wiley & Sons Ltd. Published 2020 by John Wiley & Sons Ltd.

detailed data regarding HBV serologies were not available to the FDA. However, due to these emerging data, the AASLD and IDSA recommended HBV vaccination for all susceptible individuals, testing of HBV DNA before HCV DAA therapy in anyone at risk for active viral replication, and regular monitoring of patients with HBV DNA [4,5]. These reports have also prompted several single-center and multicenter retrospective studies as well as metaanalyses to answer questions regarding the prevalence, severity, and risk factors for HBVr in the setting of HCV DAA therapy, which will be further explored in this chapter where we will describe key definitions pertaining to HBV, review recent literature on HBVr, and propose evidence-based recommendations for clinical practice.

Prevalence of HCV/HBV coinfection

The prevalence of coinfection remains unknown, but studies from the US report that about 1.4% of individual with HCV have HBsAg+ and this is about 4.1% in China [6].

Definition of HBV infection

Chronic HBV is defined as having persistent HBsAg+ or positive HBV DNA for at least six months irrespective of the results of other HBV serologies. Resolved HBV is defined as having evidence of prior HBV exposure (HBcAb+) and HBsAg+.

Definitions of HBV reactivation and clinically significant adverse events

There is no standard, agreed-upon definition of HBVr in the literature. The AASLD defines HBVr as a ≥2 log increase in HBV DNA from baseline or detection of HBV DNA greater than 100 IU/mL in patients with undetectable HBV DNA at baseline [4].

In research studies, HBVr has been defined as the appearance of quantifiable HBV DNA when HBV DNA was previously undetectable or a ≥1 log increase in HBV DNA when HBV DNA was previously detectable. Clinically significant HBVr has been defined as having concomitant alanine aminotransferase (ALT) elevation to greater than twice the upper limit of normal (>2 ULN) or the appearance of hyperbilirubinemia. With regards to timing, HBVr is generally felt to be attributable to HCV DAAs if occur-

ring during HCV therapy or for at least 12 weeks after HCV therapy completion although this definition is also not standardized. Clinically significant adverse events are defined as hepatic decompensations (jaundice, ascites, etc.), need for liver transplantation or death.

HBV reactivation among persons with chronic HBV

Several retrospective studies and metaanalyses have evaluated the risk of HBVr among HCV-infected patients undergoing DAA therapy and concomitantly coinfected with HBV.

A recent prospective study in Taiwan examined outcomes of HCV DAA therapy among 111 chronic HBV/HCV coinfected patients, none of whom were taking HBV antivirals at baseline. Among the 37 patients with no quantifiable HBV DNA at baseline, 84% became quantifiable consistent with HBVr (about half of the cases occurred during HCV therapy and half during follow-up). The majority of patients with HBVr had persistently positive HBV DNA and two of 37 (5.4%) required initiation of entecavir therapy due to clinically significant HBVr. One of those patients (2.7%) developed symptoms of malaise and jaundice and had a peak total bilirubin of 2.4 mg/dL which later normalized with HBV therapy [7].

A retrospective study in the US Veterans Affairs (a integrated system of care for veterans, which has a large population of patients with viral hepatitis) investigated HBVr among 134 HBsAg+ patients who were not treated with HBV therapy [8]. As routine HBV DNA testing was not performed in this real-world cohort, HBVr was defined in multiple ways ranging from twofold to fourfold increase in baseline ALT or >1 log IU/mL increase in HBV DNA during or after treatment. A total of 30% of HBsAg+ patients not on HBV therapy developed possible HBVr as defined by twofold increase in ALT; this was higher among patients with cirrhosis (44%). While less common, 15% developed a fourfold increase in ALT. Although HBV DNA ascertainment was limited, HBVr occurred in at least 7% of cases when defined as having a 1 log IU/mL increase in HBV DNA. Only one patient (<1%) had clinically significant toxicity.

A metaanalysis evaluated the risk of HBVr among recent prospective and retrospective studies [9]. In a pooled analysis of 242 patients, the risk of HBVr was 24% among those with HBsAg+ and 9% when using the AASLD definition.

This risk was similar whether or not HBV DNA was quantifiable at baseline. There appeared to be no difference in reactivation risk based on cirrhosis, use of ribavirin, or the specific type of DAA regimen. Although the risk of HBVr was similar between those patients with HBV DNA below the limit of quantification and those with HBV DNA ≥20 IU/mL, the chances of developing HBVr with hepatitis was 83% more common among those with a quantifiable HBV DNA at baseline. In this metaanalysis of recent studies, three (1.2%) patients had clinically significant adverse events, two with hepatic decompensation and one with hepatic decompensation requiring transplantation.

HBV reactivation among persons with resolved HBV

Several studies have investigated HBVr among patients with resolved HBV (HBsAg-/HBcAb+). The pooled HBV reactivation rate among 901 patients was 2 (0.2%). VA studies showed a less than 1% reactivation rate, but HBV

was infrequently checked on treatment, and therefore likely underestimated the true incidence of HBVr [8]. Hepatitis B surface antibody status was not protective against HBVr.

Recommendations for clinical practice

A proposed evaluation and treatment algorithm when treating with HCV DAAs is shown in Figure 14.1. Based on the available data and guidance from professional societies [4,5], universal testing for HBsAg and HBV DNA is recommended prior to starting HCV therapy as the preponderance of evidence suggests that HBVr is quite common among those with chronic HBV and occasionally, albeit rarely, occurs with resolved HBV.

If patients are found to have chronic HBV at the outset, treatment should be guided by following standard criteria based on viral load and elevated ALT as suggested by AASLD and EASL guidelines [4,5].

Patients with no quantifiable HBV DNA prior to HCV therapy should be counseled regarding the risk of reactiva-

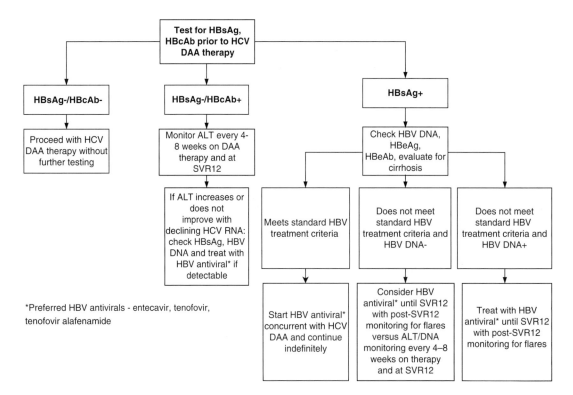

Figure 14.1 Proposed algorithm for testing and managing hepatitis B when initiating hepatitis C therapy with direct-acting antivirals.

tion and serial ALT monitoring on and after therapy versus prophylaxis. Monitoring should be performed with ALT every 4–8 weeks and significant ALT elevations or failure of ALT to improve should prompt HBV DNA testing. Although the duration of prophylaxis is not well elucidated, it is reasonable to continue for a three-month period after DAA completion. Patients with quantifiable HBV DNA who do not meet standard treatment criteria (for example, HBV viral load 200–IU/mL, normal ALT) have a higher risk of HBVr and it is reasonable to preemptively treat these patients with HBV antivirals. It should be noted that careful monitoring of ALT needs to occur after stopping HBV prophylaxis as the patients are at risk for flares with HBV therapy withdrawal; the optimal duration of that monitoring is not known. Finally, in all cases of chronic HBV therapy, prophylaxis is a safer alternative to monitoring if patient adherence with appointments or laboratory testing is expected to be problematic.

Patients with resolved HBV have a much lower risk of reactivation and should have ALT monitoring on therapy and for 3–6 months after therapy completion as delayed flares have been reported. Patients with resolved HBV should not receive HBV antiviral prophylaxis while on HCV DAA therapy as the risk of reactivation is about 1% or less.

Patients can be counseled that reactivation, if it occurs, is very well treated with nucleos(t)ide analogs such as entecavir, tenofovir, or tenofovir alafenamide with effective viral suppression.

Conclusion

Direct-acting antiviral therapy increases the risk of HBV reactivation among patients with chronic HBV (HBsAg+) and HCV and may rarely result in serious adverse consequences such as liver decompensation requiring transplantation or death. This risk of reactivation in chronic HBV is high enough to warrant preemptive HBV antiviral therapy at the time of DAA initiation in most cases. However, it is reasonable to have a risk-benefit discussion of preemptive HBV antivirals versus careful monitoring among those with chronic HBV and an undetectable HBV DNA at baseline. Patients with resolved HBV (HBsAg-/HBcAb+) have a very low risk of reactivation and monitoring with serial

ALT is generally sufficient. The presence of HBsAb+ does not appear to be protective against reactivation. DAA regimen, use of ribavirin, and cirrhosis do not affect the risk of reactivation, but patients with a higher HBV DNA baseline viral load are at increased risk of significant hepatitis if reactivation does occur. Reactivation is generally easily treated with suppression of viral replication, but careful monitoring, prevention, and early identification are key in order to optimize clinical outcomes.

References

1. Chen G, Wang C, Chen J et al. Hepatitis B reactivation in hepatitis B and C coinfected patients treated with antiviral agents: a systematic review and meta-analysis. *Hepatology* 2017;66(1):13–26.
2. Liu CJ, Chuang WL, Lee CM et al. Peginterferon alfa-2a plus ribavirin for the treatment of dual chronic infection with hepatitis B and C viruses. *Gastroenterology* 2009;136(2):496–504 e3.
3. US Food and Drug Administration. FDA Drug Safety Communication: FDA warns about the risk of hepatitis B reactivating in some patients treated with direct-acting antivirals for hepatitis C. 2016. www.fda.gov/Drugs/DrugSafety/ucm522932.htm
4. Terrault NA, Lok ASF, McMahon BJ et al. Update on prevention, diagnosis, and treatment of chronic hepatitis B: AASLD 2018 hepatitis B guidance. *Hepatology* 2018;67(4):1560–1599.
5. European Association for the Study of the Liver. EASL 2017 Clinical Practice Guidelines on the management of hepatitis B virus infection. *Journal of Hepatology* 2017;67(2):370–398.
6. Ma AT, Feld JJ. Hepatitis B reactivation with hepatitis c treatment: bringing some clarity to the black box. *Gastroenterology* 2018;154(4):795–798.
7. Liu CJ, Chuang WL, Sheen IS et al. Efficacy of ledipasvir and sofosbuvir treatment of hcv infection in patients coinfected with HBV. *Gastroenterology* 2018;154(4):989–997.
8. Serper M, Forde KA, Kaplan DE. Rare clinically significant hepatic events and hepatitis B reactivation occur more frequently following rather than during direct-acting antiviral therapy for chronic hepatitis C: data from a national US cohort. *Journal of Viral Hepatology* 2018;25(2):187–197.
9. Mucke MM, Backus LI, Mucke VT et al. Hepatitis B virus reactivation during direct-acting antiviral therapy for hepatitis C: a systematic review and meta-analysis. *Lancet Gastroenterology and Hepatology* 2018;3(3):172–180.

Drug–drug interactions with direct-acting antivirals: when do we need to care?

Fiona Marra[1,2] and David Back[1]

[1] Department of Molecular and Clinical Pharmacology, University of Liverpool, Liverpool, UK
[2] NHS Greater Glasgow and Clyde, Glasgow, Scotland, UK

LEARNING POINTS

- With increased access to DAA treatment and the widening pool of healthcare providers treating HCV-infected patients, an understanding of drug interactions is vital in making sure patients complete treatment successfully.

- Review of all medications prior to initiating DAA therapy is essential to maintain efficacay of all the drugs involved.

- For most drugs, strategies to treat HCV can be developed but particular care is needed with carbamazepine and rifampicin which are incompatible with most antiviral therapies.

Introduction

The roll-out of direct-acting antivirals (DAA) has revolutionized treatment of HCV infection. However, there are patients who remain challenging to treat, including those with complex drug–drug interactions (DDIs). Real-world data have shown that 40% or more of patients (depending on the DAA regimen) may have clinically significant DDIs [1]. With increased access to treatment and the widening of the pool of healthcare providers treating patients, an understanding of drug interactions is vital in making sure patients complete treatment successfully [2].

Mechanisms of Drug–Drug Interactions

Cytochrome P450 (CYP) enzymes are commonly involved in the metabolism of DAAs but some DAAs can also alter CYP activity, primarily through enzyme inhibition [3]. In addition, DAAs are substrates and inhibitors of various drug transporters (e.g., P-gp; BCRP; OATP) located in the gastrointestinal tract and/or liver. Another mechanism of interaction is the alteration of gastric pH which may impact absorption of an acid-sensitive DAA. An overview of the mechanisms of drug interactions for the currently recommended DAAs is shown in Figure 15.1.

As perpetrators of DDIs, a DAA may cause increased or decreased exposure of a coadministered medication, resulting in drug levels which may either predispose to toxicity or be suboptimal with potential loss of efficacy. As victims of DDIs, the DAAs can be subject to interactions whereby the comedication increases exposure of the DAA, resulting in toxicity, or reduces it, resulting in subtherapeutic levels and potentially virologic failure.

Taking a thorough patient drug history is crucial in providing correct advice. This includes knowledge of over-the-counter preparations, contraceptives, herbal or vitamin supplements or illicit drug use. Accessing up-to-date sources of drug interaction information is vital. Individual drug labels have important but relatively limited information on interactions and therefore we need other

Clinical Dilemmas in Viral Liver Disease, Second Edition. Edited by Graham R. Foster and K. Rajender Reddy.
© 2020 John Wiley & Sons Ltd. Published 2020 by John Wiley & Sons Ltd.

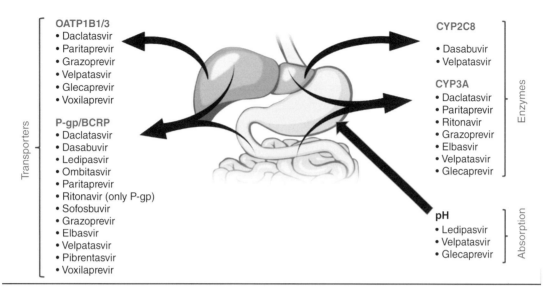

OATP1B1/3
- Daclatasvir
- Paritaprevir
- Grazoprevir
- Velpatasvir
- Glecaprevir
- Voxilaprevir

P-gp/BCRP
- Daclatasvir
- Dasabuvir
- Ledipasvir
- Ombitasvir
- Paritaprevir
- Ritonavir (only P-gp)
- Sofosbuvir
- Grazoprevir
- Elbasvir
- Velpatasvir
- Pibrentasvir
- Voxilaprevir

Transporters

CYP2C8
- Dasabuvir
- Velpatasvir

CYP3A
- Daclatasvir
- Paritaprevir
- Ritonavir
- Grazoprevir
- Elbasvir
- Velpatasvir
- Glecaprevir

Enzymes

pH
- Ledipasvir
- Velpatasvir
- Glecaprevir

Absorption

Figure 15.1 Gastrointestinal and hepatic metabolic and transporter pathways of potential drug–drug interactions with DAAs. The most common metabolic pathways involve CYP450, with transporters being either influx (e.g., OATP1B1) or efflux (e.g., P-gp; BCRP). The figure illustrates the pathways of individual DAAs. In some cases, this may involve the DAA being both a substrate and a modulator of the protein. There is also pH-dependent absorption.

resources. www.hep-druginteractions.org is recommended in both AASLD and EASL guidelines for hepatitis C treatment [4,5]. To get an overview of the pharmacology of individual drugs, readers should access the relevant prescribing information. These data are summarized in the following section.

Pharmacology of individual directly acting antivirals

Sofosbuvir and ledipasvir

Sofosbuvir is mainly renally excreted as the metabolite GS-331007. The major route of elimination of ledipasvir is biliary excretion of unchanged drug, with renal excretion being a minor pathway. Neither sofosbuvir nor ledipasvir are substrates for hepatic uptake transporters. Since both ledipasvir and sofosbuvir are transported by intestinal P-gp and BCRP, any coadministered drugs that are potent P-gp inducers, such as rifampicin, carbamazepine, and St John's wort, will decrease both sofosbuvir and ledipasvir plasma concentrations, leading to reduced therapeutic effect. Although coadministration with drugs that inhibit P-gp and/or BCRP may increase drug exposure, clinical consequences are unlikely. Ledipasvir may also be the perpetrator

of drug interactions due to inhibition of P-gp and/or BCRP, potentially increasing the absorption of coadministered drugs. Thus, caution is warranted with P-gp substrates such as digoxin and dabigatran, but also with other drugs which are transported by these proteins (e.g., amlodipine, buprenorphine). The use of rosuvastatin is not recommended (thought to be due to inhibition of hepatic OATP1B1 by ledipasvir) and interactions with other statins cannot be excluded [6].

Sofosbuvir-based regimens are contraindicated in patients being treated with the antiarrhythmic amiodarone due to the risk of life-threatening arrhythmias.

The mechanism of interaction as well as the role of other comedications is still unclear, although a direct effect of sofosbuvir and/or other DAAs on cardiomyocytes or ion channels is most likely.

Ledipasvir solubility decreases as pH increases so drugs increasing gastric pH (e.g., proton pump inhibitors) are likely to decrease concentrations of ledipasvir.

Sofosbuvir and velpatasvir

Although velpatasvir is metabolized by several CYP enzymes, most drug in plasma is as the parent. Importantly, velpatasvir is transported by P-gp and BCRP and, to a limited extent, OATP1B1. Biliary excretion is the major elimination route. Drugs that are potent P-gp or CYP inducers are contraindicated due to the decrease in sofosbuvir and/or velpatasvir exposure with potential loss of efficacy. Moderate P-gp or CYP inducers (e.g., modafinil) may also reduce velpatasvir exposure. Due to inhibition of P-gp and/or BCRP by velpatasvir, caution should be exercised with comedications with a narrow therapeutic window where an increase in drug exposure could have clinical consequences.

Velpatasvir is also susceptible to pH increases and it is important to be aware of recommendations concerning the coadministration of antacids, H2-receptor antagonists, and proton pump inhibitors [7,8].

Sofosbuvir, velpatasvir, and voxilaprevir

Voxilaprevir is metabolized by CYP3A4 but the vast majority of drug in plasma is the parent drug. Biliary excretion is the major route of elimination. Because velpatasvir and voxilaprevir are both inhibitors of P-gp, BCRP, and OATP1B1, coadministration with drugs that are substrates of these transporters may increase exposure of comedications. This means that where elevated plasma levels are associated with serious events, there may be a contraindication or requirement for dose adjustment or additional monitoring. For example, both rosuvastatin (inhibition of BCRP) and dabigatran (inhibition of P-gp) are contraindicated due to a large increase in exposure. Other P-gp substrates may need to be dose-adjusted or monitored for increased exposure. Similar caution is required with OATP1B inhibitors such as ciclosporin as voxilaprevir plasma exposure markedly increases, or with OATP1B substrates such as edoxaban.

Use of strong P-gp and/or strong CYP inducers is contraindicated due to the decrease in sofosbuvir, velpatasvir, and/or voxilaprevir exposure with potential loss of efficacy. Drugs that are moderate P-gp or CYP inducers (such as modafinil) are not recommended.

Ombitasvir/paritaprevir (+ritonavir) and dasabuvir (OBV/PTV/r) + DSV

Paritaprevir is metabolized primarily by CYP3A4 and given with low-dose ritonavir as a pharmacokinetic enhancer in combination with ombitasvir. Paritaprevir and ombitasvir are excreted predominantly in the feces. Dasabuvir is metabolized in the liver, and its predominant metabolite is cleared via biliary excretion with minimal renal clearance. Paritaprevir is primarily metabolized by CYP3A4, dasabuvir by CYP2C8, and ombitasvir undergoes hydrolysis. Transporters also play an important role, with paritaprevir inhibiting OATP1B1/B3, P-gp, and BCRP. Dasabuvir and ritonavir may also inhibit P-gp and BCRP. The presence of ritonavir gives the potential for many DDIs [9]. Also contraindicated are enzyme inducers that might compromise virologic efficacy.

Grazoprevir and elbasvir

Grazoprevir and elbasvir are partially metabolized by CYP3A4. The principal route of elimination is biliary. Grazoprevir is transported by P-gp and OATP1B1 and elbasvir by P-gp.

Since elbasvir and grazoprevir are substrates of CYP3A and P-gp, inducers of these proteins may cause a marked decrease in plasma exposure of both DAAs and are contraindicated. Strong inhibitors of CYP3A, which may markedly increase plasma concentrations, are either contraindicated or not recommended. In addition to inhibition of CYP3A, grazoprevir plasma concentrations may also be increased by inhibitors of OATP1B1. There is no effect of acid-reducing agents on either DAA.

Grazoprevir and elbasvir have low potential to affect other medications, although grazoprevir is a weak CYP3A inhibitor and elbasvir a weak inhibitor of P-gp. There needs to be some caution when coadministering drugs that use CYP3A and P-gp and have a narrow therapeutic index, or drugs with a large dose range (e.g., quetiapine) where those on higher doses may need additional monitoring.

Glecaprevir and pibrentasvir

Biliary excretion is the major route for elimination of both glecaprevir and pibrentasvir.

They are inhibitors of P-gp, BCRP, and OATP1B1. Coadministration with glecaprevir/pibrentasvir may increase the concentration of comedications that are substrates of P-gp (e.g., dabigatran etexilate), BCRP (e.g., rosuvastatin), or OATP1B1/3 (e.g., atorvastatin) leading to contraindication or dose reduction.

Glecaprevir/pibrentasvir administered with strong P-gp- and CYP3A-inducing drugs put patients at risk of virologic failure and coadministration is contraindicated. Care should be exercised with moderate inducers. Comedications that inhibit P-gp and BCRP may increase plasma exposure of glecaprevir/pibrentasvir. Similarly, OATP1B1/3 inhibitors such as ciclosporin may also increase glecaprevir concentrations. The potential for glecaprevir/pibrentasvir to affect other medications is low, although glecaprevir is a weak CYP3A inhibitor. Caution is advised when coadministering CYP3A metabolized drugs with a narrow therapeutic index or drugs with large dose ranges.

The solubility of glecaprevir decreases as pH increases and the license states no dose changes are required although caution is recommended with omeprazole doses exceeding 40 mg.

Drug–drug interaction advice for specific therapeutic areas

Antiretrovirals (ARVs)

Although HIV/HCV coinfected patients are no longer regarded as a "special" population at risk of suboptimal responses, there is an increased propensity for significant DDIs which can impact HIV and/or HCV therapy [10,11]. For most patients, DDIs associated with lifelong HIV therapy given together with short-course HCV are surmountable, particularly for the prize of complete HCV eradication. Table 15.1 outlines DDIs between DAAs and ARVs and is given to represent the information available for different drug classes at www.hep-druginteractions.org.

The protease inhibitors (PI) grazoprevir, glecaprevir, paritaprevir, and voxilaprevir are, as a class, susceptible to DDIs with drugs which are inhibitors (ritonavir or cobicistat containing) or inducers (such as efavirenz or etravirine). For example, HIV-boosted PIs and cobicistat markedly increase grazoprevir and are contraindicated, as is coadministration with efavirenz/etravirine which can be expected to lower grazoprevir (and elbasvir) exposure.

Similarly, ritonavir-boosted PIs increase glecaprevir concentrations, and nonnucleoside reverse transcriptase inhibitors (NNRTIs) (efavirenz/etravirine) reduce glecaprevir exposure and coadministration is not recommended. However, boosting with cobicistat has less of an impact with glecaprevir and coadministration (in the context of a fixed-dose integrase-containing regimen, and in the absence of HIV PIs) is permissible.

Paritaprevir-containing regimens incorporate ritonavir, which complicates the use of an HIV-boosted PI regimen. With darunavir, there is a decrease in trough concentration of ~50% and the European SPC advises that once-daily

darunavir should only be used in the absence of extensive HIV PI resistance. Coadministration with cobicistat or the NNRTIs efavirenz/etravirine is contraindicated.

Since voxilaprevir is transported by OATP1B1 and P-gp inhibition by atazanavir/r results in increased voxilaprevir exposure, this combination is contraindicated. However, once-daily darunavir (boosted with ritonavir or cobicistat) is not expected to result in clinically significant DDIs. Coadministration with efavirenz or etravirine is not recommended.

Sofosbuvir/ledipasvir, sofosbuvir/velpatasvir, and sofosbuvir/velpatasvir/voxilaprevir when combined with a tenofovir disoproxil fumarate (TDF) regimen cause increased tenofovir (TFV) exposure due to P-gp inhibition. This means that patients on a regimen containing TDF need to be monitored for renal adverse events. Lower concentrations of TFV are seen following tenofovir alafenamide (TAF) administration, and although increased TFV exposure may occur with boosted ARVs, the interaction is not clinically significant.

Although DDIs between individual antiviral agents used for treating HIV and hepatitis C may occur, there are sufficient choices to select alternative regimens to avoid interactions whilst maintaining efficacy for both treatments. Importantly, the HIV integrase inhibitors (raltegravir, dolutegravir, and bictegravir) have no or few interactions [12]. Management of therapy in this group of patients is best undertaken by prescribers with experience in both diseases.

Proton pump inhibitors (PPIs)

Some DAAs have pH-dependent solubility. This effect was first described with ledipasvir with omeprazole decreasing ledipasvir exposure. The European product license states that PPI doses comparable to omeprazole 20 mg can be administered simultaneously with sofosbuvir/ledipasvir. This effect has been extensively studied and there are conflicting data on whether it affects SVR. Real-world data have suggested slightly reduced sustained virologic response (SVR) rates in patients receiving high-dose PPIs, reinforcing the need for caution. H2-receptor antagonists can be given simultaneously or 12 hours apart at a dose not exceeding that equivalent to famotidine 40 mg.

Velpatasvir, as part of sofosbuvir/velpatasvir and sofosbuvir/velpatasvir/voxilaprevir, also has pH-dependent solubility and coadministration with PPIs is not recommended. If it is considered essential to coadminister, sofosbuvir/velpatasvir

Table 15.1 Drug–drug interactions between HCV DAAs and HIV antiretrovirals

		SOF	SOF/LDV	SOF/VEL	OBV/PTV/r + DSV	GZR/EBR	DCV	S/V/V	GLE/PIB
NRTIs	Abacavir	◆	◆	◆	◆	◆	◆	◆	◆
	Emtricitabine	◆	◆	◆	◆	◆	◆	◆	◆
	Lamivudine	◆	◆	◆	◆	◆	◆	◆	◆
	Tenofovir disoproxil fumarate (TDF)	◆	■	■	◆	◆	◆	■	◆
	Tenofovir alafenamide (TAF)	◆	◆	◆	■	◆	◆	■	◆
NNRTIs	Efavirenz	◆	■*	●	●	●	■	●	●
	Etravirine	◆	◆	●	●	●	■	●	●
	Nevirapine	◆	◆	●	●	●	■	●	●
	Rilpivirine	◆	◆	◆	■	◆	◆	◆	◆
Protease inhibitors	Atazanavir/ritonavir	◆	◆*	◆*	■	●	■	●	●
	Atazanavir/cobicistat	◆	◆*	◆*	●	●	■	●	●
	Darunavir/ritonavir	◆	◆*	◆*	■	●	◆	■*	●
	Darunavir/cobicistat	◆	◆*	◆*	●	●	■	◆*	●
	Lopinavir/ritonavir	◆	◆*	◆*	●	●	◆	●	●
Entry/Integrase inhibitors	Dolutegravir	◆	◆	◆	◆	◆	◆	◆	◆
	Elvitegravir/cobicistat/ emtricitabine/TDF	◆	■*	■*	●	●	■	■*	◆
	Elvitegravir/cobicistat/ emtricitabine/TAF	◆	◆	◆	●	●	■	◆	◆
	Maraviroc	◆	◆	◆	■	◆	◆	◆	◆
	Raltegravir	◆	◆	◆	◆	◆	◆	◆	◆

Colour legend

◆ No clinically significant interaction expected

■ Potential interaction which may require a dosage adjustment, altered timing of administration or additional monitoring

● These drugs should not be coadministered

Some drugs may require dose modifications dependent on hepatic function. Please refer to the product label for individual drugs for dosing advice. The symbol (green, amber, red) used to rank the clinical significance of the drug interaction is based on www.hep-druginteractions.org (University of Liverpool). For additional drug–drug interactions and for a more extensive range of drugs, detailed pharmacokinetic interaction data and dosage adjustments, refer to the above-mentioned website.

* Known or anticipated increase in tenofovir concentrations in regimens containing tenofovir disoproxil fumarate. Caution and frequent renal monitoring required.

DCV, daclatasvir; GLE/PIB, glecaprevir/pibrentasvir; GZR/EBR, grazoprevir/elbasvir; NNRTI, nonnucleoside reverse transcriptase inhibitor; NRTI, nucleoside reverse transcriptase inhibitor; OBV/PTV/r + DSV, ritonavir-boosted paritaprevir/ombitasvir/dasabuvir; SOF, sofosbuvir; SOF/LDV, sofosbuvir/ledipasvir; SOF/VEL, sofosbuvir/velpatasvir; S/V/V, sofosbuvir/velpatasvir/voxilaprevir.

should be taken with food and 4 hours before the PPI at maximum doses comparable to omeprazole 20 mg. Similar advice is given for sofosbuvir/velpatasvir/voxilaprevir.

Glecaprevir/pibrentasvir has pH-dependent solubility but, in this instance, it is glecaprevir that is affected and not the NS5A inhibitor pibrentasvir. However, efficacy data show that this interaction did not impact SVR and no dose adjustment is recommended although there are no data for doses higher than omeprazole 40 mg [13]. OBV/r/PTV + DSV is not impacted by PPIs [14].

In all patients on PPIs, a full drug history should be taken for appropriateness of prescribing and the PPI stopped if not necessary. H2 antagonists can be considered as a step-down mechanism if patients are struggling to manage clinically without a PPI.

Antiepileptic drugs (AEDs)

Antiepileptic drugs are often associated with drug interactions, with phenytoin, phenobarbital, and carbamazepine being CYP enzyme and P-gp inducers; they are contraindicated with all DAAs. A change to an alternative (noninteracting) antiepileptic can be considered to avoid subtherapeutic plasma levels of DAAs and risk of treatment failure. The exception may be the use of daclatasvir. There is a case report using an increased dose of daclatasvir (90 mg) in combination with oxcarbazepine and a series of cases using increased daclatasvir doses (60 mg bid) in patients receiving carbamazepine or phenytoin. Although SVR12 was achieved in these patients, there remained a reduction in DAA exposure despite the increased doses [15]. However, this strategy cannot currently be extrapolated to all DAAs without further drug interaction studies. Additionally, as most DAAs are fixed-dose combinations, increasing doses is practically difficult as well as having potential financial implications.

Antiplatelets and anticoagulants

Antiplatelets

Aspirin can be taken with all HCV DAAs. Coadministration of clopidogrel and OBV/PTV/r ± DSV should be avoided due to inhibition of formation of the active metabolite and the potential increased risk of atherothrombotic events. Although formation of the active metabolite of prasugrel is also decreased, prasugrel continues to achieve potent platelet inhibition with or without ritonavir (or cobicistat) [16].

Ticagrelor is also contraindicated with a ritonavir-containing regimen due to CYP3A4 inhibition. With other currently available DAAs, if coadministration is deemed necessary, then close monitoring of ticagrelor is prudent due to a narrow therapeutic window.

Anticoagulants

Case reports have described marked reductions in international normalized ratio (INR) in patients on warfarin starting OBV/PTV/r and DSV with ribavirin resulting in an increased warfarin dose. Close monitoring of the INR is recommended, taking into consideration the time taken for enzyme induction/deinduction to occur. There are no clinically significant interactions predicted with warfarin and other DAAs. However, fluctuations in INR values may occur in patients receiving warfarin with any HCV treatment as a result of improved liver function. Frequent monitoring is recommended [17].

The potential for interactions between HCV DAAs and direct-acting oral anticoagulants (DOACs) is complex. Rivaroxaban and apixaban, substrates of CYP3A4, P-gp, and BCRP, are contraindicated with inhibitors of both CYP3A4 and P-gp. It is recommended that OBV/PTV/r and DSV should not be used with these drugs. Other DAA regimens which are mild/moderate inhibitors are likely to have a lesser impact. However, any increase in drug levels may lead to an increased risk of bleeding and, in the absence of data, caution is recommended. A patient's individual risk of bleeding (presence of hepatic impairment, coagulopathy) should be considered before coadministration. All HCV DAA regimens have some inhibitory effect on P-gp and have the potential to increase dabigatran exposure. Coadministration of dabigatran with glecaprevir or sofosbuvir/velpatasvir/voxilaprevir resulted in an increase in dabigatran exposure, suggesting concomitant use should be avoided due to potential bleeding complications. Close monitoring is recommended if dabigatran is used with OBV/PTV/r and DSV.

Use of DOACs in patients with HCV should be individualized, assessing the interactions along with bleeding risk and prescribed therapeutic indication [18]. In cirrhotic patients with low platelets, the risk may be higher and a clinical decision regarding coadministration may have a different outcome to other patients. Some DOAC courses are 3–6 months long and options include waiting until DAA completion or switching to low molecular weight heparin.

Drugs of abuse

People who inject drugs (PWID) and those prescribed opioid substitution therapy (OST) such as methadone and buprenorphine +/- naloxone are a target group for HCV treatment given the high HCV prevalence [19]. The potential for DDIs with OST and illicit drugs should be considered when starting DAAs. Interaction studies are limited and predicting interactions from metabolic data is usually needed. Many illicit drugs are metabolized by CYP450 enzymes and therefore susceptible to drug interactions. Unfortunately, exact routes of metabolism are not always established, with the added complexity of impurities being present which may cause unexpected interactions and toxicity. Another challenge for prescribers is the novel substances being manufactured and sold with little knowledge of the chemical structure and metabolism of these substances. A thorough and nonjudgmental drug history is essential.

Synthetic opioids

There has been a significant rise in synthetic opioid deaths, particularly in the USA and Canada [20], largely caused by illicit fentanyl use. In 2016, synthetic opioids eclipsed prescription opioids as the most common drug involved in overdose deaths in the USA. In addition, synthetic opioids are increasingly found in illicit drugs supplies of heroin, cocaine, methamphetamine, and other agents. Fentanyl is metabolized by CYP3A4 and is 50–100 times more potent than morphine and therefore small increases in concentrations can have significant effects. The fentanyl license cautions on concomitant use of fentanyl with all CYP3A4 inhibitors due to increased exposure, which could increase/prolong adverse effects. Use of OBV/PTV/r +/- DSV is not recommended. Grazoprevir and glecaprevir are mild CYP3A4 inhibitors and caution is warranted. However, concentrations of illicit fentanyl vary significantly and in addition there are potent fentanyl analogs such as carfentanil, which can complicate the treatment of substance abusers [21].

Opioid substitution therapies

Methadone, administered as a combination of the R- and S-isomers, is metabolized by multiple CYP enzymes [22]. Buprenorphine is a CYP3A4 and CYP2C8 substrate and also undergoes glucuronidation [23]. There are no predicted clinically significant interactions with any of the DAA combinations and OST. Despite an increase in buprenorphine exposure with OBV/PTV/r + DSV, there were no significant changes in pharmacodynamic measurements. Daclatasvir, elbasvir/grazoprevir, glecaprevir/pibrentasvir, and sofosbuvir have all been studied in combination with methadone and buprenorphine/naloxone, with no clinically meaningful effects on the pharmacokinetics of the OST drugs or DAAs being observed.

Contraceptives

The use of contraceptives is an important aspect of HCV treatment in females of child-bearing potential [24]. Contraceptives containing ethinylestradiol (EE) are contraindicated with OBV/PTV/r and DSV, glecaprevir/pibrentasvir,

and sofosbuvir/velpatasvir/voxilaprevir due to the potential risk of ALT elevations. Interaction studies investigating safety and tolerability of coadministration of grazoprevir/elbasvir with EE and levonorgestrel reported no increased incidence of adverse effects or liver function abnormalities and concluded that this combination can be safely coadministered with oral contraceptives. Progestogen-only contraception can generally be safely used in combination with HCV DAAs with no dose adjustment required.

Conclusion

Drug–drug interactions are often unavoidable in the management of patients treated with DAAs. It is therefore vital that the potential for DDIs is considered systematically before starting a DAA regimen or when a new medication is commenced during the DAA treatment period. Stopping a comedication for the duration of the DAA or dose modification of a comedication or additional monitoring may also have to be considered. Online drug interaction databases are valuable tools to help recognize and manage patients in clinical practice.

So, when do we need to care about drug interactions? In every patient receiving a DAA!

References

1. Ottman AA, Townsend M, Hashem M et al. Incidence of drug interactions identified by clinical pharmacists in veterans initiating treatment for chronic Hepatitis C infection. *Annals of Pharmacotherapy* 2018;52(8):763–768.

2. Smolders EJ, Berden F, de Kanter C et al. The majority of hepatitis C patients treated with direct acting antivirals are at risk for relevant drug–drug interactions. *United European Gastroenterology Journal* 2017;5(5):648–657.

3. Garrison KL, German P, Mogalian E et al. The drug–drug interaction potential of antiviral agents for the treatment of chronic hepatitis C infection. *Drug Metabolism and Disposition* 2018;46(8):1212–1225.

4. www.hcvguidelines.org

5. European Association for Society of the Liver. EASL recommendations on treatment of hepatitis C 2018. *Journal of Hepatology* 2018;69(2):461–511.

6. German P, Mathias A, Brainard D et al. Drug–drug interaction profile of the fixed dose combination tablet regimen ledipasvir/sofosbuvir. *Clinical Pharmacokinetics* 2018;57(11): 1369–1383.

7. Miller MM. Sofosbuvir–velpatasvir: a single tablet treatment for hepatitis C infection of all genotypes. *American Journal of Health System Pharmacy* 2017;74(14):1045–1052.

8. Berenguer J, Gil-Martin A, Jarrin I et al. All-oral direct-acting antiviral therapy against hepatitis C virus (HCV) in human immunodeficiency virus/HCV-coinfected subjects in real-world practice: Madrid coinfection registry findings. *Hepatology* 2018;68(1):32–47.

9. King JR, Menon RM. Ombitasvir/paritaprevir/ritonavir and dasabuvir: drug interactions with antiviral agents and drugs for substance abuse. *Clinical Pharmacology in Drug Development* 2017;6(2):201–205.

10. Abutaleb A, Sherman KE. A changing paradigm: management and treatmen of the HCV/HIV co-infected patient. *Hepatology International* 2018;12(6):500–509.

11. Feng HP, Guo Z, Ross L et al. Assessment of drug interaction potential between the HCV direct-acting antiviral agents elbasvir/grazoprevir and the HIV integrase inhibitors raltegravir and dolutegravir. *Journal of Antimicrobial Chemotherapy* 2019;74:710–717.

12. Di Perri G, Calcagno A, Trentalange A et al. The clinical pharmacology of integrase inhibitors. *Expert Review of Clinical Pharmacology* 2019;12:31–44.

13. Flamm S, Reddy K, Zadeikis N et al. Efficacy and pharmacokinetics of glecaprevir and pibrentasvir with concurrent use of acid-reducing agents in patients with chronic HCV infection. *Clinical Gastroenterology and Hepatology* 2019;17(3):527–535.

14. Polepally AR, Dutta S, Hu B et al. Drug–drug interaction of omeprazole with the HCV direct-acting antiviral agents paritaprevir/ritonavir and ombitasvir with and without dasabuvir. *Clinical Pharmacology in Drug Development* 2016;5(4):269–277.

15. van Seyen M, Smolders E, van Wijngaarden P et al. Successful HCV treatment of patients on contraindicated anti-epileptic drugs: role of drug level monitoring. *Journal of Hepatology* 2019;70:552–554.

16. Brooks KM, Gordon L, Penzak S et al. Cobicistat, but not ritonavir, increases dabigatran exposure. Conference on Retroviruses and Opportunistic Infections (CROI), Seattle, February 2017, abstract 409. www.croiconference.org/sessions/cobicistat-not-ritonavir-increases-dabigatran-exposure

17. Medicines and Healthcare products Regulatory Agency. Direct-acting antivirals to treat chronic hepatitis C: risk of interaction with vitamin K antagonists and changes in INR. *Drug Safety Update* 2017;10(6):2.

18. Smolders EJ, ter Horst P, Wolters S. et al. Cardiovascular risk management and hepatitis C: combining drugs. *Clinical Pharmacokinetics* 2019;58:565–592.

19. Grebely J, Hajarizadeh B, Dore G. Direct-acting antiviral agents for HCV infection affecting people who inject drugs. *Nature Reviews Gastroenterology and Hepatology* 2018;3(11):754–767.

20. Rudd RA, Seth P, David F et al. Increases in drug and opioid-involved overdose deaths – United States, 2010–2015. *Morbidity and Mortality Weekly Report* 2016;65(5051):1445–1452.

21. O'Donnell J, Gladden R, Mattson C et al. Notes from the field: overdose deaths with carfentanil and other fentanyl analogs detected – 10 states, July 2016–June 2017. *Morbidity and Mortality Weekly Report* 2018;67(27):767–768.

22. Shiran MR, Lennard M, Iqbal M et al. Contribution of the activities of CYP3A, CYP2D6, CYP1A2 and other potential covariates to the disposition of methadone in patients undergoing methadone maintenance treatment. *British Journal of Clinical Pharmacology* 2009;67(1):29–37.

23. Elkader A, Sproule B. Buprenorphine: clinical pharmacokinetics in the treatment of opioid dependence. *Clinical Pharmacokinetics* 2005;44(7):661–680.

24. Spera AM, Eldin G, Tosone G et al. Antiviral therapy for Hepatitis C: has anything changed for pregnant/lactating women? *World Journal of Hepatology* 2016;8(12):557–565.

16 Treatment of hepatitis C in children

Maureen M. Jonas

Children's Hospital Boston, Division of Gastroenterology, Boston, MA, USA

LEARNING POINTS

- Only a minority of individuals with chronic hepatitis C are children, and liver disease is generally mild and slowly progressive in this population, but some children have advanced liver disease, and others are at risk for future complications such as cirrhosis and hepatocellular carcinoma.

- The majority of new cases of HCV infection in children are due to perinatal transmission. The likelihood of peri-natal transmission is about 5% with each pregnancy. Universal screening for hepatitis C in pregnant women has been recommended by some experts, but remains controversial.

- Children as young as 3 years of age with chronic HCV are candidates for treatment. Several interferon-sparing all-oral direct-acting antiviral (DAA) regimens are available for children 3 years and older.

Introduction

Acute hepatitis C virus (HCV) infection is not commonly detected in children, and fulminant hepatitis C has not been reported. Accordingly, there are few data regarding treatment of acute HCV in the pediatric age group. Chronic infection is generally asymptomatic during childhood, but long-term infection can lead to significant morbidity and mortality, such as cirrhosis and hepatocellular carcinoma, later in life. The proportion of HCV-infected children who will suffer these serious consequences is unknown, but several pediatric studies have demonstrated that the degree of hepatic fibrosis generally correlates with age and duration of infection [1], although progression seems to be slower than observed in those infected later in life. Understanding that HCV in children has different modes of acquisition, complications, and natural history will influence management and treatment decisions.

Principles of treatment

Vertical transmission has become the leading source of infection for children. The rate of vertical transmission averages about 5% from most studies. Universal screening of pregnant women has been a somewhat controversial topic, but recently has been recommended by an expert panel composed of members of the American Association for the Study of Liver Diseases and the Infectious Disease Society of America [2]. The change in strategy from testing only those with identifiable risk factors is supported by the higher rate of case detection, the greater likelihood of linkage of infected women to care, and the recommendations regarding obstetric practices when an HCV-infected pregnant woman is identified [3]. Universal screening has not yet been adopted by the primary obstetric professional societies, however.

Vertical transmission is associated with a high incidence of viremia and abnormal aminotransferases during the first 12 months. Of 70 infants in five European centers prospectively followed from 1990 to 1999, 93% had abnormal alanine aminotransferase (ALT) during the first 12 months, and only 19% cleared HCV RNA with normal ALT by 30 months of age [4]. Clearance of viremia was independent of sex and maternal HIV coinfection. Peak ALT greater

Clinical Dilemmas in Viral Liver Disease, Second Edition. Edited by Graham R. Foster and K. Rajender Reddy.
© 2020 John Wiley & Sons Ltd. Published 2020 by John Wiley & Sons Ltd.

than five times normal during the first 18 months and genotype 3 were more common in patients in whom viremia resolved spontaneously.

The largest pediatric natural history study to date describes a cohort of 200 HCV-infected children in Europe [5]. The majority had genotype 1b, 45% from vertical transmission and 39% from transfusion. Fifteen percent of these patients had normal ALT, and none had jaundice or extrahepatic manifestations. After follow-up of 1–17.5 years (mean 6.2), only 6% achieved sustained virologic clearance and normalization of ALT. Liver biopsies were performed in 118 of these patients at various times during follow-up; the majority (76%) had mild hepatitis and low fibrosis scores. One patient (1%) had cirrhosis and one (1%) had severe hepatitis. Greater degrees of fibrosis were seen in children older than 15 years, suggesting long-term effects of chronic HCV infection.

There have been only a few case reports of hepatocellular carcinoma associated with hepatitis C during childhood [6]. Liver transplantation for complications of chronic hepatitis C during childhood is uncommon. For these reasons, the primary indications for treatment of pediatric patients with HCV infection are prevention of future complications and the epidemiologic as well as psychosocial benefits of eradication in this young and vulnerable population.

In 2003, the Food and Drug Administration approved the combination of interferon and ribavirin for the treatment of chronic HCV in children aged 3–17 years. Studies had demonstrated that response rates depended on genotype and viral load, as in adults. Several years later, in 2008, the combination of peginterferon (peg-IFN) and ribavirin was approved for children. Children with genotype 1 HCV had only about 50% likelihood of sustained virologic response [7], and had to receive 48 weeks of weekly peg-IFN injections, with all the attendant discomfort and side effects. Children with genotypes 2 or 3 HCV did somewhat better, with response rates of about 80–85% after 24 weeks of treatment [7]. Analysis of the pretreatment liver biopsies in this cohort had reaffirmed the generally mild histologic disease during childhood, but cases of marked fibrosis and even cirrhosis were observed.

Peginterferon and ribavirin remained the only treatment option until late in 2017, when two interferon-sparing oral regimens were approved for children 12 to <18 years of age.

A phase 2, multicenter, open-label, fixed-dose, combination regimen of ledipasvir 90 mg and sofosbuvir 400 mg once daily for 12 weeks was conducted in 100 ado-

lescents (aged 12–17 years) with HCV genotype 1 [8]. Eighty percent of the patients were HCV treatment naive, and 84% were infected via perinatal transmission. One patient was known to have cirrhosis, 42 patients did not have cirrhosis, and in 57 patients the cirrhosis status was not known. Ninety-eight percent of patients achieved SVR at 12 weeks (SVR12) and none had virologic failure. The two patients who did not reach SVR were lost to follow-up. No serious adverse events were reported.

The combination of sofosbuvir 400 mg once daily and weight-based ribavirin was studied in 36 adolescents (aged 12–17 years) with genotype 2 or 3 HCV [9]. The 12 patients with genotype 2 received treatment for 12 weeks and the 24 with genotype 3 HCV were treated for 24 weeks. Eighty three percent of patients were treatment naive. Forty percent of patients did not have cirrhosis; in the remainder, the cirrhosis status was not known. SVR12 was achieved in 100% of genotype 2 and 97% of genotype 3 infections. The one patient who did not achieve SVR12 was lost to follow-up but known to have achieved SVR4. A subsequent study in children as young as 3 years demonstrated similarly high SVR rates [10]. These trials led to FDA approval of these regimens for adolescents.

The combination of ledipasvir/sofosbuvir with or without ribavirin was subsequently tested in 6–11-year-old patients [11]. This was an open-label study using two combination tablets 22.5/100 mg once daily. Ninety-seven percent of children were perinatally infected and 78% were treatment naive. There were 92 children in the cohort: 88 with HCV genotype (GT) 1 (77 1a), two with GT3 and two with GT4. Two patients had cirrhosis, while the fibrosis status was unknown in 55 patients. All patients were assigned to ledipasvir/sofosbuvir for a minimum of 12 weeks. Those who were interferon experienced with cirrhosis and genotype 1 were treated for 24 weeks. Patients with genotype 3, interferon experienced, with/without cirrhosis were given ledipasvir/sofosbuvir with ribavirin for 24 weeks. The SVR12 rate was 99%. One cirrhotic patient with GT1a HCV relapsed four weeks after completing 12 weeks of therapy.

Currently, ongoing trials of children in all age groups are testing the pangenotypic, ribavirin- sparing regimens sofosbuvir/velpatasvir and glecaprevir/pibrentasvir. Those for the youngest children have required development of new formulations that allow for accurate dosing and palatability. The data from an adolescent cohort treated with eight weeks of glecaprevir/pibrentasvir demonstrated

100% SVR in 47 patients with a variety of HCV genotypes [12], and this regimen was just approved for treatment of adolescents with chronic HCV.

All of these DAA regimens have been very well tolerated in the pediatric population in clinical trials. It is anticipated that these highly efficacious and safe regimens will be available for children within the next couple of years.

The guidance published by the AASLD/IDSA recommends treatment of all HCV-infected children, when age-appropriate DAA regimens become available [2]. Specific recommendations vary by genotype, previous therapy, and cirrhosis status. Examination of a liver biopsy is not a prerequisite for treatment; it is rare to find advanced histology in young children, and the response rates are so high that baseline biopsies may provide little information regarding either likelihood of response or long-term prognosis. Exceptions are children who have clinical evidence of cirrhosis, since duration of treatment with some of these regimens may be influenced. Experience is accumulating using noninvasive assessments of hepatic fibrosis to assist with this determination [13].

General management

The general management of children and adolescents with HCV infection includes more than just antiviral therapy. Education about the infection, its natural history and modes of transmission, and risk factors for progression such as alcohol use, obesity, and other infections is critical to ensure optimal outcomes. In addition, the clinician can be of importance in dissipation of parental guilt regarding vertical transmission, and destigmatization in school and other social settings, as well as provision of other health measures such as hepatitis A and B immunization, and pregnancy prevention counseling and measures. It is also important to emphasize that children and adolescents with HCV can participate fully in school and extracurricular activities, including sports, without any more than the standard universal precautions that are already advocated for these settings.

Conclusion

The minority of individuals with chronic HCV infection are children, and most children and adolescents with this infection have clinically unapparent and histologically mild liver disease. However, some children have more advanced liver fibrosis, and it has been demonstrated that this is a progressive disease. Children as young as 3 years with chronic HCV

are candidates for treatment with DAA regimens, and pangenotypic regimens will be available for children soon.

References

1. Badizadegan K, Jonas MM, Ott MJ, Nelson SP, Perez-Atayde AR. Histopathology of the liver in children with chronic hepatitis C viral infection. *Hepatology* 1998;28:1416–1423.
2. AASLD-IDSA. Recommendations for testing, managing, and treating hepatitis C. www.hcvguidelines.org
3. Jhaveri R, Broder T, Bhattacharya D, Peters MG, Kim AY, Jonas MM. Universal screening of pregnant women for hepatitis C: the time is now. *Clinical Infectious Diseases* 2018;67:1493–1497.
4. Resti M, Jara P, Hierro L et al. Clinical features and progression of perinatally acquired hepatitis C virus infection. *Journal of Medical Virology* 2003;70(3):373–377.
5. Jara P, Resti M, Hierro L et al. Chronic hepatitis C virus infection in childhood: clinical patterns and evolution in 224 white children. *Clinical Infectious Diseases* 2003;36(3):275–280.
6. González-Peralta R, Langham Jr MR, Andres JM et al. Hepatocellular carcinoma in 2 young adolescents with chronic hepatitis C. *Journal of Pediatric Gastroenterology and Nutrition* 2009;48:630–635.
7. Schwarz KB, Gonzalez-Peralta R, Murray KF et al. The combination of ribavirin and peginterferon is superior to peginterferon and placebo for children and adolescents with chronic hepatitis C. *Gastroenterology* 2011;140:450–458.
8. Balistreri WF, Murray KF, Rosenthal P et al. The safety and effectiveness of ledipasvir-sofosbuvir in adolescents 12-17 years old with hepatitis C virus genotype 1 infection. *Hepatology* 2017;66:371–378.
9. Wirth S, Rosenthal P, Gonzalez-Peralta RP et al. Sofosbuvir and ribavirin in adolescents 12-17 years old with hepatitis C virus genotype 2 or 3 infection. *Hepatology* 2017;66(4):1102–1110.
10. Rosenthal P, Schwarz KB, Gonzalez-Peralta RP et al. Sofosbuvir and ribavirin therapy for children 3 to < 12 Years old with hepatitis C virus genotype 2 or 3 infection. *Hepatology* 2019; doi: 10.1002/hep.30821.
11. Murray KF, Balistreri WF, Bansal S et al. Safety and efficacy of ledipasvir-sofosbuvir with or without ribavirin for chronic hepatitis C in children ages 6–11. *Hepatology* 2018;68(6): 2158–2166.
12. Jonas MM, Squires RH, Rhee SM et al. Pharmacokinetics, safety and efficacy of glecaprevir/pibrentasvir in pediatric patients with genotypes 1-6 chronic HCV infection: Part 1 of the DORA study. *Hepatology* 2018;68(S1):1347A–1348A.
13. Lee CK, Perez-Atayde AR, Mitchell PD, Raza R, Afdhal NH, Jonas MM. Serum biomarkers and transient elastography as predictors of advanced liver fibrosis in a United States cohort: the Boston Children's Hospital experience. *Journal of Pediatrics* 2013;163(4):1058–1064.

17 While direct-acting antivirals are effective, are there any unique safety considerations?

Olivia Pietri[1], Félix Trottier-Tellier[1,2], and Marc Bourlière[1]

[1] Hepato-gastroenterology Department, Hospital Saint Joseph, Marseilles, France
[2] Gastroenterology Department, Hôtel-Dieu de Lévis, Lévis, Quebec, Canada

---

LEARNING POINTS

- The current direct-acting antiviral agents are safe and well tolerated.

- In patients with decompensated cirrhosis, protease inhibitors should be avoided and for those with a MELD score of >20, recovery of liver function is unusual and it may be appropriate to consider transplantation followed by therapy.

- Drug–drug interactions require consideration in a very small number of patients.

Introduction

The advent of oral direct-acting antiviral agents (DAAs) has dramatically improved hepatitis C treatment in recent years, providing a cure rate over 95% in DAA-naive patients and 96% in DAA treatment-experienced patients. Therefore, 99.8% of HCV patients can be cured either with a single or a rescue regimen regardless of HCV genotype or fibrosis stage. Only patients with decompensated cirrhosis require the addition of ribavirin. Treatment durations are short, from eight to 16 weeks. These oral treatments are generally well tolerated and safety considerations are mainly driven by drug–drug interactions (DDI) that may orientate the choice of DAA regimen for a given patient.

Safety profile of DAAs

In clinical trials, whichever DAA combination regimen is used, side effects always appear to be mild, below grade 3, and are easily manageable in HCV patients ranging from those with no fibrosis to compensated cirrhosis Child–Pugh A (Table 17.1) [1–15]. The most frequent side effects are headache, fatigue, and nausea. Studies in which placebo groups were included demonstrated that there was no significant increase in side effects [16,17]. There was also no significant laboratory abnormality. Ribavirin-containing regimens were associated with an expected increase in reported adverse events (AEs) and drug-related AEs. Tolerability was not affected by treatment duration or compensated cirrhosis.

Patients with decompensated cirrhosis or with a previous episode of decompensation should not be treated with a regimen containing a protease inhibitor. They have an expected increase in reported AEs and serious adverse events (SAEs) mainly related to end-stage liver disease events and very few patients present with premature discontinuations [18–23]. In a large Spanish registry, half of the patients with Child–Pugh B or C cirrhosis had SAEs with incident decompensation in 16%, anemia requiring transfusion in 8% and grade 3/4 infection in 8%, all significantly higher than side effects in patients with Child–Pugh A cirrhosis [23]. DAA combinations achieve a high HCV cure rate in patients with advanced cirrhosis associated with

Clinical Dilemmas in Viral Liver Disease, Second Edition. Edited by Graham R. Foster and K. Rajender Reddy.
© 2020 John Wiley & Sons Ltd. Published 2020 by John Wiley & Sons Ltd.

Table 17.1 More frequent side effects observed in phase 2/3 trials and real life related to various DAA combinations in patients without decompensated cirrhosis

	SOF/SIM	SOF/DCV	SOF/LDV	PrOD/PrO	GZR/EBR	SOF/VEL	GLE/PIB	SOF/VEL/VOX
SAE	1–5% (C)	1–6% (C)	2–5%	1–3%	2.4%	2%	2–8% (C)	2.4%
SAE/drugs discontinuation	0–3% (C)	0%	<1%	<1%	<1%	<1%	<1%	<0.1%
Drug-related SAE	0%	0%	<1%	<1%	<1%	0%	<1%	0%
Headache	14–20% (C)	20%	23%	11–30%	18%	29%	17–14% (C)	26%
Fatigue	12–20% (C)	19%	29%	7–30%	16%	21%	14–19% (C)	22%
Nausea	15–11% (C)	12%	13%	9–19%	8%	11%	9% (C)	15%
Insomnia	9% (RL)	6%	12%	4–16%	4%	8%		6%
Diarrhea		9%	8%				8% (C)	18%
Pruritus	5–14% (C)		5%					
Rash	6–16% (C)		7%					
Arthralgia		5%	7%			6%		4%
ALT elevation grade 3							<1%	<1%
Lipase >3 × ULN						<1%		1.5%
Hyperglycemia >2.5 g/L								2.6%

ALT, alanine aminotransferase; C, Clinical trial; DCV, daclatasvir; EBR, elbasvir; GLE, glecaprevir; GZR, grazoprevir; LDV, ledipasvir; PIB, pibrentasvir; PrO, paritaprevir/ritonavir plus ombitasvir; PrOD, paritaprevir/ritonavir plus ombitasvir plus dasabuvir; RL, real life; SAE, serious adverse events; SIM, simprevir; SOF, sofosbuvir; ULN, upper limit of normal; VEL, velpatasvir; VOX, voxilaprevir.

improvements in fibrosis and liver function (Child–Pugh and model for end-stage liver disease [MELD] scores) and a lower incidence of clinical events including hepatocellular carcinoma (HCC) and deaths [19]. Moreover, several studies demonstrated that patients with advanced cirrhosis on the liver transplant waiting list can be delisted following viral clearance with sustained remission in almost 25% of the patients [20,23–25].

In regression analysis, a baseline MELD score of ≥18 was found to be predictive of death with high specificity and no patient with a MELD score >20 on the waiting list has been delisted. Given the efficacy of DAA therapy in liver transplant recipients, it may be recommended that for patients with decompensated cirrhosis awaiting a liver transplant with a MELD score > 8, consideration should be given to treating HCV post transplantation [26].

Patients with early chronic kidney disease (CKD) stage 1–3 can be treated safely with any DAA combination [27,28]. Patients with CKD stage 4 and 5 or on dialysis can be treated safely with at least three different regimens: paritaprevir boosted with ritonavir plus ombitasvir with or without dasabuvir or grazoprevir plus elbasvir for patients with genotype 1 and 4 infection or with the pangenotypic combination of glecaprevir and pibrentasvir [29–32]. Sofosbuvir-containing regimens should be used with caution in CKD stage 4 or 5 patients only if the above alternative safe regimens are not available.

Significant drug–drug interactions*

Drug–drug interactions (DDI) are the major issue to discuss with any DAA combination. However, only a few medications are contraindicated with a given combination. Potential interactions that may require a dosage adjustment, altered timing of administration or additional monitoring are much more frequent. Due to the numerous and complex DDIs, a thorough DDI risk assessment prior to starting therapy and before starting other medications during treatment is mandatory. This information can be easily found through websites such as www.hep-druginteractions.org from the University of Liverpool where recommendations are regularly updated [33].

A few drugs are always contraindicated with all DAA combinations due to the fact that they are potent inducing agents of cytochrome P450 (CYP) or P-glycoprotein (P-gp), transporters of almost all DAAs. These drugs can significantly reduce the concentration of DAA and therefore induce high risk of virologic failure (Table 17.2). Contraindication of drugs with DAAs is more frequent when we use a DAA combination including a NS3/4 protease inhibitor (Table 17.3).

_____

* Drug-drug interactions and their underlying mechanisms are discussed in more detail in Chapter 15, p.86.

Table 17.2 Drugs that are contraindicated with any DAA regimen

Amobarbital
Carbamazepine
Lumacaftor/Ivacaftor
Oxcarbazepine
Phenobarbital
Phenytoin
Primidone
Rifampicin
St John's wort

Sofosbuvir is transported by P-gp. Other potential interactions may occur with rifabutin, rifapentine, and modafinil.

Real-life data demonstrated arrhythmias, even life threatening, with the combination of Sofosbuvir-containing regimen with amiodarone [34]. Bradycardia has been observed within a few hours to days after starting the DAA but cases have been reported up to two weeks after initiating DAA treatment [35]. The exact mechanism of interaction is still unclear. Several mechanisms have been proposed involving P-gp inhibition, protein-binding displacement and direct

Table 17.3 Drugs that are contraindicated with at least one DAA regimen

Drugs	SOF	DCV	PrO± (D)	SOF/LDV	GZR/EBR	GLE/PIB	SOF/VEL	SOF/VEL/VOX
Acalabrutinib			N	TM	TM	TM	TM	TM
Alfuzosin			N					
Aliskiren		TM	N	TM		N		TM
Amiodarone	N	N	N	N	TM	TM	N	N
Apixaban		TM	N	TM	TM	TM	TM	TM
Astemizole			N			TM		
Atazanavir		TM	TM		N	N		N
Atorvastatin		TM	N	TM	TM	N	TM	N
Axitinib			N		PWI	PWI		
Bosentan		TM	N		N	N	N	N
Bosutinib			N		TM	TM		
Budenoside			N					
Ciclosporin		TM			N	TM		N
Cisapride			N	TM	TM	TM		
Clarithromycin		TM	N			PWI		PWI
Clopidogrel			N					
Cobicistat (with ATV or DRV)		TM	N	TM	N	TM		TM
Conivaptan		N	N					
Dabigatran		TM	TM	TM	TM	N	TM	N
Darunavir			TM		N	N		TM
Dexamethasone		N	TM		TM	TM		TM
Dextropropoxyphene			N					
Dihydroergotamine			N	TM	TM	TM		
Disopyramide			N					
Dofetilide			N					
Domperidone			N			TM		
Dronedarone	N	N	N	N	TM	TM	N	N
Edoxaban		TM	TM	TM	TM	TM	TM	N
Efavirenz		TM	N	TM	N	N	N	N
Eletriptan			N					
Eligustat			N		TM	TM		
Eltrombopag		TM			N	N	PWI	N
Elvitegravir/cobi/FTC/TAF		TM	N		N			
Elvitegravir/cobi/FTC/TDF		TM	N	TM	N		TM	TM
Eplerenone			N	TM	TM	TM		

(continued)

Table 17.3 (continued)

Drugs	SOF	DCV	PrO± (D)	SOF/LDV	GZR/EBR	GLE/PIB	SOF/VEL	SOF/VEL/VOX
Ergometrine (ergonovine)			N	TM	TM	TM		
Ergotamine			N	TM	TM	TM		
Erlotinib		TM	N	TM	TM	TM	TM	TM
Eslicarbazepine		N	N	N	N	N	N	N
Ethinylestradiol			N			N		N
Etonogestrel (vaginal ring)			N			N		N
Etravirine		TM	N		N	N	N	N
Everolimus		TM	N	TM	TM	TM	TM	TM
Flibanserin			N		TM	TM		
Fluticasone			N					
Fluvastatin		TM	TM	TM	TM	TM	TM	N
Fosamprenavir		TM	TM		N	N		N
Halofantrine			N					
Imatinib			TM		TM	TM	TM	N
Indinavir		TM	N		N	N		N
Irinotecan		TM	TM	TM	TM	TM	TM	N
Itraconazole		TM	N					
Ivabradine			N					
Ketoconazole		TM	N		TM	TM		
Lapatinib		TM	TM	TM	TM	TM	TM	N
Lercanidipine			N					
Levonorgestrel			N			N	PWI	N
Lopinavir			N	TM	N	N		N
Lovastatin		TM	N	TM	TM	N	TM	N
Lumefantrine			N					
Methotrexate		TM			TM	TM	TM	N
Methylergonovine			N	TM	TM	TM		
Midazolam (oral)			N	TM	TM			
Mitoxantrone		TM	TM	TM	TM	TM	TM	N
Modafinil	TM	TM	TM	TM	N	TM	N	N
Mometasone			N					
Naloxegol			N					
Nelfinavir	N		TM		N	N		N
Nevirapine		TM	N		N	N	N	N
Nilotinib		TM	TM		TM	TM	TM	N
Pimozide			N	N	N	N		
Pitavastatin		TM	TM	TM		TM	TM	N
Posaconazole		TM	N			TM		
Quetiapine			N		TM	TM		
Quinidine		TM	N	TM	TM	TM	TM	TM
Ranolazine		TM	N	TM	TM	TM		TM
Rifabutin	N	N	TM	N	N	N	N	N
Rifapentine	N	N	TM	N	N	N	N	N
Riociguat			N					
Ritonavir		TM	N		N	N		TM
Rivaroxaban		TM	N	TM	TM	TM	TM	TM
Rosuvastatin		TM	TM	N	TM	TM	TM	N
Rufinamide	N	N	TM	N	TM	TM	N	N
Salmeterol			N					
Saquinavir		TM	N		N	N		N

Table 17.3 (continued)

Drugs	SOF	DCV	PrO± (D)	SOF/LDV	GZR/EBR	GLE/PIB	SOF/VEL	SOF/VEL/VOX
Sildenafil (pulmonary Hyper)			N					
Silodosin		TM	N	TM	TM	TM	TM	TM
Simvastatin		TM	N	TM	TM	N	TM	N
Sirolimus			N		TM	TM		TM
Sulfasalazine		TM				TM	TM	N
Tacrolimus			N		TM	TM		TM
Telithromycin		TM	N	TM	TM	TM		TM
Terfenadine			N			TM		
Ticagrelor		TM	N	TM	TM	TM	TM	TM
Tipranavir	N	TM	N	N	N	N	N	N
Triamcinolone			N					
Triazolam			N					
Troleandomycin		TM	TM		N	N	TM	N
Vinblastine			TM		TM	N	TM	N
Vincristine			TM		TM	N	TM	N
Voriconazole		TM	N					

ATV, atazanavir; DCV, daclatasvir; DRV, darunavir; FTC, emtricitabine; GLE/PIB, glecaprevir/pibrentasvir, GZR/ELB, grazoprevir/elbasvir, N, contraindicated; PrOD, paritaprevir/ritonavir plus ombitasvir plus dasabuvir, PWI, potential weak interaction; SOF, sofosbuvir; SOF/LDV, sofosbuvir/ledipasvir, SOF/VEL, sofosbuvir/velpatasvir, SOF/VEL/VOX, sofosbuvir/velpatasvir/voxilaprevir; TAF, tenofovir alafenamide; TDF, tenofovir disoproxil fumarate; TTM, treatment monitoring.

effects of sofosbuvir or other DAAs on cardiomyocytes or ion channels [36]. The role of other medication such as beta-blockers has also been suggested. Because of the long half-life of amiodarone, an interaction is possible for several months after discontinuation of amiodarone. Therefore, waiting at least three months after amiodarone discontinuation before initiating a sofosbuvir-containing regimen appears to be safe. Due to reports of cardiac toxicity with sofosbuvir in the absence of amiodarone, caution should be exercised with other antiarrhythmics.

Ledipasvir is transported by intestinal P-gp and breast cancer resistance protein (BCRP). Ledipasvir may also lead to DDI by inhibiting P-gp and or BCRP, with potential increase of intestinal absorption of the coadministered drug. Therefore, caution is warranted with well-studied P-gp substrates such as digoxin and dabigatran but also with all drugs which are in part transported by these proteins. The use of rosuvastatin is also not recommended because of a potential inhibition of hepatic organic anion transporting protein (OATP) by ledipasvir. It is important to monitor for statin-related adverse reactions. Ledipasvir solubility decreases as pH increases, so drugs that increase gastric pH are likely to decrease concentration of ledipasvir.

H2-receptor antagonists and proton pomp inhibitors (PPI) should be given simultaneously at a low single daily dose (famotidine 40 mg or omeprazole 20 mg) in order to avoid loss of efficacy.

A recent metaanalysis of 32 684 patients treated with DAAs demonstrated a significantly increased risk of failure to achieve cure in HCV–infected patients taking PPI compared with non-PPI users [37]. However, data about dose and frequency are frequently missing and this limits data interpretation. Before prescribing a DAA, the prescriber should always consider whether PPI therapy is indicated for these patients and withdraw PPI therapy in the absence of indication.

Daclatasvir is a substrate of CYP3A4 and a substrate and inhibitor of P-gp. In addition, it is an inhibitor of OATP1B1 and BRCP. Some inhibitors of CYP3A4 increase the plasma level of daclatasvir and dose adjustment is therefore recommended in cases of coadministration [38].

Velpatasvir is metabolized *in vitro* by CYP2B6, CYP2C8, and CYP3A4. Velpatasvir is transported by P-gp and BRCP and to a limited extent by OATP 1B1. There are some drugs that are moderate P-gp or CYP inducers, such as modafinil, that can reduce velpatasvir exposure. Velpatasvir solubility decreases as gastric PH increases. Therefore, PPI coadministration should be cautious and follow some rules. The rule for coadministration is that sofosbuvir/velpatasvir should be given with food and taken four hours before the PPI as a maximum dose comparable to omeprazole 20 mg.

Voxilaprevir is given in combination with sofosbuvir and velpatasvir. It is metabolized by CYP3A4 and inhibits P-gp, BCRP, OATPB1, and OATPB3. Rosuvastatin is contraindicated because of a 19-fold increase in plasma exposure of the statin likely attributed more to the BCRP transporters. Dabigatran is contraindicated because of a near threefold increase in AUC caused by P-gp inhibition by both velpatasvir and voxilaprevir. Similar caution is required with OATP1B inhibitors such as ciclosporin or with OATP1B substrates such as edoxaban. Both drugs are not recommended with voxilaprevir-containing regimens. Drugs that are moderate P-gp or CYP inducers such as modafinil, oxcarbazepine and others are also not recommended. The use of ethinylestradiol-containing contraception is contraindicated because of the risk of alanine aminotransferase (ALT) elevations.

Ritonavir-boosted paritaprevir, ombitasvir (ritonavir plus ombitasvir), and ritonavir plus ombitasvir plus dasabuvir are primarily metabolized by CYP3A4, whereas dasabuvir is primarily metabolized by CYP2C8, and ombitasvir undergoes hydrolysis. However, both ombitasvir and dasabuvir can be metabolized by CYP3A4. Transporters seem to play an important role in the disposition of these drugs, with paritaprevir inhibiting OATP1B1/B3, P-gp, and BCRP. Dasabuvir and ritonavir may also inhibit P-gp and BCRP. Given the metabolic profile of the drugs and the presence of ritonavir, there is a potential for many DDIs. Ritonavir is a strong inhibitor of CYP 3A4 and coadministration with drugs metabolized by this enzyme may markedly increased plasma concentration. Several drugs are therefore contraindicated with ritonavir plus ombitasvir or ritonavir plus ombitasvir with dasabuvir (see Table 17.3).

Grazoprevir and elbasvir are available in a fixed-dose combination. Grazoprevir is transported by P-gp and OATP1B1, while elbasvir is a substrate for P-gp. Both drugs are substrates of CYP3A and P-gp. Strong inhibitors of CYP3 that may markedly increase plasma concentrations are either not recommended or contraindicated (see Table 17.3). The potential for grazoprevir/elbasvir to affect other medications is relatively low, although grazoprevir is a weak CYP3A inhibitor (approximately 30% increase in

midazolam exposure) and elbasvir a weak inhibitor of P-gp. Caution is recommended when grazoprevir/elbasvir is administered with drugs that use CYP3A and P-gp in their metabolic pathway, especially in the presence of drugs with a narrow therapeutic index such as tacrolimus, some statins, dabigatran, ticagrelor, or drugs with large ranges such as quetiapine, where those on higher doses may need additional monitoring, dose reduction, and/or ECG.

Glecaprevir and pibrentasvir are inhibitors of P-gp, BCRP, OATP1B1, and OATP1B3. Coadministration with glecaprevir/pibrentasvir may increase the concentration of comedications that are substrates of P-gp such as dabigatran, of BCRP such as rosuvastatin or of OATP1B1/3 such as atorvastatin or simvastatin, which are contraindicated. For other P-gp, BCRP, or OATP1B1/3 substrates, dose adjustment should be considered. Coadministration with other potent inducers is contraindicated. A similar effect cannot be ruled out with moderate inducers and coadministration of these drugs is not recommended. Comedications that inhibit P-gp and BCRP may increase plasma exposure of glecaprevir/pibrentasvir. Similarly, OATP1B1/3 inhibitors, such as ciclosporin, darunavir, and lopinavir, may also increase glecaprevir concentrations.

The potential for glecaprevir/pibrentasvir to affect other medications is relatively low, although glecaprevir is a weak CYP3A inhibitor (approximately 27% increase in midazolam exposure). Caution is recommended when drugs that use CYP3A are given with glecaprevir/pibrentasvir in the presence of a narrow therapeutic index such as tacrolimus or drugs with large ranges such as quetiapine, whereas patients on higher doses may need additional monitoring, dose reduction, and/or ECG.

For women of childbearing age, concomitant use with ethinylestradiol-containing contraception is contraindicated because of the risk of ALT elevations. Progestogen-containing contraception is permitted.

Similar to other DAAs, the solubility of glecaprevir decreases as pH increases. Cmax of glecaprevir decreases on average by 64% when coadministered with omeprazole 40 mg. The license states that no dose changes are recommended. However, prescribing doses of omeprazole greater than 40 mg or equivalent with glecaprevir/pibrentasvir has not been studied and may lead to a greater decrease in glecaprevir concentrations.

Drug–drug interactions are a key consideration in the treatment of HIV/HCV-coinfected patients. Close attention must be paid to anti-HIV drugs that are contra-indicated, not recommended or require dose adjustment with particular DAA regimens. sofosbuvir, ledipasvir or daclatasvir can be used with any current antiretroviral regimens. However, some renal monitoring should be done when ledipasvir is used with antiretroviral regimens using tenofovir disoproxil fumarate (TDF) in combination with a pharmacokinetic enhancer (ritonavir or cobicistat) and monitoring or drug dose reduction may be necessary when daclatasvir is used with nonnucleoside reverse transcriptase inhibitors (NNRTIs) or some protease inhibitors (atazanavir).

Velpatasvir should not be given with some NNRTIs (efavirenz, etravirine, and nevirapine). Efavirenz induces a 50% decrease in velpatasvir exposure.

In coinfected patients sofosbuvir/velpatasvir/voxilaprevir is not recommended with some NNRTIS due to velpatasvir interaction but also with some protease inhibitors including atazanavir/ritonavir or cobicistat and lopinavir/ritonavir. Caution is required with twice-daily darunavir/ritonavir and darunavir/cobicistat as there are no data.

Combinations of ritonavir plus ombitasvir or ritonavir plus ombitasvir dasabuvir are not easy regimens to use in coinfected patients. NNRTIs are contraindicated, except rilpivirine that can be used cautiously with repeated ECGs. Atazanavir and darunavir should be taken without ritonavir and other protease inhibitors are contraindicated. Cobicistat-containing regimens should not be used because of the additional boosting effect.

The combination of grazoprevir/elbasvir is not easy to use in coinfected patients. Only nucleoside reverse transcriptase inhibitors (NRTIs) can be used with rilpivirine, raltegravir, dolutegravir, and maraviroc. glecaprevir/pibrentasvir can be used in coinfected patients only with those receiving NRTIs and/or entry/integrase inhibitors. Protease inhibitors and NNRTIs are contraindicated with glecaprevir/pibrentasvir because of an expected reduction in plasma exposure of glecaprevir/pibrentasvir.

As recommended by the EASL guidelines, "Patients should be educated on the importance of adherence to therapy, following the dosing recommendations and reporting the use of over-the-counter medications, medications bought via the internet, and use of party or recreational drugs that may lead to potential unknown DDI" [33].

Conclusion

Direct-acting antivirals have very few safety considerations. Adverse events are usually mild and easily managed. Serious adverse events are rare and real-life data so far were unable to disclose any new safety issue. Drug–drug interactions are the major issue regarding the choice of DAA regimen so a thorough DDI risk assessment should be carried out prior to starting therapy and monitoring of any new drug added during treatment is mandatory.

References

1. Kwo P, Gitlin N, Nahass R et al. Simeprevir plus sofosbuvir (12 and 8 weeks) in hepatitis C virus genotype 1–infected patients without cirrhosis:OPTIMIST–1, a phase 3, randomized study. *Hepatology* 2016;64:370–380.
2. Lawitz E, Matusow G, DeJesus E et al. Simeprevir plus sofosbuvir in patients with chronic hepatitis C virus genotype 1 infection and cirrhosis:a phase 3 study (OPTIMIST–2). *Hepatology* 2016;64:360–369.
3. Sulkowski MS, Vargas HE, di Bisceglie AM et al. Effectiveness of simeprevir plus sofosbuvir, with or without ribavirin, in real–world patients with HCV genotype 1 infection. *Gastroenterology* 2016;150:419–429.
4. Nelson DR, Cooper JN, Lalezari JP et al. All-oral 12-week treatment with daclatasvir plus sofosbuvir in patients with hepatitis C virus genotype 3 infection: ALLY-3 phase III study. *Hepatology* 2015;61:1127–1135.
5. Pol S, Bourliere M, Lucier S et al. Safety and efficacy of daclatasvir–sofosbuvir in HCV genotype 1 mono-infected patients. *Journal of Hepatology* 2017;66:39–47.
6. Alqahtani SA, Afdhal N, Zeuzem S et al. Safety and tolerability of ledipasvir/sofosbuvir with and without ribavirin in patients with chronic hepatitis C virus genotype 1 infection: analysis of phase III ION trials. *Hepatology* 2015;62:25–30.
7. Dusheiko GM, Manns MP, Vierling JM et al. Safety and tolerability of Grazoprevir/Elbasvir in patients with chronic hepatitis C (HCV) infection: integrated analysis of phase 2–3 trials. *Hepatology* 2015;62 (Suppl):562A.
8. Kramer JR, Puenpatom A, Erickson KF et al. Real-world effectiveness of elbasvir/grazoprevir in HCV-infected patients in the US veterans affairs healthcare system. *Journal of Viral Hepatology* 2018;25:1270–1279.
9. Feld JJ, Jacobson IM, Hezode C et al. Sofosbuvir and velpatasvir for HCV genotype 1, 2, 4, 5, and 6 infection. *New England Journal of Medicine* 2015;373:2599–2607.
10. Foster GR, Afdhal N, Roberts SK et al. Sofosbuvir and velpatasvir for HCV genotype 2 and 3 infection. *New England Journal of Medicine* 2015;373:2608–2617.

11. Puoti M, Foster GR, Wang S et al. High SVR12 with 8-week and 12-week glecaprevir/pibrentasvir therapy: an integrated analysis of HCV genotype 1–6 patients without cirrhosis. *Journal of Hepatology.*2018;69:293–300.

12. Forns X, Lee SS, Valdes J et al. Glecaprevir plus pibrentasvir for chronic hepatitis C virus genotype 1, 2, 4, 5, or 6 infection in adults with compensated cirrhosis (EXPEDITION-1): a single-arm, open-label, multicentre phase 3 trial. *Lancet Infectious Diseases* 2017;17:1062–1068.

13. Bourliere M, Gordon SC, Flamm SL et al. Sofosbuvir, velpatasvir, and voxilaprevir for previously treated HCV infection. *New England Journal of Medicine* 2017;376:2134–2146.

14. Jacobson IM, Lawitz E, Gane EJ et al. Efficacy of 8 weeks of sofosbuvir, velpatasvir, and voxilaprevir in patients with chronic HCV infection: 2 phase 3 randomized trials. *Gastroenterology* 2017;153:113–122.

15. Ahmed H, Abushouk AI, Menshawy A et al. Safety and efficacy of ombitasvir/paritaprevir/ritonavir and dasabuvir with or without ribavirin for treatment of hepatitis C virus genotype 1: a systematic review and meta-analysis. *Clinical Drug Investigation* 2017;37:1009–1023.

16. Bourliere M, Gordon SC, Schiff ER et al. Sofosbuvir–velpatasvir–voxilaprevir after blinded placebo in NS5A-inhibitor-experienced patients with chronic hepatitis C in the Phase 3 POLARIS-1 study. *Lancet Gastroenterology and Hepatology* 2018;3:559–565.

17. Bourliere M, Bronowicki JP, de Ledinghen V et al. Ledipasvir–sofosbuvir with or without ribavirin to treat patients with HCV genotype 1 infection and cirrhosis non-responsive to previous protease-inhibitor therapy:a randomised, double-blind, phase 2 trial (SIRIUS). *The Lancet Infectious Diseases* 2015;15:397–404.

18. Charlton M, Everson GT, Flamm SL et al. Ledipasvir and sofosbuvir plus ribavirin for treatment of HCV infection in patients with advanced liver disease. *Gastroenterology* 2015;149:649–659.

19. Foster GR, Irving WL, Cheung MC et al. Impact of direct acting antiviral therapy in patients with chronic hepatitis C and decompensated cirrhosis. *Journal of Hepatology* 2016;64: 1224–1231.

20. Belli LS, Berenguer M, Cortesi PA et al. Delisting of liver transplant candidates with chronic hepatitis C after viral eradication: a European study. *Journal of Hepatology* 2016;65:524–531.

21. Manns M, Samuel D, Gane EJ et al. Ledipasvir and sofosbuvir plus ribavirin in patients with genotype 1 or 4 hepatitis C virus infection and advanced liver disease:a multicentre, open-label, randomised, phase 2 trial. *Lancet Infectious Diseases* 2016;16:685–697.

22. Curry MP, O'Leary JG, Bzowej N et al. Sofosbuvir and velpatasvir for HCV in Patients with decompensated cirrhosis. *New England Journal of Medicine* 2015;373:2618–2628.

23. Fernandez Carrillo C, Lens S, Llop E et al. Treatment of hepatitis C virus infection in patients with cirrhosis and predictive value of model for end-stage liver disease: analysis of data from the Hepa-C registry. *Hepatology* 2017;65:1810–1822.

24. Perricone G, Duvoux C, Berenguer M et al. Delisting HCV-infected liver transplant candidates who improved after viral eradication: outcome 2 years after delisting. *Liver International* 2018;38:2170–2177.

25. Belli LS, Perricone G, Adam R et al. Impact of DAAs on liver transplantation: major effects on the evolution of indications and results. An ELITA study based on the ELTR registry. *Journal of Hepatology* 2018;69:810–817.

26. Bunchorntavakul C, Reddy KR. Treat chronic hepatitis C virus infection in decompensated cirrhosis – pre- or post-liver transplantation? The ironic conundrum in the era of effective and well-tolerated therapy. *Journal of Viral Hepatology* 2016;23:408–418.

27. Kao CC, Lin YS, Chu HC, Fang TC, Wu MS, Kang YN. Association of renal function and direct-acting antiviral agents for Hcv: a network metaanalysis. *Journal of Clinical Medicine* 2018;7:ii.

28. Butt AA, Ren Y, Puenpatom A, Arduino JM, Kumar R, Abou-Samra AB. HCV treatment initiation in persons with chronic kidney disease in the directly acting antiviral agents era: results from ERCHIVES. *Liver International* 2018;38: 1411–1417.

29. Pockros PJ, Reddy KR, Mantry PS et al. Efficacy of direct-acting antiviral combination for patients with hepatitis C virus genotype 1 infection and severe renal impairment or end-stage renal disease. *Gastroenterology* 2016;150:1590–1598.

30. Munoz-Gomez R, Rincon D, Ahumada A et al. Therapy with ombitasvir/paritaprevir/ritonavir plus dasabuvir is effective and safe for the treatment of genotypes 1 and 4 hepatitis C virus (HCV) infection in patients with severe renal impairment: a multicentre experience. *Journal of Viral Hepatology* 2017;24:464–471.

31. Roth D, Nelson DR, Bruchfeld A et al. Grazoprevir plus elbasvir in treatment-naive and treatment-experienced patients with hepatitis C virus genotype 1 infection and stage 4–5 chronic kidney disease (the C-SURFER study): a combination phase 3 study. *Lancet* 2015;386:1537–1545.

32. Gane E, Lawitz E, Pugatch D et al. Glecaprevir and pibrentasvir in patients with HCV and severe renal impairment. *New England Journal of Medicine* 2017;377:1448–1455.

33. European Association for the Study of the Liver. EASL Recommendations on Treatment of hepatitis C 2018. *Journal of Hepatology* 2018;69:461–511.

34. Fontaine H, Lazarus A, Pol S et al. Bradyarrhythmias associated with sofosbuvir treatment. *New England Journal of Medicine* 2015;373:1886–1888.

35. Renet S, Chaumais MC, Antonini T et al. Extreme bradycardia after first doses of sofosbuvir and daclatasvir in

patients receiving amiodarone: 2 cases including a rechallenge. *Gastroenterology* 2015;149:1378–1380 e1.

36. Yu Y, Liu F, He L et al. Human induced pluripotent stem cell-derived cardiomyocytes reveal bradycardiac effects caused by co-administration of sofosbuvir and amiodarone. *Assay and Drug Development Technologies* 2018;16:222–229.

37. Wijarnpreecha K, Chesdachai S, Thongprayoon C, Jaruvongvanich V, Ungprasert P, Cheungpasitporn W. Efficacy and safety of direct-acting antivirals in hepatitis C virus-infected patients taking proton pump inhibitors. *Journal of Clinical and Translational Hepatology* 2017;5:327–334.

38. European Association for the Study of the Liver. EASL recommendations on treatment of hepatitis C 2016. *Journal of Hepatology* 2017;66:153–194.

Harm reduction strategies to prevent new infections and reinfections among people who inject drugs: how effective are they?

Jason Grebely and Marianne Martinello

The Kirby Institute, UNSW Sydney, Sydney, Australia

LEARNING POINTS

- People with ongoing injecting drug use and inadequate access to sterile needles/syringes are at risk of HCV infection and reinfection.

- Harm reduction strategies, including opioid substitution therapy and high-coverage needle and syringe programs (adequate sterile needles/syringes to cover all injections), are effective for the prevention of HCV infection.

- HCV reinfection should be discussed prior to, during, and following DAA therapy.

- Following successful DAA therapy, individuals with ongoing risk behaviors for potential transmission and reinfection should have annual follow-up, including liver function tests and HCV RNA testing.

- Clinicians should include discussions of HCV transmission, risk of reinfection, and strategies to minimize the risk of reinfection in patient education.

- Retreatment for reinfection should be offered, without stigma or discrimination.

Introduction

Among the 71 million people living with hepatitis C virus (HCV) infection, 6.1 million (8.5%) are people who have recently injected drugs (PWID) [1]. Almost one-quarter of new HCV infections are related to unsterile needle and syringe sharing among PWID. This is despite evidence for

and availability of harm reduction interventions, such as opioid substitution therapy (OST) and needle and syringe programs (NSP), in reducing the risk of HCV acquisition [2]. In some jurisdictions, such as the United States, there has been an increase in the number of new HCV infections, in part related to a rise in opioid use and inadequate access to both OST and NSP.

With the availability of direct-acting antiviral (DAA) therapy, there has been an increased uptake of HCV therapy globally, including among people with ongoing injecting drug use. DAA treatment has been demonstrated to be effective in people receiving OST and people who have recently used or injected drugs [3]. However, given that successful HCV treatment does not provide protection against reinfection, clinicians will encounter patients with ongoing risk behaviors for HCV (re)acquisition. As such, clinicians and patients must understand the risk factors for acquisition of HCV (re)infection, conduct appropriate clinical testing to detect HCV reinfection, and optimize strategies to prevent both HCV primary infection and reinfection [4]. However, a key premise is that as treatment is broadened to people with ongoing risk behaviors, reinfection will occur. Strategies to prevent reinfection should be the same as those implemented to prevent primary infection, including access to sterile needles and syringes and OST. Among people with HCV reinfection following successful treatment, DAA retreatment should be offered, without stigma or discrimination.

Clinical Dilemmas in Viral Liver Disease, Second Edition. Edited by Graham R. Foster and K. Rajender Reddy.
© 2020 John Wiley & Sons Ltd. Published 2020 by John Wiley & Sons Ltd.

Risk factors for HCV acquisition among people who inject drugs

Globally, there were an estimated 1.75 million new cases of HCV infection in 2015, with 23% of infections resulting from unsterile needle and syringe sharing among people with ongoing injecting drug use.

The rate of HCV infection among PWID varies considerably, from 2% to 66% per annum [5]. Among PWID, a number of individual and structural factors are associated with HCV acquisition including younger age, female gender, ethnicity, unstable housing, sex work, imprisonment, recent initiation to injecting, frequent injecting, cocaine/methamphetamine injecting, having a partner who injects, injecting network membership, requiring help injecting, and borrowing needles and syringes [6,7].

As DAA treatment scale-up expands among populations with ongoing risk behaviors for reacquisition, it is essential to acknowledge that HCV reinfection can and will occur. The rate of HCV reinfection among PWID ranges from 0% to 5% per annum, with higher incidence among people with ongoing injecting drug use (5–22% per annum) [8,9]. The rate of reinfection will depend on the study population (and risk behaviors for HCV acquisition), the HCV RNA prevalence in the population, the population-level incidence of HCV infection, and the coverage of harm reduction programs (e.g., OST and NSP). Although there are fewer data on factors associated with reinfection among PWID, needle and syringe sharing, more frequent injecting and cocaine/methamphetamine injecting have been associated with an increased risk of HCV reinfection [10].

While these factors are important for understanding the context around the risk of HCV (re)infection, it is the sharing of unsterile needles and syringes that is of paramount importance. As such, in many settings, structural barriers to ensuring access to clean needles and syringes must be addressed. Clinicians need to be aware of the risks for HCV acquisition and provide education to patients prior to, during, and following treatment about the potential for reinfection, reinforcing the importance of using sterile needles and syringes for all injections. An awareness of individual factors should assist clinicians in identifying patients requiring intensified education efforts. However, these factors should not be used as criteria for withholding DAA therapy among people with ongoing injecting drug use.

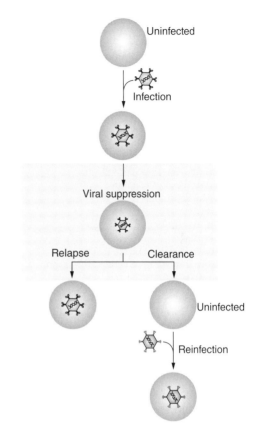

Figure 18.1 HCV reinfection following treatment. Reinfection, after treatment-induced clearance, is the detection of an HCV strain which was heterologous to that detected before recurrence. Colors represent different viral strains, sizes represent relative abundance of the virus, and gray areas represent treatment. Source: Adapted from Cunningham EB et al. [8].

Definitions of viral relapse and reinfection

Patients with undetectable HCV RNA following the completion of HCV therapy are considered to have an *end of treatment response. Sustained virologic response* (SVR) is defined as having undetectable HCV RNA at 12 weeks following treatment and is equivalent to viral cure. Among patients with an end of treatment response, the subsequent detection of HCV RNA is often referred to as *viral recurrence.* Among participants with posttreatment viral recurrence, HCV sequencing can be performed to distinguish *viral relapse* (detection of an HCV strain which is similar to the HCV strain prior to treatment due to virologic failure of therapy) from *reinfection* (detection of an HCV strain which is substantially different from the HCV strain prior to treatment).

Clinically, there are some practical strategies that can be used to characterize HCV reinfection. Given the low rate of viral relapse following cure with DAA treatment (<1% of patients with an SVR will have viral relapse following currently available DAA therapies), the detection of HCV RNA following SVR is likely to be due to reinfection. If HCV genotyping was performed prior to the initiation of HCV DAA therapy, repeating the HCV genotype at the time of suspected reinfection will provide insight into whether reinfection with a different HCV genotype (e.g., 1a to 3a) or subtype (1a to 1b) has occurred. Among people reexposed to the same genotype (e.g., 1a to 1a), HCV sequencing (either Sanger or next-generation sequencing) can be performed in some laboratories to distinguish viral relapse from reinfection. HCV sequencing can be used to determine whether the HCV strains prior to and following treatment were similar (viral relapse) or different (reinfection) by comparing the divergence in the sequences (based on genetic distance-based cut-offs for HCV reinfection and HCV viral relapse or phylogenetic tree construction). However, among individuals with apparent viral relapse and ongoing risk behavior, excluding the possibility that reinfection has occurred from the same source as the initial infection is difficult.

Strategies to reduce HCV (re)infection among PWID

Efforts directed at addressing, preventing, and managing HCV reinfection should be incorporated into individual and population-level HCV strategies, with multicomponent interventions likely to be most effective [4,11].At an individual level, prior to initiating DAA therapy, an assessment of HCV reinfection risk should be performed by the treating clinician. Management options include acknowledging populations with potential reinfection risk, education and counseling regarding HCV transmission and drug use (particularly the importance of using sterile needles/syringes), optimizing access to harm reduction services (including sterile injecting equipment) [11–14],

treating the individual, their injecting (or sexual) partner and people in their injecting network [15], management of medical and psychiatric comorbidities [12], posttreatment surveillance [16], and rapid retreatment of reinfection. At a population level, appropriate healthcare provision with universal access to care and treatment (including broad availability of NSP and OST), political will, adequate funding (for both DAA therapy and harm reduction programs), and alleviation of the stigma associated with HCV infection and drug use should assist in efforts to reduce HCV primary and reinfection incidence.

Harm reduction services

Harm reduction services are critical for prevention of HCV primary infection and reinfection. OST with methadone or buprenorphine is effective for the management of opioid dependence [17]. OST is associated with a 50% reduction in HCV acquisition risk, while combined OST and high-coverage NSP (defined as adequate sterile needles/syringes to cover all injections) are associated with a 74% reduction in HCV acquisition risk [14]. Given the benefits of preventing both HIV and HCV infections, NSPs are recognized as one of the most cost-effective public health interventions.

Interventions that combine harm reduction and DAA treatment scale-up appear to deliver the greatest benefit in reducing HCV viremic prevalence and interrupting transmission. Modeling has suggested that higher harm reduction coverage (NSP and OST) allows for lower DAA treatment uptake among PWID to achieve reductions in HCV prevalence, given the additional benefit derived from preventing new infections [18]. While a combined strategy appears to be cost-effective [19] and is supported by modeling [18] and empiric evidence [13,20], global coverage of OST and NSP interventions is low [21]. Less than 1% of PWID reside in countries with high coverage of both NSP and OST [21]. Lack of political will, stigma, discrimination, and criminalization have reduced accessibility and limited coverage in many jurisdictions. Implementation of evidence-based harm reduction programs is necessary to reduce primary HCV infection and reinfection following treatment among PWID.

Integrated care

Hepatitis C virus treatment for PWID should be integrated into existing services, concurrently managing substance misuse, mental health, and other medical comorbidities.

Lower HCV reinfection risk has been observed among recent PWID receiving OST and mental health counseling services [12]. The provision of HCV services within existing models of care (such as drug treatment clinics, harm reduction services, prisons, general practitioners, homelessness services) compared to referral to traditional tertiary hospital clinics may more effectively facilitate the ongoing healthcare needs of PWID and reduce the risk of (re)infection. Acknowledgment of the individual circumstances of PWID as opposed to rigid criteria will aid in the success of long-term HCV management strategies and drug user health overall.

Education and counseling

Education and counseling can reduce high-risk injecting behaviors among people with HCV infection [22,23]. Injecting risk behaviors do not increase following the initiation of HCV therapy. However, it is important for healthcare providers, peer support workers, and community drug user organizations to provide education and counseling to PWID commencing DAA about the potential risks of HCV reinfection (most importantly, the sharing of unsterile needles/syringes). Community-based drug user organizations should also be involved in the design and implementation of programs to educate PWID about the risk of HCV infection and strategies to prevent HCV reinfection.

It is also critical that healthcare providers are educated about best practices for the prevention and management of HCV infection among PWID. Some practitioners remain unwilling to treat HCV infection among people with ongoing injecting drug use given concerns of reinfection, adherence, and medication cost [24]. However, given the available data, concerns regarding reinfection should not be a deterrent to HCV treatment.

Posttreatment surveillance and treatment of reinfection

People at risk for HCV reinfection should have at least annual monitoring with HCV RNA and alanine aminotransferase (ALT) [5,25,26]. However, monitoring for reinfection following HCV treatment is not standardized and may be infrequent; in a Scottish cohort, only 61% of PWID were screened at least once in 4.5 years of post-SVR follow-up [27]. While the optimal testing interval for detection of (clinically significant) reinfection is unknown, more frequent testing may identify a greater number of reinfections

[16], providing the potential for earlier retreatment. Routine posttreatment surveillance and adherence to international guidelines should ensure that reinfection is diagnosed within the first year of reacquisition.

One of the barriers to testing for reinfection may be jurisdictional limitations on DAA access, driven largely by the current high prices of treatment [28,29]. DAA retreatment should be made available to all people with reinfection, without stigma or discrimination. Key healthcare bodies and medical societies should consider implicit recommendations regarding retreatment of reinfection to help facilitate reimbursement by payers.

An additional barrier to testing may be the number of competing health, family, financial or drug use priorities. A monitoring and diagnostic algorithm which incorporates rapid point-of-care HCV RNA testing [30,31] conducted in settings appropriate to and frequently utilized by PWID may facilitate testing, diagnosis, and expedient retreatment of reinfection.

Screening and targeted strategies in high-risk populations

All PWID should be screened for HCV with anti-HCV antibody [5,25,26]. In the context of ongoing injection drug use, 6–12-monthly screening should be performed with anti-HCV antibody to assess for incident primary infection and with HCV RNA to assess for reinfection [5,7,25,26]. Certain populations, including young PWID and incarcerated PWID, may require targeted screening and interventions to prevent ongoing transmission and reinfection. High incidence among young adult and incarcerated PWID highlights the importance of treating the individual within the context of their injecting (and sexual) network to gain the greatest individual and population-level benefit.

Stigma, discrimination, and criminalization of drug use

Criminalization of drug use and restrictive drug law enforcement policies hinder access to and provision of HCV prevention services, which in turn may drive increased risk behaviors (including needle and syringe sharing) and HCV transmission [32]. In jurisdictions with repressive drug policies, PWID may end up in prison, where the risk of HCV (re)infection is often high and prevention measures are absent.

Treatment as prevention and the impact of reinfection

Mathematical modeling suggests that substantial reductions in HCV incidence and prevalence could be achieved by targeted DAA treatment scale-up amongst those at highest risk of ongoing transmission [33]. Despite the cost of DAA therapy, treating recent PWID with early liver disease appears to be cost-effective compared to delaying until cirrhosis, given the reduction in liver-related complications and additional benefit of averting reinfection [34].

Rapid DAA treatment scale-up among PWID will be required to gain the greatest population-level benefit. Given high efficacy, rapid scale-up of DAA therapy (>8% per year) among PWID will markedly increase the population susceptible to HCV reinfection in the short term [35]. While initially this will lead to an increase in the number of people with HCV reinfection, as the HCV RNA prevalence decreases overall, the number with reinfection will also decrease. The incidence of HCV reinfection following DAA-based treatment needs careful evaluation. Sufficient follow-up time with regular HCV RNA testing post treatment will be required to appropriately evaluate reinfection incidence.

Practical approaches to prevent HCV infection and reinfection among PWID

- *Assess risk behaviors among people at risk for HCV infection and prior to, during or following DAA treatment and provide HCV education about potential risks.* Understanding participants who are most at risk of HCV infection and reinfection will facilitate increased education and ensure that interventions are optimized to prevent HCV infection and reinfection. Patients should be educated about the factors which place them at increased risk of HCV infection and reinfection, in particular the sharing of unsterile needles/syringes. Also, strategies to minimize risk of infection and reinfection should be discussed.
- *Assess and optimize access to harm reduction interventions.* Opioid substitution therapy has been shown to reduce the risk of HCV infection and reinfection and should be offered to people who are opioid dependent and interested in receiving treatment. Also, access to sterile needles and syringes should be optimized. However, access to such programs should not be a requirement to receive DAA therapy.
- *HCV testing should be performed annually in people at risk for infection and people who have successfully cleared HCV infection.* Individuals with ongoing risk behaviors for potential transmission and reinfection should have annual follow-up, including liver function tests and HCV RNA testing.
- *Retreatment for reinfection should be offered, without stigma or discrimination.*

References

1. Grebely J, Larney S, Peacock A et al. Global, regional, and country-level estimates of hepatitis C infection among people who have recently injected drugs. *Addiction* 2019;114:150–166.
2. Platt L, Minozzi S, Reed J et al. Needle and syringe programmes and opioid substitution therapy for preventing HCV transmission among people who inject drugs: findings from a Cochrane Review and meta-analysis. *Addiction* 2018;113:545–563.
3. Hajarizadeh B, Cunningham EB, Reid H, Law M, Dore GJ, Grebely J. Direct-acting antiviral treatment for hepatitis C among people who use or inject drugs: a systematic review and meta-analysis. *Lancet Gastroenterology and Hepatology* 2018;3:754–767.
4. Martinello M, Dore GJ, Matthews GV, Grebely J. Strategies to reduce hepatitis C virus reinfection in people who inject drugs. *Infectious Disease Clinics of North America* 2018;32:371–393.
5. Grebely J, Robaeys G, Bruggmann P et al. Recommendations for the management of hepatitis C virus infection among people who inject drugs. *International Journal on Drug Policy* 2015;26:1028–1038.
6. Grebely J, Dore GJ. Prevention of hepatitis C virus in injecting drug users: a narrow window of opportunity. *Journal of Infectious Diseases* 2011;203:571–574.
7. Martinello M, Hajarizadeh B, Grebely J, Dore GJ, Matthews GV. Management of acute HCV infection in the era of direct-acting antiviral therapy. *Nature Reviews Gastroenterology and Hepatology* 2018;15:412–424.
8. Cunningham EB, Applegate TL, Lloyd AR, Dore GJ, Grebely J. Mixed HCV infection and reinfection in people who inject drugs – impact on therapy. *Nature Reviews Gastroenterology and Hepatology* 2015;12:218–230.
9. Martinello M, Hajarizadeh B, Grebely J, Dore GJ, Matthews GV. HCV cure and reinfection among people with HIV/HCV coinfection and people who inject drugs. *Current HIV/AIDS Reports* 2017;14:110–121.
10. Young J, Rossi C, Gill J et al. Risk factors for hepatitis C virus reinfection after sustained virologic response in patients co-infected with HIV. *Clinical Infectious Diseases* 2017;64:1154–1162.

11. Hagan H, Pouget ER, Des Jarlais DC. A systematic review and meta-analysis of interventions to prevent hepatitis C virus infection in people who inject drugs. *Journal of Infectious Diseases* 2011;204:74–83.

12. Islam N, Krajden M, Shoveller J et al. Incidence, risk factors, and prevention of hepatitis C reinfection: a population-based cohort study. *Lancet Gastroenterology and Hepatology* 2017; 2:200–210.

13. Palmateer NE, Taylor A, Goldberg DJ et al. Rapid decline in HCV incidence among people who inject drugs associated with national scale-up in coverage of a combination of harm reduction interventions. *PLoS One* 2014;9:e104515.

14. Platt L, Minozzi S, Reed J et al. Needle and syringe programmes and opioid substitution therapy for preventing HCV transmission among people who inject drugs: findings from a Cochrane Review and meta-analysis. *Addiction 2017*8;113:545–563.

15. Hellard M, Rolls DA, Sacks-Davis R et al. The impact of injecting networks on hepatitis C transmission and treatment in people who inject drugs. *Hepatology* 2014;60:1861–1870.

16. Vickerman P, Grebely J, Dore GJ et al. The more you look, the more you find: effects of hepatitis C virus testing interval on reinfection incidence and clearance and implications for future vaccine study design. *Journal of Infectious Diseases* 2012;205:1342–1350.

17. Mattick RP, Breen C, Kimber J, Davoli M. Buprenorphine maintenance versus placebo or methadone maintenance for opioid dependence. *Cochrane Database of Systematic Reviews* 2014;2:CD002207.

18. Ward Z, Platt L, Sweeney S et al. Impact of current and scaled-up levels of hepatitis C prevention and treatment interventions for people who inject drugs in three UK settings – what is required to achieve the WHO's HCV elimination targets? *Addiction* 2018; doi: 10.1111/add.14217.

19. Kwon JA, Anderson J, Kerr CC et al. Estimating the cost-effectiveness of needle–syringe programs in Australia. *AIDS* 2012;26:2201–2210.

20. Morris MD, Shiboski S, Bruneau J et al. Geographic differences in temporal incidence trends of hepatitis C virus infection among people who inject drugs: the InC3 Collaboration. *Clinical Infectious Diseases* 2017;64:860–869.

21. Larney S, Peacock A, Leung J et al. Global, regional, and country-level coverage of interventions to prevent and manage HIV and hepatitis C among people who inject drugs: a systematic review. *Lancet Global Health* 2017;5:e1208–e1220.

22. Bruneau J, Zang G, Abrahamowicz M, Jutras-Aswad D, Daniel M, Roy E. Sustained drug use changes after hepatitis C screening and counseling among recently infected persons who inject drugs: a longitudinal study. *Clinical Infectious Diseases* 2014;58:755–761.

23. Roux P, Le Gall JM, Debrus M et al. Innovative community-based educational face-to-face intervention to reduce HIV, hepatitis C virus and other blood-borne infectious risks in difficult-to-reach people who inject drugs: results from the ANRS-AERLI intervention study. *Addiction* 2016;111:94–106.

24. Asher AK, Portillo CJ, Cooper BA, Dawson-Rose C, Vlahov D, Page KA. Clinicians' views of hepatitis C virus treatment candidacy with direct-acting antiviral regimens for people who inject drugs. *Substance Use and Misuse* 2016;51:1218–1223.

25. Recommendations for Testing, Managing, and Treating Hepatitis C. www.hcvguidelines.org/

26. Pawlotsky JM, Negro F, Aghemo A et al. EASL recommendations on treatment of hepatitis C 2018. *Journal of Hepatology* 2018;69:461–511.

27. Weir A, McLeod A, Innes H et al. Hepatitis C reinfection following treatment induced viral clearance among people who have injected drugs. *Drug and Alcohol Dependence* 2016; 165:53–60.

28. Barua S, Greenwald R, Grebely J, Dore GJ, Swan T, Taylor LE. Restrictions for Medicaid reimbursement of sofosbuvir for the treatment of hepatitis C virus infection in the United States. *Annals of Internal Medicine* 2015;163:215–223.

29. Marshall AD, Saeed S, Barrett L et al. Restrictions for reimbursement of direct-acting antiviral treatment for hepatitis C virus infection in Canada: a descriptive study. *CMAJ Open* 2016;4:E605–E614.

30. Grebely J, Lamoury FMJ, Hajarizadeh B et al. Evaluation of the Xpert HCV Viral Load point-of-care assay from venepuncture-collected and finger-stick capillary whole-blood samples: a cohort study. *Lancet Gastroenterology and Hepatology* 2017;2:514–520.

31. Hayes B, Briceno A, Asher A et al. Preference, acceptability and implications of the rapid hepatitis C screening test among high-risk young people who inject drugs. *BMC Public Health* 2014;14:645.

32. Grebely J, Dore GJ, Morin S, Rockstroh JK, Klein MB. Elimination of HCV as a public health concern among people who inject drugs by 2030 – what will it take to get there? *Journal of the International AIDS Society* 2017;20:22146.

33. Hickman M, de Angelis D, Vickerman P, Hutchinson S, Martin NK. Hepatitis C virus treatment as prevention in people who inject drugs: testing the evidence. *Current Opinion in Infectious Diseases* 2015;28:576–582.

34. Scott N, McBryde ES, Thompson A, Doyle JS, Hellard ME. Treatment scale-up to achieve global HCV incidence and mortality elimination targets: a cost-effectiveness model. *Gut* 2017;66:1507–1515.

35. Razavi H. Reducing a country's HCV disease burden. Presented at the 4th International Symposium on Hepatitis in Substance Users (INHSU 2015), Sydney, Australia, 2015.

19 Hepatitis C virus therapy in advanced liver disease: treat or transplant and treat?

Chalermrat Bunchorntavakul[1] and K. Rajender Reddy[2]

[1] Division of Gastroenterology and Hepatology, Department of Internal Medicine Rajavithi Hospital, College of Medicine, Rangsit University, Bangkok, Thailand

[2] Department of Medicine, Division of Gastroenterology and Hepatology, University of Pennsylvania, Philadelphia, PA, USA

LEARNING POINTS

- DAA therapy is safe and effective in patients with decompensated cirrhosis, with slightly lower SVR rates, particularly in those with Child–Pugh class C, as compared to noncirrhotic patients.

- Most patients who achieve viral eradication have an improvement in hepatic function and MELD score, but some may retain features of hepatic decompensation where quality of life is still poor and the chance of getting a liver transplant for such patients may be further delayed due to the improvement in their MELD score.

- While drug–drug interations are managed, DAA therapy in liver transplant recipients is associated with higher SVR rates compared to treatment in those with decompensated cirrhosis.

- Predictors for nonimprovement of hepatic function following pre-liver transplant treatment include Child–Pugh class C, MELD >15–20, age ≥65 years, BMI >25 kg/m^2, severe portal hypertension, serum ALT >60 U/L, albumin <3.5 g/dL and sodium <135 mEq/L.

- The decision to treat HCV in patients with decompensated cirrhosis in the context of liver transplant should be individualized. In general, patients with MELD <15 should be treated before liver transplant while those with MELD >20 should be transplanted first and treated after. Treatment for those with MELD 15–20 should be individualized based on clinical and laboratory predictors of response or nonresponse.

- Treatment strategy also is dependent on factors such as availability or nonavailability of liver transplant, the prevalent MELD at which they are transplanted in a given country, and the availability and use of HCV donors that can facilitate earlier transplant in untreated patients.

Introduction

Although effective therapies for chronic hepatitis C (HCV) are currently available, it is still predicted that the number of cases of HCV-related cirrhosis and hepatocellular carcinoma (HCC) requiring liver transplantation (LT) will continue to rise through the decades [1,2]. Among HCV patients with decompensated cirrhosis, the availability of highly effective direct-acting antivirals (DAA) therapy provides a great opportunity for HCV cure in patients who were previously ineligible for interferon-based treatment. Effective therapy subsequently leads to improvement in hepatic function (may obviate the need for LT), reduces LT waiting list mortality, and prevents post-LT HCV recurrence [1–5]. However, we now have a dilemma on the ideal timing for HCV treatment in the context of LT and this is due to issues such as only achieving partial improvement in hepatic function (MELD purgatory), being still at risk for HCC, and reducing the opportunity for achieving earlier LT by receiving a HCV+ organ [1–5].

Efficacy and safety of treatment before liver transplantation

Several DAA regimens have been evaluated in patients with decompensated cirrhosis in phase 2/3 and real-world studies, with promising outcomes. Overall, sustained virologic response in 12 weeks (SVR12) rates for sofosbuvir plus ledipasvir, daclatasvir or velpatasvir, with or without ribavirin, for 12–24 weeks for HCV genotype 1–6 were 87–96% and 56–87% in patients with Child–Turcotte–Pugh

Clinical Dilemmas in Viral Liver Disease, Second Edition. Edited by Graham R. Foster and K. Rajender Reddy.
© 2020 John Wiley & Sons Ltd. Published 2020 by John Wiley & Sons Ltd.

(CTP) class B and C, respectively [1,2,4,6–12] (Table 19.1). Notably, SVR appeared to be slightly lower in patients with genotype 3 compared to those with other genotypes. DAA treatment was well tolerated in this population and severe adverse events developed in 20–30%, mainly related to liver disease progression without additional treatment-related side effects, other than ribavirin-induced anemia. The use of protease inhibitors is contraindicated in patients with decompensated cirrhosis, because of substantially higher drug exposure, which is associated with toxicities in these patients [3].

Treatment in patients with decompensated cirrhosis awaiting a LT has two complementary goals: preventing liver graft reinfection after LT and improving liver function before LT [2]. Further, a sustained improvement in patient-reported outcomes (e.g., quality of life, physical well-being, and work productivity) has also been observed, albeit not for all [13]. Successful antiviral therapy was associated with an improvement in hepatic function in 20–60% of patients; varying degrees of improvement have been observed (although substantial improvement in model for end-stage liver disease [MELD] score of >6 points has been reported in some patients, the median improvement in MELD score was approximately -2) and may consequently lead to delisting in a proportion of patients (the chance of being delisted in various studies was 35%, 12% and 5% with MELD <16, 16–20, and >20, respectively) [1,4,14]. In a US study combining real-life data and modeling, the life expectancy benefit of treating patients with MELD >20 before LT was only less than one year [15].

Apart from MELD score, other predictors for nonimprovement of hepatic function and clinical status following pre-LT treatment include CTP class C, age ≥65 years, Body Mass Index (BMI) >25 kg/m^2, severe portal hypertension, serum alanine aminotransferase (ALT) level <60 U/L, serum albumin <3.5 g/dL (especially <2.8 g/dL) and sodium <135 mEq/L [4,8,11,14,16]. In the UK experience (n = 467), patients with age <65 years and albumin ≥3.5 g/dL had higher rates (~60%) of improvement in hepatic function after successful HCV therapy compared to those with albumin <3.5 g/dL or sodium <135 mEq/L (~40% chance) [8]. In addition, by analyzing data from four major trials of sofosbuvir-based regimens among 502 CTP-B and 120 CTP-C HCV patients, the BE3A score (1 point for each item: BMI <25, no Encephalopathy, no Ascites, serum ALT >1.5 times ULN and Albumin >3.5 g/dL) has been proposed as a predictive score to quantify the potential benefits of DAA therapy for patients with decompensated cirrhosis [16]. A BE3A score of 4–5 was associated with a 75% chance of reducing CTP score to class A, while those with a score of 0 or 1 were associated with a <5% and 25% chance of achieving CPT-A at 36 weeks following therapy, respectively [16].

Efficacy and safety of treatment after liver transplantation

Results from phase 2/3 and real-world studies demonstrated excellent SVR rates of >93% with DAA therapy in patients with post-LT HCV recurrence, including those

Table 19.1 Recommendations for HCV treatment in patients with decompensated cirrhosis

HCV genotype	Prior treatment status	Recommended regimens
HCV genotype 1, 4, 5 or 6 infection	Naive or prior IFN treatment failure	• SOF/LDV+ RBV 12–24 wk* • SOF/VEL + RBV 12–24 wk* • SOF/DCV + RBV 12–24 wk* (genotype 1 or 4 only)
	Prior SOF- or NS5A-based treatment failure	• SOF/VEL + RBV 24 wk • SOF/LDV+ RBV 24 wk (prior SOF-based treatment failure only)
HCV genotype 2 or 3 infection	Naive or prior IFN treatment failure	• SOF/VEL + RBV 12–24 wk* • SOF/DCV + RBV 12–24 wk*
	Prior SOF- or NS5A-based treatment failure	• SOF/VEL + RBV 24 wk

Ribavirin dose: initially 600 mg/day, then adjusted to 1000–1200 mg/day for SOF/LDV and SOF/DCV regimens and weight-based dosing for SOF/VEL regimens.
* Duration of treatment: 12 weeks with ribavirin and 24 weeks without ribavirin.
DCV, daclatasvir; IFN, interferon; LDV, ledipasvir; RBV, ribavirin; SOF, sofosbuvir; VEL, velpatasvir.

with cirrhosis CTP class A and fibrosing cholestatic hepatitis [4,6,10,11,17–19]. Treatment of recurrent HCV should be considered as early as clinically feasible (often within 3–6 months after LT) as SVR appeared to be reduced if advanced cirrhosis developed in the graft [4,6,10,11]. The recommended DAA regimens for LT recipients do not differ from general patients although caution should be exercised for drug–drug interactions, particularly between calcineurin inhibitors and protease inhibitors [3,4]. Notably, SVR rates are higher in LT recipients (similar to those of the non-LT population) compared to those patients with decompensated cirrhosis, especially CTP class C [1,4].

Controversies in the timing of HCV treatment of patients with decompensated cirrhosis

The decision to treat HCV in patients with decompensated cirrhosis should be individualized, together with consideration of the probability of deriving improvement in hepatic function and the expected waiting time to LT in each region (Figure 19.1) [1,2,4,7]. In patients who have a

contraindication for LT or in parts of the world where there are challenges with access to LT, HCV treatment would be ideal for all patients with decompensated cirrhosis with the hope that there would be functional and quality of life improvement, and prolonged survival, although the favorable outcomes most likely will not be seen in all. However, if LT is an option, the decision of HCV treatment is more complex and the pros and cons of treating patients with decompensated cirrhosis should be taken into consideration (Table 19.2) [1,2,4,7].

It is debated whether those with decompensated cirrhosis with MELD >20 should be treated before LT with the aim to cure and achieve functional improvement, which hopefully precludes the need for LT in some patients, or prevent post-LT recurrence, or whether such patients should be monitored until LT and treatment initiated at the time of HCV recurrence and before the development of advanced fibrosis [2]. In a modeling study, pre-LT treatment was reported to be cost-effective for patients without HCC with a MELD score ≤20, while treatment after LT was cost-effective in patients with a MELD score >20 [20]. We had previously advocated treating even those with a MELD score of 15–25 on a case-by-case basis but

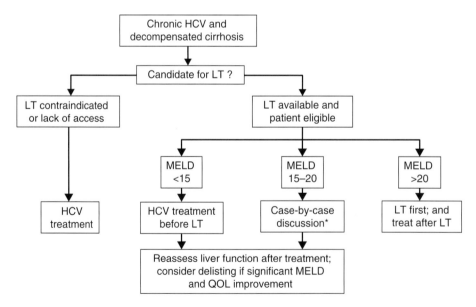

Figure 19.1 Suggested algorithm for initiating HCV therapy for patients with decompensated cirrhosis in the context of liver transplantation. Source: Modified from Bunchorntavakul and Reddy [2], with permission.
CTP, Child–Turcotte–Pugh; DAA, direct-acting antivirals; GFR, glomerular filtration rate; HCC, hepatocellular carcinoma; LT, liver transplantation; QOL, quality of life; SVR, sustained virologic response.

Table 19.2 Pros and cons of treating patients with decompensated cirrhosis before liver transplantation

Pros	Cons
• SVR is achieved in >85% of patients • Hepatic function often improves • May obviate the need for LT (up to 30% of patients) • Save an organ thus benefiting the organ pool • Prevent post-LT HCV recurrence • Fewer drug–drug interactions (compared to treating in LT recipients) • May be the only option in situations where LT is unavailable or contraindicated • May allow locoregional treatment for HCC and reduce HCC recurrence	• May eliminate or delay the opportunity to have a curative treatment (LT) of liver disease, and place the patient into "MELD purgatory" where quality of life is still poor • Still at risk of progressive liver disease and HCC • Preclude the use of HCV+ organs • Treatment after LT is associated with higher SVR rates compared to treatment in decompensated cirrhosis before LT • In those who fail therapy, exposure to NS5A inhibitors and development of viral resistance may compromise treatment options after LT

Source: Modified from Bunchorntavakul and Reddy [2], with permission.
HCC, hepatocellular carcinoma; LT, liver transplantation; MELD, model of end-stage liver disease; SVR, sustained virologic response.

have the dropped the MELD "gray zone" to 15–20; a study has evaluated changes in MELD in CPT-B and -C patients and noted that at 36 months after HCV treatment, a substantial number of patients with MELD ≥15 still remained in that category [21].

Although the currently available treatment regimens for patients with decompensated cirrhosis are associated with high SVR rates, they are still lower than those gained by treating early HCV recurrence after LT. It should be noted that the robust pangenotypic regimens (glecaprevir/pibrentasvir and voxilaprevir/sofosbuvir/velpatasvir) contain a protease inhibitor, thus contraindicating their use in those with decompensated cirrhosis [2]. For those who fail DAA therapy before LT, the occurrence of resistance-associated variants, especially for NS5A, may compromise the SVR when re-treating after LT. Further, in such cases of NS5A resistance, protease inhibitors may be challenging in LT recipients due to drug–drug interaction with calcineurin inhibitors, thus providing fewer DAA options for such patients. Even with successful HCV eradication, the quality of life is likely to improve but may not be normalized, the risk of progressive liver disease and HCC is not eliminated, and the chance of getting a LT for such patients may be further delayed due to the improvement in their MELD scores – so-called MELD purgatory [2].

Liver grafts from HCV+ donors (HCV prevalence among organ donors is 1.4–5.5%) have been underused for many years. Utilization of these organs for HCV+ candidates may shorten waiting times without a significant impact on long-term outcomes after LT [4,22,23]. In general, HCV+ livers are not ideal for HCV- or HCV+ candidates in whom HCV has been previously eradicated before LT, for both ethical and cost-effectiveness reasons [4]. In candidates with severe decompensated cirrhosis and/or with HCC in whom a long waiting time can be expected, HCV treatment before LT should be balanced against the benefit of accelerated access to LT using an HCV+ liver graft [4].

Conclusion

While we have worked for decades for effective and well-tolerated HCV therapies, we have now created a dilemma on timing of HCV therapy in the context of LT. There is an urgent need to identify robust predictors of clinical response after successful HCV therapy and long-term outcomes so that we can inform our patients on what might be the expectations with treatment and if it is wise to wait till after LT to treat them [1,2]. Realistically, this dilemma may only be applicable to a small group of LT-eligible patients while the majority of patients with decompensated liver disease would be ideal candidates for DAA therapy with the expectation of improved hepatic function, quality of life, and longer survival [1,2].

References

1. Bunchorntavakul C, Reddy KR. Treat chronic hepatitis C virus infection in decompensated cirrhosis – pre- or post-liver transplantation? The ironic conundrum in the era of

effective and well-tolerated therapy. *Journal of Viral Hepatitis* 2016;23(6):408–418.

2. Bunchorntavakul C, Reddy KR. HCV therapy in decompensated cirrhosis before or after liver transplantation: a paradoxical quandary. *American Journal of Gastroenterology* 2018;113(4):449–452.

3. AASLD and IDSA. HCV Guidance: recommendations for testing and treating hepatitis C. www.hcvguidelines.org/contents.

4. Belli LS, Duvoux C, Berenguer M et al. ELITA consensus statements on the use of DAAs in liver transplant candidates and recipients. *Journal of Hepatology* 2017;67:585–602.

5. Terrault NA, McCaughan GW, Curry MP et al. International Liver Transplantation Society consensus statement on hepatitis c management in liver transplant candidates. *Transplantation* 2017;101(5).945–955.

6. Charlton M, Everson GT, Flamm SL et al. Ledipasvir and sofosbuvir plus ribavirin for treatment of HCV infection in patients with advanced liver disease. *Gastroenterology* 2015;149(3):649–659.

7. Coilly A, Roche B, Duclos-Vallee JC, Samuel D. Optimum timing of treatment for hepatitis C infection relative to liver transplantation. *Lancet Gastroenterology and Hepatology* 2016;1(2):165–172.

8. Foster GR, Irving WL, Cheung MC et al. Impact of direct acting antiviral therapy in patients with chronic hepatitis C and decompensated cirrhosis. *Journal of Hepatology* 2016; 64(6):1224–1231.

9. Kwo P, Fried MW, Reddy KR et al. Daclatasvir and sofosbuvir treatment of decompensated liver disease or post-liver transplant hepatitis C virus recurrence in patients with advanced liver disease/cirrhosis in a real-world cohort. *Hepatology Communications* 2018;2(4):354–363.

10. Manns M, Samuel D, Gane EJ et al. Ledipasvir and sofosbuvir plus ribavirin in patients with genotype 1 or 4 hepatitis C virus infection and advanced liver disease: a multicentre, open-label, randomised, phase 2 trial. *Lancet Infectious Diseases* 2016;16(6):685–697.

11. Poordad F, Schiff ER, Vierling JM et al. Daclatasvir with sofosbuvir and ribavirin for hepatitis C virus infection with advanced cirrhosis or post-liver transplantation recurrence. *Hepatology* 2016;63(5):1493–1505.

12. Takehara T, Sakamoto N, Nishiguchi S et al. Efficacy and safety of sofosbuvir-velpatasvir with or without ribavirin in HCV-infected Japanese patients with decompensated cirrhosis: an open-label phase 3 trial. *Journal of Gastroenterology* 2019; 54(1):87–95.

13. Younossi ZM, Stepanova M, Charlton M et al. Patient-reported outcomes with sofosbuvir and velpatasvir with or without ribavirin for hepatitis C virus-related decompensated cirrhosis: an exploratory analysis from the randomised, open-label ASTRAL-4 phase 3 trial. *Lancet Gastroenterology and Hepatology* 2016;1(2):122–132.

14. Belli LS, Berenguer M, Cortesi PA et al. Delisting of liver transplant candidates with chronic hepatitis C after viral eradication: a European study. *Journal of Hepatology* 2016; 65(3):524–531.

15. Chhatwal J, Samur S, Kues B, Ayer T, Roberts MS. Optimal timing of hepatitis C treatment for patients on the liver transplant waiting list. *Hepatology* 2017;65(3):777–788.

16. El-Sherif O, Jiang ZG, Tapper EB et al. Baseline factors associated with improvements in decompensated cirrhosis after direct-acting antiviral therapy for hepatitis C virus infection. *Gastroenterology* 2018;154(8):2111–2121.e8.

17. Saxena V, Khungar V, Verna EC et al. Safety and efficacy of current DAA regimens in kidney and liver transplant recipients with hepatitis C: results from the HCV-TARGET Study. *Hepatology* 2017;66:1090–1101.

18. Faisal N, Bilodeau M, Aljudaibi B et al. Sofosbuvir-based antiviral therapy is highly effective in recurrent hepatitis C in liver transplant recipients: Canadian multicenter "real-life" experience. *Transplantation* 2016;100(5):1059–1065.

19. Reau N, Kwo PY, Rhee S, Brown RS Jr, Agarwal K. Glecaprevir/pibrentasvir treatment in liver or kidney transplant patients with hepatitis C virus infection. *Hepatology* 2018;68(4):1298–1307.

20. Cortesi PA, Belli LS, Facchetti R et al. The optimal timing of hepatitis C therapy in liver transplant-eligible patients: cost-effectiveness analysis of new opportunities. *Journal of Viral Hepatitis* 2018;25(7):791–801.

21. Muir AJ, Buti M, Nahass R et al. Long-term follow-up of patients with chronic HCV infection and compensated or decompensated cirrhosis following treatment with sofosbuvir-based regimens. *Hepatology* 2016;64(S1):437A–438A.

22. Northup PG, Argo CK, Nguyen DT et al. Liver allografts from hepatitis C positive donors can offer good outcomes in hepatitis C positive recipients: a US National Transplant Registry analysis. *Transplant International* 2010;23(10):1038–1044.

23. Montenovo MI, Dick AA, Hansen RN. Donor hepatitis C sero-status does not impact survival in liver transplantation. *Annals of Transplantation* 2015;20:44–50.

20 Hepatocellular carcinoma and hepatitis C virus: which should be treated first?

Mario U. Mondelli[1,2], Andrea Lombardi[1,2], and Massimo Colombo[3]

[1] Division of Infectious Diseases II and Immunology, Department of Medical Sciences and Infectious Diseases, Fondazione IRCCS Policlinico San Matteo di Pavia, Pavia, Italy
[2] Department of Internal Medicine and Therapeutics, University of Pavia, Pavia, Italy
[3] Department of Internal Medicine, Center for Translational Research in Hepatology, Humanitas, Rozzano, Italy

---

LEARNING POINTS

- The short- and long-term effects of HCV eradication on the development of liver cancer remain in dispute and more research is needed.

- Personalized treatment taking account of liver dysfunction and HCC risk is required to optimize the benefits of therapy.

- In patients with or without a history of HCC harboring one or more liver nodules of undefined nature on contrast imaging, DAA therapy should be deferred by 6–12 months and started only after complete eradication of any HCC precursor lesion has been obtained.

Introduction

Since 2015, the widespread availability of direct-acting antivirals (DAAs) against hepatitis C virus (HCV) has radically changed the landscape of chronic hepatitis C treatment. These drugs are highly effective, well tolerated, can be taken orally, and treatment usually lasts for only about 8–12 weeks. The excellent tolerability profile allows treatment of patients with advanced liver disease, namely Child–Turcotte–Pugh (CTP) class B–C subjects, otherwise untreatable due to the risk of decompensation with former interferon (IFN)-based regimens [1].

While HCV cure leads to a significant reduction in complications associated with advanced liver disease [2], several retrospective studies and metaanalyses have reported a reduction in the risk of HCC development after successful HCV eradication, obtained with both former IFN-based regimens and new DAA-based regimens, emphasizing the importance of sustained virologic response (SVR) in reducing the risk of primary liver cancer [3–6]. Overall, in Western countries HCV infection is still the leading cause of HCC, whereas a significant number of patients with advanced liver disease remain at risk of developing HCC even after an SVR, worlwide [7].

Notwithstanding currently universal consensus on the beneficial effect of antiviral treatment in this setting [8,10], data are insufficient to suggest which must be treated first, HCC or HCV.

Treatment of HCV before tumor eradication

Hepatitis C virus cure before HCC treatment is especially relevant for those patients in the early stage (A) of the Barcelona Clinic Liver Cancer (BCLC) classification [11]. This stage enjoys several treatment options consisting of ablation, resection or transplantation. Indeed, a major advantage with HCV cure before liver transplantation is the prevention of posttransplant HCV recurrence. This has been clearly shown in patients with any genotype and compensated cirrhosis on the waiting list for liver transplantation for HCC, even when using a suboptimal regimen of sofosbuvir plus ribavirin [12]. It follows that higher proportions of posttransplant virologic responses were to be expected with the use of more efficient DAA combinations,

Clinical Dilemmas in Viral Liver Disease, Second Edition. Edited by Graham R. Foster and K. Rajender Reddy.
© 2020 John Wiley & Sons Ltd. Published 2020 by John Wiley & Sons Ltd.

as shown in one study reporting more than 75% of transplanted subjects, half of whom were beyond Milan criteria, achieving SVR with newer DAA generations [13]. Importantly, no difference in HCC recurrence rates were observed post transplant, irrespective of whether SVR was achieved before or after transplant. HCV eradication before liver transplantation may also reduce the risk of decompensation and death on the waiting list.

The potential model of end-stage liver disease (MELD) purgatory, an increase of time spent on the waiting list due to improved liver function that may occur with decompensated HCV without HCC, does not impact on HCC patients who are eligible for liver transplant through MELD exception points [14]. Moreover, viral eradication does not seem to be associated with an increased risk of dropout due to neoplastic progression in HCV/HCC patients awaiting liver transplantation, independently of tumor burden, differentiation, or microvascular invasion [15]. Of note, HCV eradication can also impact on survival after transplantation among subjects transplanted for HCC, as those persistently infected with HCV show lower posttransplant survival [16]. Moreover, selected patients achieving SVR can be referred for curative treatments as a result of improved liver function [17], although a minority of

patients with HCC can be delisted because of HCC progression. However, there is no rose without thorns, since the presence of active HCC, beside the competing risk of cancer-related mortality, is associated with a small but statistically significant decrease in SVR with DAA treatment [18–20]. Nonetheless, DAA therapy should not be denied to patients with complete response to HCC treatment. It must also be emphasized that patients with complete response to HCC therapy treated with DAA maintain a risk of HCC recurrence and require life-long HCC surveillance.

If a DAA treatment is planned before transplantation, the choice of medications must take into account liver and renal functions, which are frequently impaired in these patients. NS3 protease-containing regimens can be safely used only in patients with compensated cirrhosis but may perform better in those with renal insufficiency. The duration of DAA treatment should be as short as possible and DAA combinations achieving an SVR within 12 weeks should be preferred. Graft reinfection may be prevented in the majority of patients when a HCV RNA negative status is achieved at least four weeks before transplantation [21]. Table 20.1 summarizes the data available in the literature which highlight the advantages of HCV therapy before HCC treatment.

Table 20.1 Summary of studies investigating the impact of HCV eradication before HCC treatment

HCV First

Study	Comment
Terrault, *Transplantation* (2017)	HCV eradication before LT may reduce risk of decompensation and death on the waiting list
Curry, *Gastroenterology* (2015)	HCV eradication in the preliver transplant setting prevents recurrence of liver infection
Dumitra, *HPB* (2013)	HCV eradication before LT has been associated with higher survival in patients transplanted for HCC
Cabibbo, *J Hepatol* (2017)	Hepatic decompensation is the major driver of death in HCV-infected cirrhotic patients with successfully treated early HCC
Zanetto, *Liver Transplantation* (2017)	Viral eradication does not seem to be associated with an increased risk of dropout due to neoplastic progression in HCV-HCC patients awaiting LT
Pascasio, *J Hepatol* (2017)	HCV eradication was associated with an improvement of CTP score of HCC patients on the waiting list
Beste, *J Hepatol* (2017)	Reduced SVR rates in HCC (74.4%)
Prenner, *J Hepatol* (2017)	Reduced SVR rates in HCC (79%)
Chang, *Medicine* (2017)	Reduced SVR rates in HCC (82%)

CTP, Cihild–Turcotte–Pugh; HCC, hepatocellular carcinoma; HCV, hepatitis C virus; LT, liver transplantation; SVR, sustained virologic response.

Treatment of HCV after tumor eradication

Antiviral treatment of HCV after a cure of HCC is recommended by professional liver societies, owing to the fact that advanced hepatitis C complicated by liver cancer poses a substantial risk of lethal clinical decompensation if treatment of infection is deferred whereas the suppression of liver inflammation is thought to enhance the risk of developing *de novo* HCC [11,22]. Early attempts at achieving virus eradication using IFN-based regimens almost invariably met with limited success, due to poor uptake, tolerability, and efficacy of antiviral therapy in such a difficult-to-cure population as patients with advanced hepatitis C and a history of liver cancer. Although a per protocol analysis of 10 studies of adjuvant therapy with IFN reported a 40% reduction of tumor recurrence in this population that translated into a significantly prolonged patient survival, these optimistic findings are clouded by the lack of an intention-to-treat analysis of outcomes [6].

Following the advent of IFN-free DAA regimens, HCV eradication is now possible in virtually all patients with advanced hepatitis C, including those with a history of HCC, thereby subverting the prognosis of this fragile patient population [23]. This notwithstanding, an area of uncertainty remains regarding both efficacy and safety of this novel therapeutic regimen in patients with a history of HCC. In fact, in a recent report of veterans with advanced hepatitis C who were treated with DAAs, a history of HCC was more often collected among nonresponders than among responders (13.7% versus 4.8%, p<0.001), a finding that matches previous observations at Veteran Affairs hospitals [24]. The use of DAAs in this patient population has also raised safety concerns when unusual rates of early and severe exacerbation of tumor recurrence were reported in DAA-treated patients who exhibited a complete radiologic response to resection or radiofrequency ablation of a small tumor [8,9]. While the debate on DAA safety in these patients at risk of tumor recurrence was fueled by the lack of robust, prospectively collected controlled data, evidence is now emerging that HCC more often recurred in DAA-treated patients with cirrhosis and a preexisting liver nodule of undefined nature at imaging [25,26].

While these findings point to the presence of histologic precursors of HCC, a basis for DAA-induced exacerbation of tumor recurrence, another study tried to identify local predisposing factors that escape imaging detection like an excess tissue expression of the proangiogenetic factor angiopoietin-2 [8,27]. While these hypotheses point to a link between enhanced tumor recurrence and a disturbance of immune surveillance, caused by a swift removal of HCV which favors enhanced proliferation of sparse cancer cells in patients with a cured tumor [28], they found some credit by reports of hepatitis B and herpes virus reactivation taking place in HCV coinfected patients after DAA therapy of HCV [29,30]. Yet, with all the caveats of the retrospective design, a large multicenter study in the USA was unable to highlight any faster tumor recurrence, enhanced incidence and clinical aggressiveness of the recurrence in DAA-treated versus DAA-untreated patients [31]. This is also the message of the histologic analysis of liver resections collected in 18 hospitals in Italy where the rates of tumor cell grading, portal invasion, and satellitosis did not differ between DAA-treated and -untreated patients [32].

Finally, DAA therapy also appears to be safe in waitlisted patients who underwent either bridge therapy or downstaging with locoablative techniques, where HCV eradication proved to be clinically advantageous. In a retrospective study at a single center, in fact, not only was the risk of HCC recurrence similar in DAA-treated patients compared to those without DAA, but patients treated with DAA faced a lower risk of waitlist dropout due to tumor progression or death compared to DAA-untreated patients in adjusted weighted analysis (hazard ratio 0.30, 95% confidence interval 0.13–0.69, p=0.005) [33].

In the end, the few reports of DAA therapy associated with enhanced risk of HCC recurrence are outnumbered by studies that denied any link between DAA therapy and exacerbation of tumor recurrence, although data analysis of both positive and negative studies was clouded by relevant methodologic weaknesses due to heterogeneity of patient selection and HCC treatment coupled with the lack of prospective surveillance for HCC. This notwithstanding, reports of unusual rates of tumor recurrence might be biased by a cohort effect, as patient age, liver disease severity, response to DAA, and possibly timing and modality of cancer treatment often emerged as independent predictors of tumor recurrence.

All in all, these uncertainties make it difficult to determine meaningful recommendations for optimizing DAA therapy in this patient population. Table 20.2 summarizes the data available in the literature which highlight the advantages of HCV therapy before HCC treatment.

Table 20.2 Summary of studies investigating the impact of HCV eradication after HCC treatment

HCC First

Study	Comment
Reig, *J Hepatol* (2016)	A multicenter study in Spain showing unusual rates and severity of tumor recurrence after DAA
Conti, *J Hepatol* (2016)	A single-center study in Italy showing unusual rates and severity of tumor recurrence after DAA
El Kassas, *J Viral Hepatol* (2018)	A multicenter study in Egypt showing increased rates of tumor recurrence after DAA
Waziry, *J Hepatol* (2017)	A metaanalysis of seven initial studies denying increased tumor recurrence after DAA
Sarayia, *APT* (2018)	A metaanalysis of nine recent studies denying increased tumor recurrence after DAA
Huang, *Hepatology* (2018)	DAA therapy after HCC eradication in waitlisted patient does not affect rates and severity of tumor recurrence while reducing the rates of dropouts
Singal, *Gastroenterology* (2019)	A multicenter study in the USA showing that DAAs are not tied to tumor recurrence
Zoe Marino, *J Hepatol* (2019)	Noncharacterized liver nodules are associated to higher tumor recurrence after DAA

DAA, direct-acting antiviral; HCC, hepatocellular carcinoma.

Conclusion

In conclusion, an unequivocal answer on which must be treated first between HCV and HCC cannot be safely provided. The choice must take into account the patient's liver function, the therapeutic path chosen for HCC, and the long-term prognosis. More data are needed to evaluate the long-term effect of HCV eradication in HCC-treated subjects, to estimate the cost-effectiveness of treatment, and establish a timely and personalized approach to HCV treatment in candidates for liver transplantation for HCC. In patients with or without a history of HCC harboring one or more liver nodules of undefined nature on contrast imaging, DAA therapy should be deferred by 6–12 months and started only after complete eradication of any HCC precursor lesion has been obtained.

References

1. European Association for the Study of the Liver. EASL recommendations on treatment of hepatitis C 2018. *Journal of Hepatology* 2017;66:153–194.
2. Bruno S, Marco V Di, Iavarone M et al. Survival of patients with HCV cirrhosis and sustained virologic response is similar to the general population. *Journal of Hepatology* 2016;64:1217–1223.
3. Morgan RL, Baack B, Smith BD et al. Eradication of hepatitis C virus infection and the development of hepatocellular carcinoma. *Annals of Internal Medicine* 2013;158:329–337.
4. Kanogawa N, Ogasawara S, Chiba T et al. Sustained virologic response achieved after curative treatment of HCV-related hepatocellular carcinoma serves as an independent prognostic factor. *Journal of Gastroenterology and Hepatology* 2015;30:1197–1204.
5. Calvaruso V, Cabibbo G, Cacciola I et al. Incidence of hepatocellular carcinoma in patients with HCV-associated cirrhosis treated with direct-acting antiviral agents. *Gastroenterology* 2018;155:411–421.
6. Singal AK, Singh A, Jaganmohan S et al. Antiviral therapy reduces risk of hepatocellular carcinoma in patients with hepatitis C virus-related cirrhosis. *Clinical Gastroenterology and Hepatology* 2010;8:192–199.
7. Yang JD, Roberts LR. Hepatocellular carcinoma: a global view. *Nature Reviews Gastroenterology and Hepatology* 2010;7:448–458.
8. Reig M, Mariño Z, Perelló C et al. Unexpected early tumor recurrence in patients with hepatitis C virus-related hepatocellular carcinoma undergoing interferon-free therapy: a note of caution. *Journal of Hepatology* 2016;65:719–726.
9. Conti F, Buonfiglioli F, Scuteri A et al. Early occurrence and recurrence of hepatocellular carcinoma in HCV-related cirrhosis treated with direct-acting antivirals. *Journal of Hepatology* 2016;65:727–733.
10. Backus L, Belperio PS, Shahoumian TA et al. Impact of sustained virologic response with direct-acting antiviral treatment on mortality in patients with advanced liver disease. *Hepatology* 2019;69:487–497.
11. European Association for the Study of the Liver. EASL Clinical Practice Guidelines: Management of hepatocellular carcinoma. *Journal of Hepatology* 2018;69:182–236.
12. Curry MP, Forns X, Chung RT et al. Sofosbuvir and ribavirin prevent recurrence of hcv infection after liver transplantation: an open-label study. *Gastroenterology* 2015;148:100–107.e1.
13. Emamaullee J, Bral M, Meeberg G et al. HCV eradication with DAA therapy should be attempted prior to liver transplantation and does not impact HCC recurrence (abstract).

https://atcmeetingabstracts.com/abstract/hcv-eradication-with-daa-therapy-should-be-attempted-prior-to-liver-transplantation-and-does-not-impact-hcc-recurrence/

14. Terrault NA, McCaughan GW, Curry MP et al. International Liver Transplantation Society Consensus Statement on Hepatitis C Management in Liver Transplant Candidates. *Transplantation* 2017;101:945–955.

15. Zanetto A, Shalaby S, Vitale A et al. Dropout rate from the liver transplant waiting list because of hepatocellular carcinoma progression in hepatitis C virus–infected patients treated with direct-acting antivirals. *Liver Transplantation* 2017;23:1103–1112.

16. Dumitra S, Alabbad SI, Barkun JS et al. Hepatitis C infection and hepatocellular carcinoma in liver transplantation: a 20-year experience. *HPB* 2013;15:724–731.

17. Pascasio JM, Vinaixa C, Ferrer MT et al. Clinical outcomes of patients undergoing antiviral therapy while awaiting liver transplantation. *Journal of Hepatology* 2017;67:1168–1176.

18. Prenner SB, VanWagner LB, Flamm SL et al. Hepatocellular carcinoma decreases the chance of successful hepatitis C virus therapy with direct-acting antivirals. *Journal of Hepatology* 2017;66:1173–1181.

19. Beste LA, Green PK, Berry K et al. Effectiveness of hepatitis C antiviral treatment in a USA cohort of veteran patients with hepatocellular carcinoma. *Journal of Hepatology* 2017; 67:32–39.

20. Chang CY, Nguyen P, Le A et al. Real-world experience with interferon-free, direct acting antiviral therapies in Asian Americans with chronic hepatitis C and advanced liver disease. *Medicine* 2017;96:e6128.

21. Belli LS, Duvoux C, Berenguer M et al. ELITA consensus statements on the use of DAAs in liver transplant candidates and recipients. *Journal of Hepatology* 2017;67:585–602.

22. Cabibbo G, Petta S, Barbara M et al. Hepatic decompensation is the major driver of death in HCV-infected cirrhotic patients with successfully treated early hepatocellular carcinoma. *Journal of Hepatology* 2017;67:65–71.

23. Backus LI, Belperio PS, Shahoumian TA et al. Direct-acting antiviral sustained virologic response: impact on mortality in patients without advanced liver disease. *Hepatology* 2018;68: 827–838.

24. Ioannou GN, Green PK, Beste LA et al. Development of models estimating the risk of hepatocellular carcinoma after antiviral treatment for hepatitis C. *Journal of Hepatology* 2018;69:1088–1098.

25. Scott RA, Aithal GP, Francis ST et al. Pretreatment lesions on magnetic resonance imaging in patients with hepatitis C virus infection diagnosed with hepatocellular carcinoma after initiating direct-acting antiviral therapy. *Gastroenterology* 2018; 154:1848–1850.

26. Mariño Z, Darnell A, Lens S et al. Time association between HCV therapy and hepatocellular carcinoma emergence in patients with cirrhosis. The relevance of non-characterized nodules. *Journal of Hepatology* 2019;70:874–884.

27. Faillaci F, Marzi L, Critelli R et al. Liver angiopoietin-2 is a key predictor of de novo or recurrent hepatocellular cancer after hepatitis C virus direct-acting antivirals. *Hepatology* 2018;68:1010–1024.

28. Reig M, Boix L, Mariño Z et al. Liver cancer emergence associated with antiviral treatment: an immune surveillance failure? *Seminars in Liver Disease* 2017;37:109–118.

29. Perelló MC, Fernández-Carrillo C, Londoño MC et al. Reactivation of herpesvirus in patients with hepatitis C treated with direct-acting antiviral agents. *Clinical Gastroenterology and Hepatology* 2016;14:1662–1666.e1.

30. Collins JM, Raphael KL, Terry C et al. Hepatitis B virus reactivation during successful treatment of hepatitis C virus with sofosbuvir and simeprevir. *Clinical Infectious Diseases* 2015;61: 1304–1306.

31. Singal AG, Rich NE, Mehta N et al. Direct-acting antiviral therapy not associated with recurrence of hepatocellular carcinoma in a multicenter North American cohort study. *Gastroenterology* 2019;156:1683–1692.

32. Vitale A, Russo FP, Sposito C et al. Pathological characteristics and early post-hepatic-resection outcome of patients with hepatocellular carcinoma occurred after hepatitis C treatment with new direct-acting antivirals: a multicenter cohort study characteristics. *Journal of Hepatology* 2018;68:s15.

33. Huang AC, Mehta N, Dodge JL et al. Direct-acting antivirals do not increase the risk of hepatocellular carcinoma recurrence after local-regional therapy or liver transplant waitlist dropout. *Hepatology* 2018;68:449–461.

21

Should we incentivize patients to take hepatitis C virus therapy?

Ed Gane

University of Auckland, Auckland, New Zealand

LEARNING POINTS

- Barriers to hepatitis C elimination include low diagnosis rates and poor linkage to care in those already diagnosed.

- In marginalized patient populations, there are additional barriers including stigma associated with the diagnosis of hepatitis C and lack of access to specialists and funded treatment.

- Incentivization, either with money or with peer support or other benefits, has been demonstrated to improve testing and uptake of TB and HIV treatment in people with substance abuse.

- Pilot studies have demonstrated that incentivization can improve testing and treatment of hepatitis C in previously difficult-to-reach patient populations, including people who inject drugs and prisoners.

Introduction

The recent development of safe and highly effective oral direct-acting antiviral (DAA) therapy has seen a paradigm shift in the management of this condition and provides a means to cure HCV and prevent all complications, thereby removing this as a major public health threat. In May 2016, the World Health Organization announced the Global Hepatitis Strategy, with the goal of eliminating viral hepatitis as a major public health threat. Specific targets include a 90% reduction in new hepatitis C infections, 80% rate of treatment uptake, and a 65% reduction in liver-related deaths by 2030.

However, more than three years after the introduction of DAAs, progress towards global elimination of hepatitis C has been disappointing. In many countries with unrestricted access to fully funded DAA therapy, HCV cure rates remain well below the 7–10% needed to achieve the WHO 2030 elimination targets. This is despite an increase in diagnosis rates thanks to public awareness campaigns and community-based testing programs (including targeted testing and birth cohort screening).

The major reason for low cure rates is poor linkage to care in newly diagnosed patients. This may reflect geographic and social isolation, and lack of local expertise or funding for DAA therapy. Patients may be unaware of the availability and benefits of DAA therapy, or have competing health or social needs, which make treatment of their HCV infection a low priority. Itinerant patients may simply be unable to afford the clinic visits or prescription charges.

Even when patients do initiate treatment, psychosocial factors may result in nonadherence, loss to follow-up, and treatment failure.

The benefits to the community from successful treatment of people who inject drugs (PWID) are clear – stopping transmission, improving survival, and reducing the costs of complications and hospitalization. Cure is also associated with reduced stigma, improved quality of life, and an associated increase in productivity.

Contingency management (CM) is a form of operant conditioning that uses stimulus control and positive reinforcement to change someone's behavior. In the field of

Clinical Dilemmas in Viral Liver Disease, Second Edition. Edited by Graham R. Foster and K. Rajender Reddy.
© 2020 John Wiley & Sons Ltd. Published 2020 by John Wiley & Sons Ltd.

substance abuse, CM uses incentivization, with money or other benefits, and has been demonstrated to improve testing and treatment uptake for HIV and TB.

People who inject drugs have a high incidence of hepatitis, HIV, and TB infections and delayed diagnosis, reduced treatment uptake, and poor adherence to specific therapy [1]. Although increasing number of PWIDs are diagnosed with HCV within targeted testing programs in needle exchanges, opioid substitution therapy programs, and community addiction centers, few are linked to care, and even fewer initiate or complete treatment. Therefore, there is considerable interest in using CM or incentivization to improve diagnosis, treatment uptake, and adherence in the PWID population who have previously been difficult to engage.

A simple example of CM has been the linking of daily observed therapy (DOT) of antimicrobial therapy with methadone dispensing [2]. In a study of PWID receiving isoniazid (INH) prophylaxis following TB exposure, completion rates for INH therapy were higher in those patients randomly assigned to methadone treatment combined with directly observed preventive treatment (methadone arm) compared to those assigned to routine TB clinic referral without methadone treatment (control arm). Pulmonary tuberculosis was subsequently diagnosed in none of the patients in the methadone arm compared to 4% of the control arm. In a systematized review of 23 controlled studies evaluating the impact of incentive-based treatment approaches, adherence rates averaged almost 35% higher among patients receiving incentives compared to controls [3].

The impact of financial incentives on treatment uptake and adherence has also been studied in PWID. The incremental small cost of such incentives seems justified given the high cost of DAA therapy. In a small pilot study at a New York needle exchange, 39 injecting drug users recently diagnosed with HCV infection received either usual care plus cash incentives ($25 per visit) or usual care (which included transport to and from the clinic). Compared to those who received usual care alone, patients who received the cash incentive had higher rates of linkage to care (74% versus 40%) and treatment initiation (53% versus 10%) [4].

In a larger pilot study at Chapel Hill, different types of financial incentives were evaluated [5]. Fifty-nine patients with substance abuse disorders and HCV infection were randomized to two different types of cash incentives – either "fixed cash incentive" ($40 each scheduled visit plus bonus of $20 for each pill count demonstrating adherence of >90% plus bonus of $50 for achieving sustained virologic response [SVR]) or "lottery cash incentive" (where patients drew a card from a bag to determine whether they received $10, $50 or $100 for each milestone). Both forms of cash incentives achieved excellent results – on intention-to-treat, 95% of patients started treatment, a very high rate for PWID. Of those randomized to fixed cash incentives, 93% achieved SVR compared to 92% of those randomized to lottery cash incentives. Adherence was similar, with 92% of both groups attending all clinic visits. Pill adherence based on electronic medication monitoring (MEMSCaps) was 92% for fixed cash incentive patients who achieved SVR compared to 91% of those receiving lottery cash incentives. These results were much greater than reported previously in patients with substance abuse disorders, suggesting that cash incentives improve treatment uptake and outcome.

Additional support with peers, usually people who injected drugs in the past (peer support), has also been demonstrated to be effective in reducing stigma, increasing testing and linkage to care in patients with HIV infection, enabling them to reduce perceived stigma, improve knowledge, and enhance well-being [6].

A study conducted at Johns Hopkins Hospital evaluated whether the assignment of a dedicated peer mentor would be as successful as financial incentives in increasing HCV treatment initiation and adherence in patients with substance abuse disorders. In the CHAMPS study, 144 patients coinfected with HIV and HCV genotype 1 undergoing treatment with 12 weeks Harvoni® were randomized (1:2:2) to either usual care (nurse supervision only) or usual care plus peer-mentors (trained HIV+ peers previously cured from HCV and recruited from active support groups in the clinic), or usual care plus cash incentives (escalating cash incentives up to a maximum of $230, contingent on clinic attendance). The primary endpoint, initiation of Harvoni, was higher in both the peer mentor (88%) and cash incentive (77%) groups compared to usual care (66%). SVR rates after randomization were also higher in both the peer mentor (76%) and cash incentive (69%) groups compared to usual care (61%). However, in those patients who actually started Harvoni, SVR rates were similar across the three groups (91%, 90%, and 91% respectively) [7].

The prison population consists of marginalized individuals with a very high prevalence of HCV infection and a high rate of HCV transmission. Targeted "test and treat" campaigns in prisons should improve prisoner well-being and as a "treatment-as-prevention" initiative should accelerate national HCV elimination programs. The availability of well-tolerated DAAs should allow effective treatment in this hard-to-reach population. However, the stigma associated with HCV infection and illicit drug use has hindered uptake of testing and treatment within prisons. Therefore, incentivizing testing and treatment in prisons would seem worthwhile. In the United Kingdom, NHS England financially incentivize the regional Operational Delivery Networks (ODNs) to establish links with prisons to facilitate identification and treatment of HCV cases in the prison population in their region [8]. An innovative incentive-based test and treat study in Australia pays prisoners directly. More than 30 000 prisoners have been recruited into the SToP-C study, of whom approximately 25% have HCV infection. A $10 payment is provided for each study visit (including testing, counseling, and treatment) as reimbursement for their time. This money is deposited into the participant's individual bank account and used to buy items from the prison stores.

In addition to improving diagnosis and treatment uptake in high-risk populations such as PWID and prisoners, there has been recent interest in the role of incentives in national screening programs. In the extremely successful Egyptian National HCV Elimination Project, HCV testing is incentivized by combining with free health assessments including diabetes and hypertension.

In New Zealand, a community-based HepC elimination campaign includes financial incentives for both general practitioners (GPs) and patients. GPs receive $100 per patient started on treatment which is designed to supplement the government subsidy for each visit. Patients can also apply for government funding to cover any ancillary expenses during treatment such as food, travel, or GP fees. In the first three years of this initiative, the proportion of patients treated in the community has increased steadily from less than 5% to more than 60%.

Conclusion

In summary, contingency management approaches, including financial incentives for testing and treatment, may help increase HCV diagnosis rates and linkage to care in both the marginalized PWID and prisoners and also the wider population.

References

1. Arnsten J, Demas A, Farzadegan H et al. Antiretroviral therapy adherence and viral suppression in HIV-infected drug users: comparison of self-report and electronic monitoring. *Clinical Infectious Diseases* 2001;33:1417–1423.
2. Batki S, Gruber V, Bradley J et al. A controlled trial of methadone treatment combined with directly observed isoniazid for tuberculosis prevention in injection drug users. *Drug and Alcohol Dependence* 2002;66:283–293.
3. Herrmann E, Matusiewicz A, Stitzer M et al. Contingency management interventions for HIV, tuberculosis, and hepatitis control among individuals with substance use disorders: a systematized review. *Journal of Substance Abuse Treatment* 2017;17:117–125.
4. Norton B, Singh R, Agyemang L, Litwin A. Contingency management improves HCV linkage and treatment outcomes in persons who inject drugs: a pilot study. www.eiseverywhere.com/file_uploads/3ec71e35a4212210edcc74b7bd715909_163_BriannaNorton.pdf
5. Wohl D, Allmon A, Evon D, et al. Financial incentives for adherence to HCV clinical care and treatment: a randomized trial of two strategies. *Open Forum Infectious Diseases* 2017;4:ofx095
6. Marino P, Simoni JM, Silverstein LB. Peer support to promote medication adherence among people living with HIV/AIDS: the benefits to peers. *Social Work in Health Care* 2007;45:67–80.
7. Sulkowski M, Ward K, Falade-Nwulia O et al. Randomized controlled trial of cash incentives or peer mentors to improve HCV linkage and treatment among HIV/HCV coinfected persons who inject drugs: the CHAMPS Study. *Journal of Hepatology* 2017;66:S543–S750.
8. Public Health England. National engagement event for bloodborne virus (BBV) opt-out testing in prisons in England. Kia Oval, London, 30 November 2017.

22

Treating prisoners with hepatitis C: should we do it and how?

Seth Francis-Graham and William Rosenberg

Institute for Liver and Digestive Health, Division of Medicine, University College London, London, UK

LEARNING POINTS

- Testing and treating people with HCV in prisons is an important component of any elimination plan.

- Training is essential and if multiple agencies are to be used to deliver training, it is crucial that their messages are coordinated to ensure consistency.

- It is essential that any health initiative is supported by prison staff. Securing the support of the governors is essential and prison staff engagement should be incentivized.[xbl][xkpt]

- Opt-out testing is important but needs to be appropriately developed and approved to avoid coercion. An offer that presents testing as the default but also provides a verbal sense-check for consent may be a suitable middle ground and a written script should be used as a guide and combined with detailed staff training on the concept of "opt-out" and informed consent.

- Easy-to-use therapies are essential and pre- and post-treatment testing should be minimized.

Introduction

With the advent of second-generation direct-acting antiviral treatments (DAAs), which are oral, short course, well tolerated, and highly effective (>95%), the feasibility of large-scale case detection and treatment of chronic hepatitis C (CHCV) has become a reality [1]. Focus has fallen on the target of elimination, solidified by the UK's support of the WHO Global Health Sector Strategy on Viral Hepatitis [2].

For elimination to be achieved, widespread testing combined with rapid treatment needs to be in place, supported by harm reduction measures to prevent new infection [3]. However, more work is required to develop robust care pathways that effectively detect infection, which is often asymptomatic [1], and then quickly progress patients to treatment and cure.

Two options for case detection present themselves. Policymakers could consider universal screening; however, such an approach would be cost-intensive and only cost-effective if population prevalence is high and treatment widespread. Another option is to focus screening on population groups at increased risk of infection, increasing the likelihood of finding cases and reducing the cost per case detected. In the USA, universal screening was rejected in favour of birth cohort screening, in light of the high prevalence of infection amongst "baby boomers" [4]. The UK is taking a similar approach, targeting testing amongst high-risk groups.

In the UK, the most common route of HCV transmission is via injecting drug use (IDU). In England, IDU is cited as a risk in around 90% of all laboratory reports where risk factors have been disclosed [3]. Consequently, HCV is reported as being most prevalent in present or "ever" injectors in the UK. The criminalization of drug use and the relationship between drug dependency and crime both mean that people who inject drugs (PWID) pass through the prison estate [5]. Therefore, testing in prisons should reveal a high prevalence of HCV. Furthermore, patients' detention in prison should offer an ideal opportunity to

Clinical Dilemmas in Viral Liver Disease, Second Edition. Edited by Graham R. Foster and K. Rajender Reddy.
© 2020 John Wiley & Sons Ltd. Published 2020 by John Wiley & Sons Ltd.

provide treatment, or at the very least information and linkage to care, before they reengage with potentially chaotic lifestyles in the community.

Response

Opt-out testing for HIV in the antenatal setting was introduced in the 1990s and has been widely credited as being successful in diagnosing infection [6]. A similar approach might prove effective in the prison setting, with people being tested on entry into the prison estate for HCV, hepatitis B (HBV), and the human immunodeficiency virus (HIV), unless they explicitly decline.

In 2013, a multiagency meeting including Public Health England (PHE), NHS England (NHSE), and Her Majesty's Prison and Probation Service (HMPPS) formally agreed to implement an opt-out blood-borne virus (BBV) test strategy in prison. Phased implementation began during 2014, with 11 "pathfinder prisons" introducing opt-out testing. PHE developed and disseminated guidance notes. However, this guidance afforded commissioners and healthcare providers significant flexibility [7].

Guidance primarily focused on testing (Figure 22.1). However, no explicit information was provided about what comprises an "opt-out" offer and how that offer should be delivered. Additionally, no prescriptive instructions were provided on referral and treatment. Instead, the guidance presented a "wishlist" of ideals. These included the fact that short sentences, release, or transfer should not be a barrier to treatment; that treatment should be delivered within prison; and that care pathways should include access to other relevant services (i.e., mental health and drug and alcohol treatment) [7].

NHS operational delivery networks (ODNs) (networks set up to coordinate the assessment and treatment of HCV), established in 2016, were encouraged to innovate models of care delivery within prisons. However, OD's faced their own challenges, having been assigned minimum and maximum treatment targets, enforced by financial penalties [8]. They were also required to restrict access to treatment to those at greatest risk of harm, mainly those with the most advanced disease [8]. Ideals on how treatment should be delivered, set out by PHE, did not take account of these restrictions and many ODNs had little experience of working with the prison estate.

In March 2015, PHE published a questionnaire-based evaluation of the opt-out program, reporting a doubling of HCV testing (from 11% between January and December 2013 to 21% between April and September 2014) [7]. An additional 14 prisons implemented testing as a second wave in 2014–15, and a further eight in a tertiary wave in 2015. Similar questionnaire-based evaluative activities were undertaken, focused on linkage to care (for phase 2 pathfinders) [9] and treatment effectiveness (for phase 3 pathfinders) [10].

During phase 2 and phase 3 evaluations, PHE began to report that the lack of standardization of opt-out testing and linkage to care may have inhibited performance, with few prisons reporting that they adhered to established BBV pathway algorithms [9]. However, following phase 1, the NHS had increasingly taken over program implementation, with PHE taking an "advisory" role. Full roll-out across the rest of the English estate continued, unguided by an evidence-based model of best practice or intensive national coordination, with universal implementation achieved in March 2018.

Challenges and solutions

Several challenges presented themselves following the implementation of opt-out BBV testing and the associated HCV pathways of care.

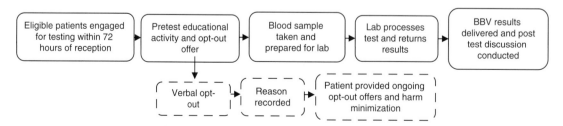

Figure 22.1 Opt-out BBV test algorithm, as recommended by Public Health England in collaboration with NHS England and the Her Majesty's Prison and Probation Service.

Staff training

As implementation switched from piloting activities to roll-out, it became apparent that stakeholders lacked awareness of each other. Prison health teams had little understanding of HCV treatment and ODNs had little understanding of how prison health teams operated or might be enabled to deliver services [8].

Confusion was increased by the involvement of multiple agencies in delivering training. Different agencies emphasized different aspects of care and, at times, provided contradictory messages. This led to situations where an ODN had developed a care pathway with one group of prison nurses, whilst a separate organization had established a different pathway with another group working in the same prison. There was also a general lack of clarity about the goal of elimination and an exaggerated focus on opt-out testing, making treatment and cure seem like an afterthought.

Finally, although commitment to implement opt-out testing existed amongst HMPPS commissioners, little information had filtered down to prison governors or staff and HMPPS ran no training for prison officers. This oversight was significant, as health services are entirely dependent on prison officers to unlock prisoners and escort them to clinics. When news did reach prison management, the opt-out strategy was frequently viewed as "one more" health initiative that they would have to facilitate, costing additional time, money, and personnel [8].

Solution

All stakeholders need to share a common goal of elimination. This requires that they communicate and understand one another's roles. If multiple agencies are to be used to deliver training, it is crucial that their messages are coordinated to ensure consistency. Finally, it is essential that any health initiative is supported by prison staff. Securing the support of the governors is essential and prison staff engagement should be incentivized.

The opt-out

The lack of prescriptive instruction on what constitutes an opt-out offer and how to deliver it became the "elephant in the room" during meetings on HCV elimination. This oversight stemmed from the way interventions are frequently recycled in commissioning.

Inspiration to make testing "opt-out" came from the success of opt-out antenatal HIV testing. However, it is wrong to assume that making testing "opt-out" for BBVs within prison will necessarily have the same effect, as prison clinics and antenatal clinics are very different contexts. PHE and NHSE should have explored how "opt-out" is thought to increase engagement with testing. If they had done this, they would have discovered the "default effect", a theory from behavioral economics which suggests that for any decision, most people will stick with the default option [11].

Some psychologists believe the default effect works because individuals interpret the default option as an implicit recommendation [11]. Most mothers, concerned about the health of their newborn baby, are likely to accept an apparent recommendation from a trusted medical authority. In contrast, a large proportion of freshly incarcerated people are likely to feel some level of animosity or distrust towards "the state" and in turn healthcare staff offering a test.

This is not to say that opt-out testing within prison cannot be effective. An implicit recommendation is just one of many ways in which opt-out is thought to increase uptake. The point is that "opt-out" is a social intervention and therefore its success or failure hinges on the social and physical context in which it is implemented [12].

Solution

Policy makers need to spend more time engaging with the underpinning theories of opt-out and consider how they can use these to maximize testing.

Opt-out and informed consent

Without consensus on what an opt-out offer involves, evaluative work suggested significant variation in delivery, from "opt-in" to mandatory testing (Figure 22.2). Reports that health workers misinterpreted what is meant by opt-out and told prisoners that they must be tested are concerning but relatively easy to address via training.

More challenging are concerns that the social context of prison itself could lead to large numbers of prisoners assuming that testing for HCV is mandatory. Prisoners have much of their autonomy stripped away and the prison setting is one where coercion and mandatory instructions are commonplace.

In this environment, policymakers must think carefully about the wording used to offer testing [13]. Telling someone that you are going to test them unless they decline may inadvertently encourage prisoners to decline, whereas

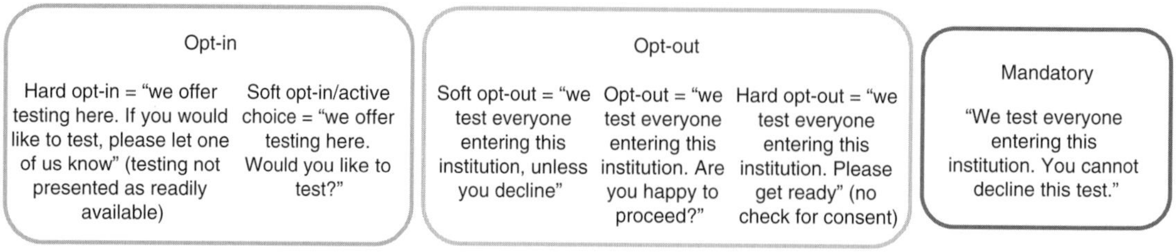

Figure 22.2 Different types of test offer, from a hard opt-in approach, where testing is not presented as readily available to the patient, to a mandatory test offer, where a patient is explicitly told they cannot decline the test. Authors recommend the middle opt-out approach, where testing is presented as the default option, but a "sense-check" for consent is also administered.

a "hard opt-out" offer (see Figure 22.2), where there is potential ambiguity about the nature of testing, could be perceived as mandatory by many prisoners. Work by Rosen et al. within a US prison, for example, found that less than 40% of prisoners understood they could refuse an opt-out HIV test [13].

Solution

More evidence is required to determine how, and whether, opt-out can be delivered within prison in a manner that ensures high engagement, whilst respecting principles of informed consent. An offer that presents testing as the default, but also provides a verbal sense-check for consent, may be a suitable middle ground [14]. To reduce offer variability, a written script should be used as a guide and combined with detailed staff training on the concept of "opt-out" and informed consent.

When to offer

It is advisable for all health teams to offer testing soon after reception, to prevent attrition due to release or transfer. Two clinics present themselves as opportune: "first reception" (a clinic hosted on the night someone enters the prison) and "second reception" (usually held within 72 hours of someone entering the prison) [15].

First reception is time pressured and a bewildering time for prisoners. The introduction of HCV testing here has met with strong opposition. Arguments cite a lack of time and that prisoners are not in the right frame of mind to test (having likely spent a long and stressful day at court). Additionally, a relatively high proportion of new receptions may suffer from unchecked mental health issues and substance withdrawal and therefore may lack the capacity to provide consent [16,17].

Second reception is usually less time pressured and designed to allow a longer interaction. However, any delay in engaging new receptions will likely result in some attrition in remand prisons (which hold short-stay sentenced and unsentenced prisoners). This is further frustrated by failure of prisoners to attend second-day screening [18]. Common reasons include the clinic being cancelled because of incidents (lockdown, emergencies), officers not being able to facilitate the clinic, and prisoners refusing to attend (a particular problem if second day is run at the same time as "association," which is prisoners' free time out of their cell to catch up with friends, make phone calls, and have a shower).

Solution

Testing is recommended for either first- or second-day screening, depending on the specific circumstances of each prison. Training prisons (holding long-stay prisoners), which receive high levels of clinic attendance, may get away with offering testing only at second day. However, remand prisons should consider offering testing at first night and second day, to balance risk of release and capacity to consent. Reception-based testing should also be supported by a "catch-up" test program, for those who have missed testing or who have tested and subsequently put themselves at risk.

Diagnosis and assessment

Initially, diagnosis and assessment involved sequential antibody then molecular RNA testing to confirm chronic infection [19]. Following a provisional diagnosis, phlebotomy was required to assess liver function and many ODNs recommended transient elastography to assess liver fibrosis. Problems with venous access meant that some patients required a specialist phlebotomist and prisons that lacked access to a FibroScan® found it difficult to assess liver fibrosis and struggled to bring scanners into prisons or transport prisoners to hospital clinics for assessment.

Solution

With the development and availability of accurate serologic tests for fibrosis, such as the enhanced liver fibrosis test [20,21], all tests required to assess a patient's infection and disease status can be achieved from a single blood draw, with results available within 1–2 days.

Linkage to care

Reliance on ODN staff to visit the prison, explain test results, link patients into care, and administer treatment is unnecessary and adds vulnerability to the pathway. Staffing changes (requiring fresh security clearance), prison incidents, and lockdowns can all prevent ODN staff from entering the prison. Furthermore, finding patients within the prison can be challenging for outside staff. These factors lead to unnecessary delays and risk significant attrition. Prison health staff are capable of conducting assessment and linkage to care, as well as delivering DAA treatments with minimal supervision from their local ODN.

Solution

Close collaboration between prison health services and the local liver unit is important, particularly in terms of the management of cirrhosis, which requires specialist hepatology input. However, this should not become an unnecessarily dependent relationship. It is better to invest in training of prison staff, so that they can offer and conduct assessment tests, explain results, link patients into care, and administer treatment with minimal supervision, as they have greater access to patients.

Treatment

NHSE treatment policies mandated that ODNs should discuss all cases at multidisciplinary team (MDT) meetings, to determine the need for treatment and specify what drugs should be used [8]. This requires communication of detailed information from the prison team to the MDT.

Many prisoners are also prescribed a range of medications that may interact with DAAs. The inclusion of pharmacists in the ODN MDTs helps identify drug–drug interactions and recommend alternative treatments, but changes in treatment are often difficult to institute within prison.

Early HCV treatment regimens enforced by NHSE through the ODNs prescribed genotype-specific treatments, some of which incorporated ribavirin, comprising different dosing regimens and lasting for different durations. This complexity proved daunting for prison healthcare teams. Furthermore, NHSE reimbursed ODNs after they reported treatment outcomes. This proved to be particularly challenging in the prison population, where transfer and release make it hard to perform follow-up testing to confirm sustained viral response (SVR) (i.e., cure).

Solution

The advent of ribavirin-free, once-per-day, pangenotypic regimens has made treatment much easier to manage in prisons. Prisons should be enabled to make preferential use of these drugs. Removal of the requirement for SVR48 blood tests by NHSE has made it easier to confirm treatment outcomes.

Referral

Difficulties with managing referrals from prisons can disrupt continuity of care. In remand prisons, where patients cycle rapidly in and out of custody, not all prisoners can be treated within the prison. Furthermore, the timing of release can often be unpredictable, especially for those prisoners awaiting sentencing (i.e., "on remand").

There is often considerable uncertainty around the destination of domicile after release and once patients are released, prison health staff often struggle to access this information.

Finally, there is often uncertainty around the point-of-care contact in the community for patients, making it challenging for the patient to then attempt to reengage with care post release, whilst simultaneously trying to reorder other parts of their life [22].

Solution

It is important to recognize that diagnosis and education, with or without onward referral, empowers patients and is a valuable experience. However, considerable work is required to make patient referral from prison robust. A two-pronged approach is required: reinforcing institutional support so that patients are followed up in the community whilst empowering patients to also follow up with care.

To do this, prison health teams, ODNs, courts, prison services, and probation services should collaborate to triangulate institutional support for continued HCV care during a patient's transition. A platform should be designed to help do this (such as an interactive map providing contact information for each service within a geographic area).

To help patients to reengage with care, an HCV health card, containing key clinical information about a patient's disease status and contact information, could be developed so that they can directly self-refer to an ODN. This would allow patients to easily access care, holding all the information they would need to commence treatment.

Conclusion

Prisons represent an ideal setting in which to diagnose and cure HCV. The higher prevalence of infection amongst prisoners and the proximity of patients, testing resources, and healthcare workers capable of delivering treatment justify intensive efforts to test and treat people in prison.

However, lessons learnt in UK prisons have highlighted the need to implement prescriptive testing strategies and link these to simple investigation and treatment pathways that are well understood, widely accepted, and invested in by prison staff and healthcare workers alike.

It is vital that prisoners perceive the offer of testing and treatment as advantageous and not controlling. Prison care pathways also need to utilize new and evolving testing and treatment regimens, that are simpler and better able to facilitate the rapid progression of patients from diagnosis to cure. With greater pragmatism on the part of those funding care pathways, the elimination of HCV amongst prisoners could become an achievable goal.

Acknowledgments

SF-G and WMR are members of the UCL NIHR Health Protection Research Unit. WMR is a NIHR Senior Investigator.

References

1. Cramp ME, Rosenberg W, Ryder S et al. Modelling the impact of improving screening and treatment of chronic hepatitis C virus infection on future hepatocellular carcinoma rates and liver-related mortality. *BMC Gastroenterology* 2014;14:137.

2. World Health Organization. Global Health Sector Strategy on Viral Hepatitis 2016–2021. www.who.int/hepatitis/strategy 2016-2021/ghss-hep/en/

3. Public Health England. Hepatitis C in England 2018 report. www.hcvaction.org.uk/sites/default/files/resources/HCV_IN_THE_UK_2018_UK.pdf

4. Moore KJ, Gauri A, Koru-Sengul T. Prevalence and sociodemographic disparities of hepatitis C in baby boomers and the US adult population. *Journal of Infection and Public Health* 2019;12(1):32–36.

5. Brunsden A. Hepatitis C in prisons: evolving toward decency through adequate medical care and public health reform. *Public Law and Legal Theory Research Paper Series* 2006;54(7–2):465.

6. British HIV Association. UK National Guidelines for HIV Testing 2008. www.bhiva.org/HIV-testing-guidelines

7. Public Health England. Blood-borne Virus Opt-Out Testing in Prisons: Preliminary Evaluation of Pathfinder Programme, Phase 1, April–September 2014. London: Public Health England.

8. Hepatitis C Coalition. Report on Operational Delivery Network Visits. www.hcvaction.org.uk/resource/hepatitis-c-coalition-report-operational-delivery-network-visits

9. Public Health England. BBV bulletin: Special Edition. Issue 11. https://assets.publishing.service.gov.uk/government/uploads/system/uploads/attachment_data/file/560863/BBV_bulletin_October_2016.pdf

10. Public Health England. BBV bulletin: Special Edition. Issue 13. https://assets.publishing.service.gov.uk/government/uploads/system/uploads/attachment_data/file/666850/BBV_bulletin_Dec_2017.pdf

11. Johnson EJ, Goldstein DG. Defaults and donation decisions. *Transplantation* 2004;78(12):1–4.

12. Pawson R, Tilley N. Realistic Evaluation. London: Sage, 1997.

13. Rosen DL, Golin C, Grodensky C et al. Opt-out HIV testing in prison: informed and voluntary? *AIDS Care* 2015;27(5):545–554.

14. Francis-Graham S, Ekeke N, Nelson C et al. Understanding how, why, for whom, and under what circumstances opt-out blood- borne virus testing programmes work to increase test engagement and uptake within prison: a rapid-realist review. *BMC Health Services Research* 2019;19(1):1–18.

15. Offender Health Research Network. An Evaluation of the Reception Screening Process Used within Prisons in England and Wales. www.ohrn.nhs.uk/OHRNResearch/RecepScreen.pdf

16. Kavasery R, Maru DSR, Sylla LN, et al. A prospective controlled trial of routine opt-out HIV testing in a men's jail. *PLoS One* 2009;11:e8056.

17. Kavasery R, Maru DSR, Cornman-Homonoff J et al. Routine opt-out HIV testing strategies in a female jail setting: a prospective controlled trial. *PLoS One* 2009;4(11):e7648.

18. Rumble C, Pevalin D, O'Moore E. Routine testing for blood-borne viruses in prisons: a systematic review. *European Journal of Public Health* 2015;25(6):1078–1088.

19. Gupta, E, Bajpai M, Choudhary A. Hepatitis C virus; screening, diagnosis and interpretation of laboratory assays. *Asian Journal of Transfusion Science* 2014;8(1):19–25.

20. Friedrich-Rust M, Rosenberg W, Parkes J et al. Comparison of ELF, FibroTest and FibroScan for the non-invasive assessment of liver fibrosis. *BMC Gastroenterology* 2010;10(103):1–8.

21. Rosenberg WMC, Voelker M, Thiel R et al. Serum markers detect the presence of liver fibrosis: a cohort study. *Gastroenterology* 2004;127(6):1704–1713.

22. Binswanger IA, Nowels C, Corsi K et al. 'From the prison door right to the sidewalk, everything went downhill.' A qualitative study of the health experiences of recently released inmates. *International Journal of Law and Psychiatry* 2011;34:249–255.

23 Use of hepatitis C virus-positive organs for uninfected recipients in the era of effective and safe direct-acting antivirals: pros and cons

Sirina Ekpanyapong and K. Rajender Reddy

Department of Medicine, Division of Gastroenterology and Hepatology, University of Pennsylvania, Philadelphia, PA, USA

LEARNING POINTS

- Increasing numbers of HCV-positive organs are being retrieved from young individuals who unfortunately die from opioid drug overdose and the use of such organs in HCV-infected and uninfected individuals is increasing and has helped to decrease waiting list time, morbidity, and mortality.

- The effectiveness and safety of pangenotypic DAAs, that allow for their use successfully in the posttransplant period, have enhanced confidence among the transplant community in using HCV-positive organs.

- HCV-positive organs may be anti-HCV antibody positive but nucleic acid test (NAT) positive or negative. Proper serologic categorization is essential to define the risk of transmission to the recipient. A NAT-positive donor should be precisely characterized as viremic in order to define the risk of transmission. Major concerns in transplanting HCV-positive organs into uninfected recipients are the hepatic and extrahepatic complications of posttransplant HCV infection, nonapproval of HCV therapy by payers or healthcare agencies, HCV treatment failures, graft failures, and drug–drug interactions between DAAs and immunosuppressive agents.

- There are currently no policies or regulations on transplantation of HCV-viremic organs into HCV-negative recipients, while there is ongoing debate on whether such a strategy should be pursued as standard of care or if it should be done under regulatory oversight and transparent patient education.

Introduction

Scarcity of donor organs and long waiting times are major issues in achieving solid organ transplantation while potential recipients remain at high risk for considerable morbidity and mortality. Average waiting times for kidney transplantation in the United States usually exceed 3–5 years, resulting in an approximate 5% mortality per year among waitlisted candidates [1,2]. Ironically, in the era of organ shortage, more than 500 good-quality kidneys from deceased donors with hepatitis C (HCV) infection are unfortunately discarded annually [1,3]. Introduction of pangenotypic direct-acting antiviral agents (DAA) for the treatment of HCV infection, with cure rates exceeding 95%, has created a potential for increase in the numbers of kidney transplantations by making HCV-infected kidneys available for HCV-negative recipients. HCV-viremic donors are commonly from the "baby boomer" population in the US (born 1945–1965) where there has been a high prevalence of HCV infection, and those often acutely infected young people who inject drugs (PWID) [4].

Over the past decade, the death rate from drug overdose in the United States has been increasing, especially from opioid use among the young PWID. High-incidence regions include the North Eastern, Mid-Western, and Southern US [5]. Accordingly, the New England Organ Bank (NEOB) reported a 254% increase in organ donors who died as a consequence of drug overdose from the year 2012 to 2016,

Clinical Dilemmas in Viral Liver Disease, Second Edition. Edited by Graham R. Foster and K. Rajender Reddy.
© 2020 John Wiley & Sons Ltd. Published 2020 by John Wiley & Sons Ltd.

and a 300% increase in transplants from HCV-positive donors. The characteristics of the NEOB organ donors were that they were young (average age 33 years), male (60%), and white (86%) [6], reflecting the shift toward retrieving more HCV-infected organs from the young PWID population and less from the "baby boomer" population.

Definitions

In December 2014, the Organ Procurement and Transplantation Network (OPTN) updated its policy in that donors be screened with HCV NAT in addition to anti-HCV testing [7]. HCV infection is diagnosed by serologic testing (e.g., enzyme immunoassays [EIAs]) which can detect HCV antibodies (anti-HCV) within 2–6 months after exposure, but cannot differentiate between active HCV infection and resolved infection. Nucleic acid testing (NAT) for the detection of HCV RNA using polymerase chain reaction (PCR), branched DNA signal amplification, and transcription-mediated amplification (TMA), which can detect HCV RNA as early as 5–7 days after exposure, remains the gold standard for diagnosing active HCV infection [8]. A precise understanding of the various serologic patterns and the potential risk for transmission is provided in Table 23.1 [4,9].

Use of organs from HCV-positive donors in HCV-negative recipients

Kidney transplantatio

Kidney transplantation (KT) is considered the best treatment strategy for end-stage renal disease (ESRD). However, waiting times are over five years in many regions of the United States. While the number of HCV-seropositive kidneys transplanted into HCV-seropositive recipients increased to 334.7 kidneys/year during 2014–2016, utilization rates for HCV-seropositive kidneys remained low [10]. This also reflects that the HCV-seropositive kidney from deceased donors are five times more likely to be discarded than non-HCV organs [11]. Posttransplant HCV complications, both hepatic (e.g., cirrhosis, fibrosing cholestatic hepatitis) and extrahepatic manifestations (e.g., glomerulonephritis which can cause graft injury), are reasons for major reluctance in using HCV-positive organs [1]. However, an observational study from 1990 to 2007 (n = 468, mean follow-up 74.5 months) noted good long-term outcome of HCV-positive recipients transplanted with kidneys from HCV-positive donors (not necessarily viremic because of NAT not being routine testing in that era) in terms of patient survival, graft survival, and liver disease [12].

Because of the high efficacy of DAA therapy currently and with more unfortunate deaths from drug overdose in young individuals, the potential for KT from HCV-positive donors to HCV-negative recipients presented a new opportunity to expand the donor pool. A single-group, pilot trial at the University of Pennsylvania (THINKER) that sought to determine the safety and efficacy of KT from HCV genotype 1 viremic donors into HCV-negative recipients, followed by elbasvir/grazoprevir treatment (n = 10). noted excellent allograft function with 100% cure rate of HCV infection [3]. Another open-label single-center trial at Johns Hopkins University (EXPANDER) to study safety and efficacy outcomes following the use of genotype 1–3

Table 23.1 Interpretation of HCV donor test results and risks for transmission

Anti-HCV	HCV NAT	Suggested terminology	Interpretation	Transmission risk
+	+	Anti-HCV positive, viremic donor	Active HCV infection	High
+	-	Anti-HCV positive, nonviremic donor	Cleared/treated infection or false-positive antibody	Low-intermediate risk of transmission (varies by donor age, gender, recent history of intravenous drug use, and timing of NAT in donor)
-	+	Anti-HCV negative, viremic donor	Acute infection (window period)	High
-	-	Anti-HCV negative, nonviremic donor	No HCV infection	None

HCV, hepatitis C virus; NAT, nucleic acid testing.

viremic donors in 10 HCV-negative recipients and treating them with elbasvir/grazoprevir (sofosbuvir added in genotype 2–3) found no treatment-related adverse events, with sustained virologic response (SVR)12 achieved in all patients [13]. Further, long-term benefits at 12 months, compared with those receiving an HCV uninfected organ, have been demonstrated with regard to renal function and quality of life with such a strategy [2]. The strategy of using HCV-infected kidneys for HCV-infected recipients has also been shown to be cost-effective by decreasing time on hemodialysis [14].

Regardless, it is too early to draw conclusions for broader adoption of this strategy, as large prospective studies are needed and should be conducted with full disclosure to the recipient about the potential consequences of progressive liver disease and other HCV infection consequences, in the event that HCV infection cannot be cured, either because the therapy has failed and there is no rescue therapy or drug could not be procured, after "deliberately" causing an infection. Further, genotype subtypes 1a and 3 have been notorious in leading to DAA therapy failure in the few cases of relapse; these genotypes have been encountered relatively more often in the donor population and thus awareness of potential failure of HCV therapy post transplant is essential and needs to be well discussed with the recipients [15]

Liver transplantation

The paradigm of using HCV-infected organs in uninfected individuals has not reached the same stage as in the renal transplant population for a few reasons: a good number of the HCV-infected organs are targeted to recipients who have ongoing and untreated HCV infection with the rationale for not treating them being the concern of placing them in MELD "purgatory"; untreated primary liver cancer patients with ongoing HCV infection; and finally those donors infected with HCV infection may have significant liver disease, making them unsuitable for use as grafts. Previous reports on outcomes in HCV-positive recipients have largely been confined to those receiving HCV-positive organs relative to those transplanted with uninfected organs. Prior to the advent of DAA therapy, the challenge in the population of HCV-positive recipients had been progressive liver disease, including the infrequently encountered entity of fibrosing cholestatic hepatitis, due to the inability to treat HCV successfully with the suboptimally effective and tolerable interferon-based regimens.

A multivariate analysis on HCV-positive liver transplant (LT) recipients from 1994 to 2008 (n = 934) demonstrated no difference in overall patient survival between those receiving HCV-positive and HCV-negative donor livers (adjusted hazard ratio [HR] 1.176 vs 1.165; p=0.91) [16]. Although the proportion of HCV-positive LT recipients receiving an HCV-positive donor liver is increasing, data on intentional transplantation of HCV-positive livers into HCV-negative recipients are still lacking [17]. In a prospective study of non-HCV liver recipients receiving grafts from HCV antibody-positive/NAT-negative donors between 2016 and 2017 (n = 25), the incidence of HCV transmission was 16% (4/25). Three patients (75%) were treated with DAA (two achieving SVR and one achieving an end-of-treatment response) [18].

Although the newly developed pangenotypic DAAs have high efficacy and safety profiles from up-to-date clinical trials, some concerns about drug–drug interactions with the various regimens, and severe renal insufficiency after transplantation contraindicating the use of sofosbuvir, may limit the choice of DAA therapy.

Heart and lung transplantation

Previous data on cardiac transplants in HCV-positive recipients had yielded poor results and thus dampened the enthusiasm of transplant centers to offer a transplant to such individuals [19]. However, with the advent of HCV DAA therapy, there is now more reason to consider transplantation with infected organs, in both infected and uninfected cardiac transplant recipients. A pilot study in 2016–2017 on transplanting HCV-positive hearts into HCV-uninfected or previously treated recipients (n = 13, genotype 1a/1b/3) noted that 9/13 patients (69%) developed HCV viremia after transplantation; eight patients completed DAA treatment and achieved SVR12 and with good tolerability [20]. Another pilot study on transplanting HCV-infected hearts into HCV-negative recipients followed by DAA therapy (USHER trial) reported, preliminarily, outcome of good SVR and allograft function and none of the serious adverse effects were related to HCV treatment [21].

In lung transplantation, current practice largely is to use HCV-infected donor lungs in only HCV-positive recipients, although this has not been broadly adopted by all centers [22]. Unique problems in postlung transplantation include higher-intensity immunosuppression and patients can rarely be initiated on oral therapy immediately. The University of Alberta Hospital reported a case series of lung transplantation from five HCV-viremic donors (geno-type 1a/1b/2) into negative recipients between 2016 and 2017. Despite posttransplant complications resulting in delayed initiation of DAA therapy (24–94 days), all recipients achieved SVR without HCV or DAA-related adverse effects [22]. It is important to recognize that HCV may not be successfully treated with initial therapy, as noted in the Toronto experience with lung transplantation where there was a relapse in two patients and one had early fibrosing cholestatic hepatitis [23].

Treatment and ethical concerns

Important potential risks from transplanting HCV-positive organs into uninfected recipients include hepatic and extrahepatic complications of HCV infection, treatment failures particularly if there is transmission of HCV infection from a graft with resistance-associated substitutions (RAS), graft failures, and sexual transmission of HCV to a partner [4]. Although the available data suggest minimal risks, particularly with being able to intervene early with HCV therapy, more information is needed in the setting of

intentional HCV transmission. Unique considerations should apply to previously treated or self-cleared recipients who are receiving organs from HCV-viremic donors. Recipients should be counseled that their responses and types of HCV treatment may be different from their previous regimens [4]. However, current pangenotypic DAA regimens effectively treat those with prior treatment failure with or without the presence of RAS [4].

Managing DAA treatment in the posttransplant setting requires additional considerations on drug–drug interactions (DDI), renal dysfunction, and organ-specific protocols. Potential DDIs such as protease inhibitors with calcineurin inhibitors are of concern and need vigilant monitoring [24]. Common concomitant medications such as proton pump inhibitors (PPI) and statins may need dose adjustment. Prompt treatment should be delivered in the perioperative or early posttransplant period at time of first positive NAT. Available data on pros and cons of using HCV-positive organs for uninfected recipients in this new DAA era are outlined in Table 23.2.

Currently, there is no OPTN policy or regulation on transplanting HCV-viremic organs into non-HCV-viremic

Table 23.2 Pros and cons of using HCV-positive organs for uninfected recipients in the era of effective DAAs

Pros	Cons
• Reducing organ shortage and mortality for patients on the waitlist	• Transmission risk:

• Reducing cost of caring (e.g., hemodialysis) while on long-term kidney transplant waitlists due to more rapid HCV-positive organ transplantation	• Universal from HCV-viremic donor
	   • 73% (range 14–96%) in KT from anti-HCV-positive donor [26]
	   • 25% in heart transplantation from anti-HCV-positive donor [27]
	   • 16% in liver transplantation from anti-HCV-positive donor [18]

• Transplant organs are from young donors, with few comorbidities (mostly PWID), thus organ quality is generally good	• The PWID population has higher prevalence of genotype 1a and 3 [15]. Both these have challenges with HCV therapy and have risk of relapse, albeit low. If treatment post transplant is unsuccessful, genotype 3-associated infection has a greater likelihood of progression to cirrhosis and HCC
• Approved pangenotypic DAAs are effective and safe after transplantation and immunosuppression does not limit the effectiveness of DAAs for HCV treatment [29]	• Donor organ may bring in a resistant HCV strain. • Access to DAAs is currently limited in some countries due to the high cost • Severe renal dysfunction after transplantation can restrict the use of sofosbuvir-based regimens
• Current pangenotypic DAA regimens can provide successful therapy to patients with prior treatment failure with or without the presence of resistance-associated substitutions (RAS) [4]	• Ribavirin regimens may not be applicable in patients with anemia • Many drug–drug interactions need to be monitored for, after transplantation • Patients with heart or lung transplantation may need prolonged intubation; no formulations or published data for nasogastric tube administration of DAAs
• Good allograft function and HCV treatment outcome without serious adverse effects, as noted in pilot studies	• Insufficient data on outcomes regarding graft survival, hepatic, and nonhepatic comorbidities in this setting

Source: Modified from references [4,25–29].

DAA, direct-acting antiviral agents; HCC, hepatocellular carcinoma; HCV, hepatitis C virus; KT, kidney transplantation; PWID, people who inject drugs.

recipients, which leads to open-ended questions for each transplant center. There has been discussion on whether such studies should require collaboration with pharmaceutical companies or insurance providers in order to ensure prompt HCV treatment in the posttransplant period. Appropriate recipient selection should be those individuals who are most likely to suffer clinical deterioration while on the waitlist, as the risk of mortality on the waitlist may outweigh the risk from donor-derived HCV infection [1].

Current and future perspectives

Deceased donor organs from HCV-viremic individuals represent an underutilized resource. In this pangenotypic DAA era, HCV eradication is readily achievable and with less drug toxicity, and this has led to the new paradigm of transplanting HCV-viremic organs into uninfected recipients. As a result of tremendous advances in HCV therapy, an increasing number of HCV-positive individuals in the general population are likely to be screened and cured, HCV-seropositive donors are more likely to become HCV-RNA negative (HCV-nonviremic donor), and their grafts might be offered to uninfected recipients. Further, the rising epidemic of opioid abuse and deaths in young individuals is likely to perpetuate the availability of HCV-positive organs unless the epidemic is curbed, while on a positive note, these organs have paradoxically helped those in need of a transplant. There are clinical trials at some transplant centers addressing outcomes and safety of such a strategy in larger numbers of recipients. Failure of HCV therapy to rescue a graft is a potential threat to the ubiquitous adoption of the strategy of "deliberately" infecting a recipient and then treating the infection.

Further prospective studies are needed in order to assess the risk versus benefit of using these HCV-infected organs for uninfected recipients, which then may result in ubiquitous changes in our clinical practice.

References

1. Reese PP, Abt PL, Blumberg EA, Goldberg DS. Transplanting hepatitis C-Positive kidneys. *New England Journal of Medicine* 2015;373(4):303–305.
2. Reese PP, Abt PL, Blumberg EA et al. Twelve-month outcomes after transplant of hepatitis C-infected kidneys into uninfected recipients: a single-group trial. *Annals of Internal Medicine* 2018;169(5):273–81.
3. Goldberg DS, Abt PL, Blumberg EA, Van Deerlin VM, Levine M, Reddy KR, et al. Trial of Transplantation of HCV-Infected Kidneys into Uninfected Recipients. *New England Journal of Medicine* 2017;376(24):2394–2395.
4. Levitsky J, Formica RN, Bloom RD et al. The American Society of Transplantation Consensus Conference on the Use of Hepatitis C Viremic Donors in Solid Organ Transplantation. *American Journal of Transplantation* 2017;17(11):2790–2802.
5. Rudd RA, Aleshire N, Zibbell JE, Gladden RM. Increases in drug and opioid overdose deaths – United States, 2000–2014. *Morbidity and Mortality Weekly Report* 2016;64(50-51): 1378–1382.
6. Glazier AK, Delmonico FL, Koh HK. Organ donation in the era of the opioid crisis: a clinical strategy to maximize transplantation. *Transplantation* 2017;101(11):2652–2654.
7. OPTN Policy 2.0 Deceased Donor Organ Procurement. https://optn.transplant.hrsa.gov/media/1200/optn_policies.pdf
8. Kamili S, Drobeniuc J, Araujo AC, Hayden TM. Laboratory diagnostics for hepatitis C virus infection. *Clinical Infectious Diseases* 2012;55 Suppl 1:S43–48.
9. Mullis CE, Laeyendecker O, Reynolds SJ et al. High frequency of false-positive hepatitis C virus enzyme-linked immunosorbent assay in Rakai, Uganda. *Clinical Infectious Diseases* 2013;57(12):1747–1750.
10. Li AA, Cholankeril G, Cheng XS et al. Underutilization of hepatitis C Virus seropositive donor kidneys in the United States in the current opioid epidemic and direct-acting antiviral era. *Diseases* 2018;6(3):ii.
11. Mohan S, Chiles MC, Patzer RE et al. Factors leading to the discard of deceased donor kidneys in the United States. *Kidney International* 2018;94(1):187–198.
12. Morales JM, Campistol JM, Dominguez-Gil B et al. Long-term experience with kidney transplantation from hepatitis C-positive donors into hepatitis C-positive recipients. *American Journal of Transplantation* 2010;10(11):2453–2462.
13. Durand CM, Bowring MG, Brown DM et al. Direct-acting antiviral prophylaxis in kidney transplantation from hepatitis C virus-infected donors to noninfected recipients: an open-label nonrandomized trial. *Annals of Internal Medicine* 2018;168(8):533–540.
14. Eckman MH, Woodle ES, Thakar CV, Paterno F, Sherman KE. Transplanting hepatitis C virus-infected versus uninfected kidneys into hepatitis C virus-infected recipients: a cost-effectiveness analysis. *Annals of Internal Medicine* 2018; 169(4):214–223.
15. Robaeys G, Bielen R, Azar DG, Razavi H, Nevens F. Global genotype distribution of hepatitis C viral infection among people who inject drugs. *Journal of Hepatology* 2016;65(6): 1094–1103.

16. Northup PG, Argo CK, Nguyen DT et al. Liver allografts from hepatitis C positive donors can offer good outcomes in hepatitis C positive recipients: a US National Transplant Registry analysis. *Transplant International* 2010;23(10): 1038–1044.

17. Leroy V, Dumortier J, Coilly A et al. Efficacy of sofosbuvir and daclatasvir in patients with fibrosing cholestatic hepatitis C after liver transplantation. *Clinical Gastroenterology and Hepatology* 2015;13(11):1993–2001.e1–2.

18. Bari K, Luckett K, Kaiser T et al. Hepatitis C transmission from seropositive, nonviremic donors to non-hepatitis C liver transplant recipients. *Hepatology* 2018;67(5):1673–1682.

19. Gasink LB, Blumberg EA, Localio AR, Desai SS, Israni AK, Lautenbach E. Hepatitis C virus seropositivity in organ donors and survival in heart transplant recipients. *JAMA* 2006;296(15):1843–1850.

20. Schlendorf KH, Zalawadiya S, Shah AS et al. Early outcomes using hepatitis C-positive donors for cardiac transplantation in the era of effective direct-acting anti-viral therapies. *Journal of Heart and Lung Transplantation* 2018;37(6):763–769.

21. Early Results from USHER: A Pilot Trial of Transplanting HCV-Infected Hearts into HCV-Negative Recipients Followed by Anti-Viral Therapy. https://atcmeetingabstracts.com/abstract/early-results-from-usher-a-pilot-trial-of-transplanting-hcv-infected-hearts-into-hcv-negative-recipients-followed-by-anti-viral-therapy/

22. Abdelbasit A, Hirji A, Halloran K et al. Lung transplantation from hepatitis C viremic donors to uninfected recipients. *American Journal of Respiratory and Critical Care Medicine* 2018;197(11):1492–1496.

23. Feld JJ, Humar A, Singer L et al. Lung transplantation from HCV-infected donors to HCV-uninfected recipients (abstract 223). *Hepatology* 2018;68(S1):139A–140A.

24. Kwo PY. Direct acting antiviral therapy after liver transplantation. *Current Opinion in Gastroenterology* 2016;32(3):152–158.

25. Coilly A, Samuel D. Pros and cons: usage of organs from donors infected with hepatitis C virus – revision in the direct-acting antiviral era. *Journal of Hepatology* 2016;64(1):226–231.

26. Natov SN. Transmission of viral hepatitis by kidney transplantation: donor evaluation and transplant policies (Part 2: hepatitis C virus). *Transplant Infectious Disease* 2002;4(3): 124–131.

27. Marelli D, Bresson J, Laks H et al. Hepatitis C-positive donors in heart transplantation. *American Journal of Transplantation* 2002;2(5):443–447.

28. Goldberg DS, Abt PL, Reese PP. Transplanting HCV-infected kidneys into uninfected recipients. *New England Journal of Medicine* 2017;377(11):1105.

29. Saxena V, Khungar V, Verna EC et al. Safety and efficacy of current direct-acting antiviral regimens in kidney and liver transplant recipients with hepatitis C: results from the HCV-TARGET study. *Hepatology* 2017;66(4):1090–1101.

24 Is real-life hepatitis C virus therapy as effective as in clinical trials?

Jessica Su[1] and Joseph K. Lim[2]

[1] Department of Internal Medicine, Yale University School of Medicine, New Haven, CT, USA
[2] Yale Liver Center, Section of Digestive Diseases, Yale University School of Medicine, New Haven, CT, USA

LEARNING POINTS

- Real-life HCV therapy has been shown to be effective in real-world cohorts, with rates of SVR comparable to clinical trials.
- Current HCV therapies have excellent safety profiles in real-life cohorts.
- HCV therapies have comparable effectiveness across geographical regions.
- The effectiveness of HCV therapies is preserved in special populations of HIV coinfection, post liver transplantation, and chronic kidney disease.
- While earlier data indicated that there are lower rates of SVR in patients with cirrhosis, especially decompensated cirrhosis, newer data suggest a smaller gap in SVR.
- Risk factors for treatment failure in real-life HCV therapy include drug resistance, adherence, prior treatment failure and emergence of resistance-associated substitutions (RAS), HCV subtype (genotypes 2 and 3), and cirrhosis. Selection of appropriate DAA regimen is essential.
- Shorter regimens that maintain efficacy of current DAA regimens would increase treatment adherence and efficacy of real-life HCV therapy.
- Further evidence is needed to determine the effectiveness of HCV therapy in patients with acute HCV infection, with active injection drug use, and with treatment using generic DAAs.

Clinical trials of direct-acting antiviral (DAA) regimens have shown rates of sustained virologic response (SVR) greater than 95% after completion of regimens as short as eight weeks [1] in patients without risk factors associated with DAA treatment failure, such as cirrhosis or prior treatment failure [2]. The high efficacy of DAA therapy has led to industry benchmarks of >95% SVR for development of new DAA regimens [1]. When translating clinical trials to treatment of patients with HCV in the real-world setting, it is important to look at whether the high efficacy of DAA therapies is preserved in real-world cohorts. Cohorts in clinical trials tend to be healthier and younger, with careful selection based on strict inclusion and exclusion criteria. Furthermore, most clinical trials take place in North America and Europe whereas HCV prevalence is higher in non-Western endemic regions. When considering treatment of HCV, it is also important to take into account special populations such as patients with HIV coinfection, post liver transplantation, chronic kidney disease (CKD), and compensated and decompensated cirrhosis.

Real-world observational studies have primarily examined efficacy of DAA regimens for genotypes 1–3 and in patients coinfected with HIV, while data on genotypes 4–6 are limited. These studies have reported real-world efficacy of second-generation DAAs: sofosbuvir/ledipasvir, sofosbuvir plus daclatasvir, paritaprevir/ritonavir/ombitasvir/dasabuvir, and glecaprevir plus pibrentasvir [3], and largely from established multicenter cohorts from the United States [4–9], North America/Europe [10], Italy [11], Germany [12], Saudi Arabia [13], and Spain [14]. These studies confirm that current HCV therapies have high rates of SVRs and excellent safety profiles comparable to clinical trials, across geographies and special populations (Table 24.1).

Clinical Dilemmas in Viral Liver Disease, Second Edition. Edited by Graham R. Foster and K. Rajender Reddy.
© 2020 John Wiley & Sons Ltd. Published 2020 by John Wiley & Sons Ltd.

In addition to datasets summarized in Table 24.1, a real-world cohort study from the German Hepatitis C-Registry (DHC-R) investigating the effectiveness of glecaprevir plus pibrentasvir revealed preliminary data which confirmed high rates of SVR12 (99–100%) in patients with genotypes 1–6 [15].

With regards to special populations of patients with HCV infection, overall there is preserved effectiveness of DAA regimens in patients with HIV coinfection, post liver transplantation, and CKD. In patients with HIV coinfection, several studies have shown high rates of SVR in patients with HCV genotype 1 infection treated with sofosbuvir/ledipasvir

Table 24.1 Sustained virologic response rates in key large real-world cohorts

Regimen	Author	Year	Country/region	Genotype	Cirrhosis status	SVR (%)[a]
SOF + RBV, 12 weeks	Ioannou	2016	United States (Veterans Affairs National Health Care System)	2	No cirrhosis	89.1
				2	Cirrhosis	77.3
SOF + RBV, 24 weeks	Ioannou	2016	United States (Veterans Affairs National Health Care System)	3	No cirrhosis	77.6
				3	Cirrhosis	61.9
LDV/SOF, 8 weeks	Lai	2017	United States (Kaiser)	1	No cirrhosis	94.3
	Curry	2017	United States (Trio Healthcare)	1	No cirrhosis	95.2
LDV/SOF, 8 weeks[b]	Buggisch	2018	Germany (German Hepatitis C-Registry)	1	No cirrhosis	98.5
				1	Cirrhosis	90.5
LDV/SOF, 8–12 weeks	Backus	2016	United States (Veterans Affairs National Health Care System)	1	Non decompensated	91.5
				1	Decompensated	86.1
LDV/SOF, 8-24 weeks	Ioannou	2016	United States (Veterans Affairs National Health Care System)	1	No cirrhosis	93.5
				1	Cirrhosis	90.5
LDV/SOF, 8–24 weeks	Calleja	2017	Spain (National Registry, HEPA-C)	1	No cirrhosis	96.8
				1	Cirrhosis	93.7
LDV/SOF, 12 weeks	Lai	2017	United States (Kaiser)	1	No cirrhosis	95.1
	Curry	2017	United States (Trio Healthcare)	1	No cirrhosis	94.9
	Tapper	2017	United States (Trio Healthcare)	1	No cirrhosis	95.9
LDV/SOF, 12 weeks +	Buggisch	2018	Germany (German Hepatitis C-Registry)	1	No cirrhosis	98.8
				1	Cirrhosis	94.3
LDV/SOF +/- RBV, 8–24 weeks	Terrault	2016	North America/Europe (HCV-TARGET)	1	No cirrhosis	97.7
				1	Cirrhosis	93.5
				1	Nondecompensated	97.4
				1	Decompensated	89.8
				1	Cirrhosis	90.6
LDV/SOF + RBV, 8–24 weeks	Calleja	2017	Spain (National Registry, HEPA-C)	1	No cirrhosis	98.1
				1	Cirrhosis	95.2
LDV/SOF +/- RBV, 12–24 weeks	Sanai	2018	Saudi Arabia (Systematic Observatory Liver Disease registry)	4	No cirrhosis	93.3
				4	Compensated cirrhosis	93.3
				4	Decompensated cirrhosis	89.6

(continued)

Table 24.1 (Continued)

Regimen	Author	Year	Country/region	Genotype	Cirrhosis status	SVR (%)[a]
LDV/SOF + RBV, 12 weeks	Backus	2016	United States (Veterans Affairs National Health Care System)	1	Nondecompensated	92.3
				1	Decompensated	91.5
LDV/SOF + RBV, 12–24 weeks	Ioannou	2016	United States (Veterans Affairs National Health Care System)	1	No cirrhosis	95.6
				1	Cirrhosis	89.4
LDV/SOF + RBV, 12 weeks	Ioannou	2016	United States (Veterans Affairs National Health Care System)	3	No cirrhosis	84.8
				3	Cirrhosis	65.3
	Ioannou	2016	United States (Veterans Affairs National Health Care System)	4	No cirrhosis	90.3
				4	Cirrhosis	80.0
PrOD, 12 weeks	Ioannou	2016	United States (Veterans Affairs National Health Care System)	1	No cirrhosis	94.8
				1	Cirrhosis	95.7
PrOD, 12 weeks	Backus	2016	United States (Veterans Affairs National Health Care System)	1	Nondecompensated	98
				1	Decompensated	100 (2/2)
PrOD, 12–24 weeks	Calleja	2017	Spain (National Registry, HEPA-C)	1	No cirrhosis	96.1
				1	Cirrhosis	93.4
PrOD + RBV, 12–24 weeks	Calleja	2017	Spain (National Registry, HEPA-C)	1	No cirrhosis	98.7
				1	Cirrhosis	97.1
PrOD + RBV, 12 weeks	Ioannou	2016	United States (Veterans Affairs National Health Care System)	1	No cirrhosis	92.1
				1	Cirrhosis	93.4
PrOD + RBV, 12 weeks	Backus	2016	United States (Veterans Affairs National Health Care System)	1	Nondecompensated	95.7
				1	Decompensated	87.5
PrOD + RBV, 12 weeks	Ioannou	2016	United States (Veterans Affairs National Health Care System)	4	No cirrhosis	95.5
				4	Cirrhosis	100
GLE/PIB, 8–16 weeks (per protocol analysis)	D'Ambrosio	2018	Italy	1	No cirrhosis or compensated Child–Pugh A	100
				2	No cirrhosis or compensated Child–Pugh A	98.2
				3	No cirrhosis or compensated Child–Pugh A	95.8
				4	No cirrhosis or compensated Child–Pugh A	100
				1,2,3,4	Compensated cirrhosis (METAVIR F4)	100 (4/4)

[a] Intention to treat analysis unless otherwise specified.
[b] Per protocol analysis.
GLE, glecaprevir; LDV, ledipasvir; PIB, pibrentasvir; PrOD, paritaprevir, ritonavir, ombitasvir, dasabuvir; RBV, ribavirin; SOF, sofosbuvir.

[5,8,12]. In patients with status post liver transplantation, there has been no significant difference in terms of SVR rates [8]. In patients with CKD, DAA therapy effectiveness is preserved in real-world cohorts even in patients with estimated glomerular filtration rate (eGFR) <30 mL/min/1.73m^2 [11].

In patients with cirrhosis, particularly decompensated cirrhosis, initial data suggested that SVR rates are lower compared to patients without cirrhosis. Ioannou et al. found that the gap in SVR between cirrhotic and noncirrhotic patients was greater in genotypes 2 and 3 patients compared to genotype 1 when treated with sofosbuvir/ledipasvir and paritaprevir/ritonavir/ombitasvir/dasabuvir regimens, supporting the high effectiveness of these regimens for treatment of HCV in cirrhotic genotype 1-infected patients and relatively poor effectiveness of sofosbuvir and sofosbuvir/ledipasvir regimens in cirrhotic patients with genotype 2 and 3 infection respectively [4]. However, more recent large real-world cohorts have found high rates of SVR12 similar to rates in clinical trials. Calleja et al. reported that their Spanish real-world cohort experienced high rates of SVR12 without statistically significant decrease in patients with cirrhosis [14], although these rates may be higher compared to studies from the United States [4,5] due to a difference in proportion of patients with black race, which was associated with lower SVR. Sanai et al. found that in patients with HCV genotype 4 infection treated with sofosbuvir/ledipasvir, no difference in SVR was observed between patients with advanced fibrosis or compensated cirrhosis (SVR12 93.3%), although lower SVR12 (89.6%) was observed in patients with decompensated cirrhosis [13].

Real-life HCV therapy has been shown to be highly effective in real-world cohorts, particularly in patients with HCV genotype 1, although there are subgroups in which lower SVR12 has been reported, including patients with cirrhosis, black race, prior DAA failure, and genotype 3 infection. Concurrent use of proton pump inhibitors, especially at higher doses, has also been associated with lower SVR [10,16]. Differences in SVR rates between clinical trials and real-world cohorts may also in part reflect a comparison between "per protocol" and "intent-to-treat" estimates of SVR through the exclusion of real-world patients with early discontinuation or lack of follow-up for evaluation of SVR accounted for in several real-world cohorts by exclusion of patients who had early discontinuation or lack of follow-up for evaluation of SVR

[5,11,12]. Further assessment of the impact of treatment adherence, drug–drug interactions, and treatment completion in real-world studies is needed. Other factors which have been identified as predictive of SVR12 include normal albumin [4,10,14], normal total bilirubin [4,10], and normal BMI [5].

In conclusion, data from real-life cohorts have shown that current HCV therapies with DAA regimens have high SVR rates comparable to clinical trials, with excellent safety profiles. The effectiveness of HCV therapies is preserved across geographies and among special populations, with the exception of decompensated cirrhosis. However, there are still several aspects of HCV therapy requiring more real-world data to determine effectiveness in patients with acute HCV infection, in people who inject drugs, and with treatment using generic DAA in Western countries. There are some studies of real-world cohorts treated with generic oral DAA regimens, which reported SVR rates ranging from 92% to 98% [2], but most of these data are derived from licensed generic formulations used in India, China, or Egypt. Continued efforts to acquire data on real-life effectiveness of HCV therapies will be important in addressing challenges to HCV eradication.

References

1. AALD/IDSA HCV Guidance Panel. HCV Guidance: Recommendations for Testing, Managing, and Treating Hepatitis C. www.hcvguidelines.org

2. Baumert TF, Berg T, Lim JK, Nelson DR. Status of direct-acting antiviral therapy for HCV infection and remaining challenges. *Gastroenterology* 2019;156:431–445.

3. Hezode C. Treatment of hepatitis C: results in real life. *Liver International* 2018;38:21–27.

4. Ioannou GN, Beste LA, Chang MF et al. Effectiveness of sofosbuvir, ledipasvir/sofosbuvir, and paritaprevir/ritonavir/ombitasvir/dasabuvir regimens for treatment of patients with hepatitis C in the Veterans Affairs National Health Care System. *Gastroenterology* 2016;151:457–471.e5.

5. Backus LI, Belperio PS, Shahoumian TA, Loomis TP, Mole LA. Comparative effectiveness of ledipasvir/sofosbuvir +/- ribavirin vs. ombitasvir/paritaprevir/ritonavir + dasabuvir +/- ribavirin in 6961 genotype 1 patients treated in routine medical practice. *Alimentary Pharmacology and Therapeutics* 2016;44(4):400–410.

6. Lai JB, Witt MA, Pauly MP et al. Eight- or 12-week treatment of hepatitis C with ledipasvir/sofosbuvir: real-world experience in a large integrated health system. *Drugs* 2017;77(3):313–318.

7. Curry MP, Tapper EB, Bacon B et al. Effectiveness of 8- or 12- weeks of ledipasvir and sofosbuvir in real-world treatment-naïve, genotype 1 hepatitis C infected patients. *Alimentary Pharmacology and Therapeutics* 2017;46(5):540–548.

8. Tapper EB, Bacon BR, Curry MP et al. Real-world effectiveness for 12 weeks of ledipasvir-sofosbuvir for genotype 1 hepatitis C: the Trio Health Study. *Journal of Viral Hepatitis* 2017;24(1):22–27.

9. Backus LI, Belperio PS, Shahoumian TA, Loomis TP, Mole LA. Real-world effectiveness of ledipasvir/sofosbuvir in 4,365 treatment-naïve, genotype 1 hepatitis C-infected patients. *Journal of Hepatology* 2016;64(2):405–414.

10. Terrault NA, Zeuzem S, di Bisceglie AM et al. Effectiveness of ledipasvir-sofosbuvir combination in patients with hepatitis C virus infection and factors associated with sustained virologic response. *Gastroenterology* 2016;151:1131–1140.e5.

11. D'Ambrosio R, Pasulo L, Puoti M et al. Real-life effectiveness and safety of glecaprevir/pibrentasvir in 723 patients with chronic hepatitis C. *Journal of Heaptology* 2019;70:379–387.

12. Buggisch P, Vermehren J, Mauss S et al. Real-world effectiveness of 8-week treatment with ledipasvir/sofosbuvir in chronic hepatitis C. *Journal of Hepatology* 2018;68:663–671.

13. Sanai FM, Altraif IH, Alswat K et al. Real life efficacy of ledipasvir/sofosbuvir in hepatitis C genotype 4-infected patients with advanced liver fibrosis and decompensated cirrhosis. *Journal of Infection* 2018;76:536–542.

14. Calleja JL, Crespo J, Rincon D et al. Effectiveness, safety, and clinical outcomes of direct-acting antiviral therapy in HCV genotype 1 infection: results from a Spanish real-world cohort. *Journal of Hepatology* 2017;66(6):1138–1148.

15. Berg T, Naumann U, Stoehr A et al. First real-world data on safety and effectiveness of glecaprevir/ pibrentasvir for the treatment of patients with chronic hepatitis C virus infection: data from the German Hepatitis C-Registry. *Journal of Hepatology* 2019;68, suppl 1:S37.

16. Tapper EB, Bacon BR, Curry MP et al. Evaluation of proton pump inhibitor use on treatment outcomes with ledipasvir and sofobuvir in a real-world cohort study. *Hepatology* 2016;64(6):1893–1899.

Section 2: HBV, HDV, and HEV

Management of acute hepatitis B infection: when should we offer antiviral therapy?

Emma Hathorn and David J. Mutimer

Liver Unit, University Hospitals NHS Foundation Trust, Birmingham, UK

LEARNING POINTS

- Acute hepatitis B infection in adults is usually subclinical and self-limiting, with the majority of individuals achieving spontaneous clearance and lifelong immunity,

- Antiviral therapy may have a role in severe acute HBV, defined as coagulopathy (INR >1.5) or a protracted course (persistent symptoms or marked jaundice for >4 weeks), to prevent development of acute liver failure,

- Antiviral therapy has no proven role in acute HBV infection to prevent the development of chronic infection.

Introduction

Hepatitis B vaccination has led to a decline in the incidence of acute hepatitis B virus (HBV) infection. Between 2007 and 2016, the overall rate of reported acute HBV infection fell from 1.2 to 0.6 per 100 000 population in Europe [1]. Acute infection is usually asymptomatic and self-limiting but 30–50% of infected adults will develop jaundice [2]. The majority will achieve a sufficient immune response to enable clearance of the virus and will acquire protective levels of hepatitis B surface antibody (anti-HBs) with lifelong immunity. However, significant complications can occur, including fulminant hepatitis (2%) and chronic infection (1–27%) [3,4].

Fulminant hepatitis is defined by the development of liver failure (high international normalized ratio [INR] and hepatic encephalopathy) which can necessitate liver

transplantation or result in death [4]. The overall mortality rate across all severity of acute HBV is estimated to be 1% but of those who develop fulminant hepatitis, transplant-free survival rates as low as 26% have been reported [5].

Chronic HBV infection is defined by persistence of hepatitis B surface antigen (HBsAg) for more than six months. The main determinant of progression to chronicity is age at the time of infection. The risk of chronic infection if the acute infection occurs at birth is as high as 90% in contrast to only 1–5% of individuals infected in adulthood [6]. Immunosuppressed patients are also at risk of chronicity instead of immune-mediated resolution of infection. Chronic infection carries a 13.5% lifetime risk of liver cirrhosis and 5% risk of hepatocellular cancer [7,8]. For individuals who develop compensated cirrhosis related to chronic HBV infection, there is an additional risk of decompensation (3–5% per year), hepatocellular cancer (2–8% per year), and death (3–4% per year) [9].

This chapter will discuss the potential role of antiviral therapy in the management of acute HBV infection in order to prevent fulminant hepatitis and/or to prevent evolution to chronic hepatitis B.

Rationale for treatment of acute HBV infection

The primary aim of antiviral therapy for acute HBV is to prevent acute liver failure. In severe infection, an improvement in liver function may obviate the need for liver trans-

Clinical Dilemmas in Viral Liver Disease, Second Edition. Edited by Graham R. Foster and K. Rajender Reddy.
© 2020 John Wiley & Sons Ltd. Published 2020 by John Wiley & Sons Ltd.

plantation. Secondary goals include the prevention of evolution to chronic infection and amelioration of symptoms. However, it is important to remember that only 1–5% of individuals infected in adulthood progress to chronic infection, and the majority will experience subclinical infection.

Viral kinetics of acute HBV infection

The viral kinetics and clinical correlations of acute HBV infection were well described in seven patients who were part of a single-source outbreak of acute HBV in London [10]. Initial rise in viral titer was rapid (minimum estimated doubling time 2.2–5.8 days, mean 3.7 +/- 1.5 days) and a peak serum HBV titer of almost 10^{10} was reached within 80 days of inoculation (Figure 25.1). Subsequent clearance of HBV appeared multiphasic, with initial steeper decline (mean half-life of 3.7 +/- 1.2 days) followed by more gradual reduction in HBV DNA titers (mean half-life of 12 +/-6 days).

The onset of clinical symptoms (lethargy, malaise, myalgia, headache) occurred at about the time of peak serum HBV DNA or the first phase of viral decline and this also coincided with the initial rise in alanine aminotransferase (ALT) (see Figure 25.1). The onset of jaundice occurred 2–6 weeks after the peak in serum HBV DNA, by which time symptoms were resolving and HBV DNA levels had substantially fallen by up to 5 $\log_{10}$ copies/mL. Peak ALT was observed 14 +/- 6 days after peak viral levels and remained elevated during the final phase of viral decay. In this case series, faster viral doubling time correlated with severity of acute infection.

Antiviral options for acute HBV infection

Hepatitis B is a noncytopathic virus and fulminant hepatitis occurs as a result of an enhanced immune response to viral replication within the host. Early studies explored the benefit of treatment with type 1 interferons. A randomized controlled trial compared three weeks of recombinant interferon-alpha (n = 67) at a dose of 3 million units or 10 million units to placebo (n = 33) in 100 patients with acute hepatitis B [11]. Patients with fulminant hepatitis were excluded. A significantly shorter duration of signs and symptoms of acute hepatitis was observed in patients receiving low-dose interferon but no data were reported on short-term mortality. No patient remained hepatitis B surface antigen positive so an impact on progression to chronic infection could not be assessed. Therefore, though interferon may have been tolerated, its role in the management of acute HBV infection was unproven.

More recent studies have explored the role of nucleoside/nucleotide inhibitors of HBV DNA polymerase (lamivudine, entecavir, tenofovir) that primarily interrupt viral replication through DNA chain termination and result in rapid reduction of detectable serum HBV DNA. This may prove clinically advantageous if early viral burden determines the course of acute infection.

Antiviral therapy to improve liver function in acute HBV

Treatment of severe acute HBV

Three randomized controlled trials have investigated lamivudine for the treatment of severe acute hepatitis B.

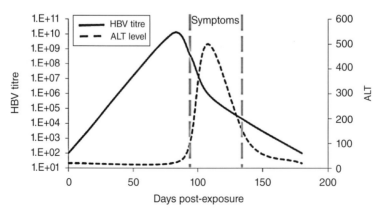

Figure 25.1 Viral and biochemical characteristics of acute hepatitis B.

The first, from India, compared 100 mg lamivudine daily for three months (n = 31) versus placebo (n = 40) in patients with acute hepatitis B infection and serum bilirubin >5 mg/dL (85.5 μmol/L) [12]. Whilst HBV DNA titers were significantly lower in the lamivudine-treated group at week 4 (3.7 log copies/mL versus 4.3 log copies/mL; p=0.037), levels were not significantly different at time points thereafter, even when patients with more severe infection were analyzed separately. The authors concluded a lack of efficacy but, like many studies of this condition, the study appears to have been underpowered to demonstrate a possible treatment benefit.

A more recent trial from centers across Germany randomized 40 patients with severe, nonfulminant acute HBV infection (ALT >10 × upper limit of normal [ULN], bilirubin >85 μmol/L, prothrombin time >50%) to receive either lamivudine 100 mg daily until four weeks after loss of HBsAg or maximum 24 weeks treatment (n = 18) versus placebo (n = 17) initiated within eight days of diagnosis [13]. No patients progressed to liver failure and all but one achieved a bilirubin of <34.2 μmol/L(primary endpoint). There was no significant difference reported in time to primary endpoint, time to ALT normalization or time to HBsAg loss although median time endpoints were shorter in the treatment arm.

A randomized trial from China demonstrated a significant survival advantage in favor of lamivudine in patients with severe acute HBV infection [14]. In this study, 80 patients were randomly assigned to treatment (n = 40) or control group (n = 40). Mortality was significantly lower in the lamivudine-treated group (7.5% [3/40] versus 25.0% [10/40], p=0.034). Additionally, the incidence of liver failure was significantly lower in patients who received treatment within a week compared to those who did not (8.7% [2/23] versus 35.3% [6/17], p=0.038).

Thus, whilst robust, adequately powered randomized controlled trials are lacking, some data suggest that early use of lamivudine may prevent acute liver failure and reduce mortality in severe acute HBV infection.

Treatment of fulminant acute HBV

No randomized controlled trials have been performed in patients with fulminant liver failure related to HBV infection but several retrospective cohort studies do suggest reduced mortality with antiviral treatment in this setting. Mortality was compared in a Chinese retrospective cohort study of 40 treated patients with fulminant hepatitis B and 40 matched historical controls [15]. Significantly lower mortality was observed in the lamivudine-treated group (63.2% [28/40] versus 84.6% [39/40], p=0.032). These findings are consistent with a large Japanese case series (n = 33) of consecutive patients with fulminant hepatitis B who did not undergo liver transplantation [16]. Lamivudine was started in only 10 patients within three days of diagnosis but a survival advantage with treatment was still observed (70% survival versus 26%). There were no differences in clinical parameters at diagnosis between patients who received and did not receive treatment and the rationale for treatment in the 10 selected cases is unclear. However, age ≥45, systemic inflammatory response syndrome (as a marker of advanced disease) and nonadministration of lamivudine were associated with death. Another case series suggests survival benefit may be lost once advanced hepatic encephalopathy (grade 3 or 4) is established [17].

Antiviral therapy to prevent chronic infection in acute HBV

Acute infection in immunocompetent adults is associated with a high rate of spontaneous viral clearance regardless of cohort studied although variation is reported across e-antigen status and HBV genotype. This makes evaluation of the impact of antiviral therapy on natural history in clinical trials challenging. A recent open-label study in Romania randomized 200 patients with severe acute hepatitis B to receive either lamivudine 100 mg/day (n = 69), entecavir 0.5 mg/day (n = 21) or no antiviral therapy (standard of care, n = 110) [18]. The primary endpoint was HBsAg to HBsAb seroconversion by 24 weeks. Treatment with lamivudine was associated with a lower rate of seroconversion (n = 7/69, 10%; entecavir n = 9/21, 43%; no antiviral n = 25/110, 23%) and with lower rate of HBsAg clearance without antibody development (n = 16/69, 23%; entecavir n = 11/21, 52%; no antiviral n = 43/110, 39%). No difference was observed in the proportion of people who developed chronic HBV infection when entecavir was used compared to no antiviral. A possible negative impact of lamivudine on HBsAg clearance had previously been reported in a study which compared lamivudine with placebo in severe acute hepatitis (92.5% versus 97.5%) [12].

Therefore data do not currently support the use of antiviral treatment to prevent evolution of acute to chronic HBV infection in nonimmunosuppressed patients with severe hepatitis.

Discussion

The subclinical nature of acute HBV infection and high rate of spontaneous viral clearance make it difficult to design robust, controlled studies to determine the role of antiviral therapy. Furthermore, fulminant hepatitis B is rare, making clinical trials challenging. In 2017, a Cochrane review of pharmacologic interventions for acute hepatitis B infection concluded that, based on very low-quality evidence due to risk of bias, small sample size and wide confidence intervals, there was no evidence of benefit with any intervention in acute HBV infection [19]. A metaanalysis could not be performed but odds ratio (OR) and rate ratio with 95% confidence interval (CI) were reported for short-term mortality and the proportion of people who progressed to chronic infection. There was no difference in short-term mortality across any comparison (lamivudine versus placebo or no intervention OR 1.29, 95% CI 0.33–4.99, n = 250; lamivudine versus entecavir OR 1.23, 95% CI 0.13–11.65, n = 90; entecavir versus no intervention OR 1.05, 95% CI 0.12–9.47, n = 131) and no included trial reported progression to fulminant infection.

However, some individual trial data and reported series suggest that selected patients with very severe hepatitis and early fulminant liver failure may derive some benefit from prompt initiation of nucleoside analogs. When balanced against the lack of difference in adverse events in people who receive lamivudine, placebo or no intervention and its low cost, there appears little to challenge the current guidance from the European Association for the Study of the Liver (EASL) that recommends nucleoside/nucleotide analogs only for those patients with severe acute hepatitis B in addition to consideration of liver transplantation [20]. There is, however, no good evidence to support the use of antiviral therapy to prevent progression to chronicity, with pooled data from the Cochrane review suggesting a higher rate of progression in those patients who received lamivudine when compared to placebo or no intervention (OR 1.99, 95% CI 1.05–3.77, n = 285) and to entecavir (OR 3.64, 95% CI 1.31–10.13, n = 90).

Conclusion

In conclusion, the role of antiviral therapy in acute HBV infection remains unproven but treatment should be considered for those patients with severe acute hepatitis B, defined by coagulopathy (INR >1.5) or a protracted course (persistent symptoms or marked jaundice for >4 weeks), in conjunction with consideration of liver transplantation.

References

1. ECDC. Annual Epidemiological Report for 2016: Hepatitis B. https://ecdc.europa.eu/sites/portal/files/documents/AER_for_2016-hepatitis-B-rev1.PDF
2. McMahon BJ, Alward WLM, Hall DB et al. Acute hepatitis B virus infection: relation of age to the clinical expression of disease and subsequent development of the carrier state. *Journal of Infectious Diseases* 1985;151:599–603.
3. Leen CL, Davison SM, Flegg PJ, Mandal BK. Seven years' experience of acute hepatitis B in a regional department of infectious diseases and tropical medicine. *Journal of Infection* 1989;18(3):257–263.
4. Tillman HL, Patel K. Therapy of acute and fulminant hepatitis. *Intervirology* 2014;57(3-4):181–188.
5. Lee HC. Acute liver failure related to hepatitis B virus. *Hepatology Research* 2008;38(S1):S9–S13.
6. Fattovich G. Natural history of hepatitis B. *Journal of Hepatology* 2003;39:S50–S58.
7. Yang YF, Zhao W, Zhong YD, Xia HM, Shen L, Zhang N. Interferon therapy in chornic hepatitis B reduces progression to cirrhosis and hepatocellular carcinoma: a meta-analysis. *Journal of Viral Hepatitis* 2009;16(4):265–271.
8. Thiele M, Gluud LL, Fialla AD, Dahl EK, Krag A. Large variations in risk of hepatocellular carcinoma and mortality in treatment naïve hepatitis B patients: systematic review with meta-analyses. *PLoS One* 2014;9(9):e107177.
9. Chu CM, Liaw YF. Hepatitis B virus-related cirrhosis: natural history and treatment. *Seminars in Liver Disease* 2006; 26(2):142–152.
10. Whalley SA, Murray JM, Brown D et al. Kinetics of acute hepatitis B virus infection in humans. *Journal of Experimental Medicine* 2001;193(7):847–853.
11. Tassopoulos NC, Koutelou MG, Polychronaki H, Hadziyannis SJ. Recombinant interferon-alpha therapy for acute hepatitis B: a randomised, double-blind, placebo-controlled trial. *Journal of Viral Hepatitis* 1997;4:387–394.
12. Kumar M, Satapathy S, Monga R et al. A randomised controlled trial of lamivudine to treat acute hepatitis B. *Hepatology* 2007;45(1):97–101.

13. Wiegand J, Wedemeyer H, Franke A et al. Treatment of severe, nonfulminant acute hepatitis B with lamivudine vs placebo: a prospective randomised double-blinded multi-centre trial. *Journal of Viral Hepatitis* 2014;21(10): 744–750.

14. Yu JW, Sun LJ, Zhao YH, Kang P, Li SC. The study of efficacy of lamivudine in patients with severe acute hepatitis B. *Digestive Diseases and Sciences* 2010;55:755–783.

15. Yu JW, Sun LJ, Yan BZ, Kang P, Zhao ZH. Lamivudine treatment is associated with improved survival in fulminant hepatitis B. *Liver International* 2011;31:499–506.

16. Miyake Y, Iwasaki Y, Takaki A et al. Lamivudine treatment improves prognosis of fulminant hepatitis B. *Internal Medicine* 2008;47(14):1293–1299.

17. Wang C, Zhao P, Liu W et al. Acute liver failure caused by severe acute hepatitis B: a case series from a multi-centre investigation. *Annals of Clinical Microbiology and Antimicrobials* 2014;13:23.

18. Streinu-Cercel A, Sandulescu O, Stefan M, Streinu-Cercel A. Treatment with lamivudine and entecavir in severe acute hepatitis B. *Indian Journal of Medical Microbiology* 2016; 34(2):166–172.

19. Mantzoukis K, Rodríguez-Perálvarez M, Buzzetti E et al. Pharmacological interventions for acute hepatitis B infection. *Cochrane Database of Systematic Reviews* 2017;3: CD011645.

20. EASL. Clinical Practice Guidelines on the management of hepatitis B virus infection. https://easl.eu/wp-content/uploads/2018/10/HepB-English-report.pdf

26 Rethinking the inactive carrier state: management of patients with low-replicative HBeAg-negative chronic hepatitis B and normal liver enzymes

María Buti[1,2], Mar Riveiro-Barciela[1,2], and Rafael Esteban[1,2]

[1]Liver Unit, Department of Internal Medicine, Hospital Universitari Vall d'Hebron, Universitat Autònoma de Barcelona, Barcelona, Spain

[2]Centro de Investigación Biomédica en Red de Enfermedades Hepáticas y Digestivas (CIBERehd), Instituto de Salud Carlos III, Madrid, Spain

LEARNING POINTS

- Low-level HBV replication with normal liver function tests is best regarded as *HBeAg-negative chronic hepatitis B infection* to reflect the presence of the infection and the lack of liver disease. The term "inactive carrier" should be discarded.

- Patients with HBeAg-negative chronic hepatitis B infection are at low risk of liver disease when compared to those with active disease, although the risk is greater than in uninfected people and reactivation is common if immunosuppression is introduced.

- Levels of HBsAg and hepatitis B core-related antigen may be helpful in distinguishing those with HBeAg-negative chronic hepatitis B infection who are likely to develop progressive disease and those who are unlikely to do so, although neither test in isolation is entirely satisfactory.

- It is not clear whether emerging drugs for chronic HBV infection should be targeted at these individuals.

Introduction

An estimated 340 million individuals worldwide are chronically infected with the hepatitis B virus (HBV). Most of them are hepatitis B e antigen (HBeAg) negative and have varying degrees of liver fibrosis. The severity of their condition ranges from the inactive carrier state to chronic active hepatitis, liver cirrhosis, decompensated liver disease, and hepatocellular carcinoma (HCC) (Table 26.1) [1].

Inactive carrier (IC) state is defined based on a lack of HBeAg in serum, presence of antibodies against HBeAg (anti-HBe), undetectable or low (<2000 IU/mL) HBV DNA levels, and normal alanine aminotransferase (ALT) levels for more than six months. Characteristically, these patients have mild or no liver disease and a low risk of progression to cirrhosis or HCC if they remain in this phase [1]. The European Association for the Study of the Liver (EASL) 2017 clinical practice guidelines on the management of HBV infection have adopted a new term for the inactive carrier state. It is now named *HBeAg-negative chronic hepatitis B infection* to reflect the presence of the infection and the lack of liver disease.

HBeAg-negative chronic hepatitis B (CHB) patients cannot always be easily categorized into the different stages of infection or disease. In a large study performed in the United States including 1390 adults and using biochemical and serologic markers, 233 (17%) patients were classified as having HBeAg-negative CHB, 318 (23%) as ICs, and 524 (38%) were in a gray area based on elevated serum ALT with low levels of HBV DNA (<10 000 IU/mL), and were considered *indeterminant*. Most of them remained indeterminant in a subsequent analysis [2]. These findings illustrate the difficulty of categorizing patients with chronic HBV infection/disease,

Clinical Dilemmas in Viral Liver Disease, Second Edition. Edited by Graham R. Foster and K. Rajender Reddy.
© 2020 John Wiley & Sons Ltd. Published 2020 by John Wiley & Sons Ltd.

Table 26.1 Summary of the risk of clinical events in subjects with HBeAg-negative chronic hepatitis B infection with normal ALT and HBV DNA <20 000 IU/mL

Country/ reference	Number	Genotype	Follow-up, years	Liver fibrosis	Treatment criteria[a]	LR death	HCC	HBsAg loss
HBV inactive carriers (normal ALT and HBV DNA <2000 IU/mL)								
Taiwan [18]	1932	NA	12.9	NA	NA	11 (0.6%)	16 (0.8%)	NA
China [5]	244	NA	3.7	7 (2.9%)	20 (8.2%)	0 (0%)	0 (0%)	NA
USA [22]	146	B and C	8	NA	13 (8.9%)	0 (0%)	2 (1.4%)	13 (8.9%)
France [16]	109	NA	5.7	NA	NA	NA	NA	11 (3.5%)
Portugal [23]	100	A and D	4.6	0 (0%)	10 (10%)	0 (0%)	0 (0%)	4 (4%)
Taiwan [9]	777	B and C	1.5	32 (4.1%)[b]	63 (6.4%)[c]	NA	15 (1.9%)	154 (19.8%)
Japan [17]	388	B and C	2.8	0 (0%)[b]	75 (19.3 %)	0 (0%)	0 (0%)	NA
Italy [15]	87	D	4.8	NA	3 (3.4%)	0 (0%)	0 (0%)	19 (21.8%)
Thailand [10]	200	NA	2	NA	NA	NA	NA	15 (7.5%)
HBeAg-negative chronic hepatitis B infection with normal ALT and HBV DNA between 2000 and 20 000 IU/mL								
China [5]	117	NA	3.7	3 (2.6%)	29 (24.8%)	0 (0%)	0 (0%)	NA
Italy [15]	46	D	4.8	1 (2.2%)	1 (2.2%)	0 (0%)	0 (0%)	0 (0%)

[a] Treatment criteria following the EASL 2017 clinical practice guidelines on the management of HBV infection.
[b] Patients who developed liver cirrhosis.
[c] Data from patients with normal baseline ALT levels and HBV DNA <2000 IU/mL who showed HBV DNA >20 000 or HBV DNA >2000 plus abnormal ALT during follow-up.
CHB, chronic hepatitis B; HCC, hepatocellular carcinoma; LR, liver-related; NA, not available.

an important task as the management and treatment indications differ according to the infection stage.

In recent years, new parameters and data have emerged to optimize the management of chronic HBV patients, particularly ICs. These advances are placing the inactive carrier state in a new light and may help to better define it. In this review, we analyze the role of ALT levels, HBV DNA levels, presence of fibrosis, noninvasive tools, and new markers to facilitate the diagnosis of ICs.

Definition of normal ALT levels

Traditionally, ALT levels that fall below the laboratory upper limit of normality, usually 40 IU/mL, have been considered normal, without applying separate criteria for men and women. The American Association for the Study of Liver Diseases (AASLD) guidelines have adopted a new estimate for normal ALT levels, placing the upper limit at 35 IU/L for men and 25 IU/L for women [3]. These limits are lower than the previous one, but they better identify true ICs after excluding causes other than HBV infection (e.g., fatty liver disease, alcohol-associated liver disease, drug-induced liver injury), particularly in cases of recurrent or persistent ALT elevation. Of note, different results

have been described in repeat testing of the same sample [4,5]. This might prompt clinicians to repeat test when a single ALT elevation is near the cut-off for treatment.

Hepatitis B virus DNA levels

Serum HBV DNA below 2000 IU/mL is the rule in ICs, but occasional fluctuations of one or two logarithms around this cut-off are sometimes observed [1]. For this reason, consecutive serum HBV DNA and ALT determinations (i.e., at least three or four determinations in the first year after diagnosis) are needed to distinguish between active and inactive HBV carriers and avoid misclassification of the infection phase due to spontaneous HBV DNA and ALT fluctuations. Nearly two-thirds of patients with IC features at baseline were confirmed to be true ICs after one year of follow-up, whereas the remaining patients with fluctuating virologic and biochemical activity were classified as HBeAg-negative CHB patients or indeterminants [6,7]. In ICs, HBV DNA occasionally falls between 2000 IU/mL and 20 000 IU/mL, but this is usually accompanied by persistently normal ALT levels; hence it is important to monitor these patients to appropriately categorize them [1].

Serum HBsAg levels

HBsAg has been proposed as a marker to differentiate between chronic infection and chronic hepatitis. Usually, HBsAg levels are higher in HBeAg-positive than HBeAg-negative patients [8]. In HBeAg-negative patients infected by genotype D, low levels of HBsAg (<1000 IU/mL) and HBV DNA (≤2000 IU/mL) in a single determination identify ICs as effectively as one year of ALT and HBV DNA monitoring [6]. In a large community-based study including 1529 well-characterized inactive or active HBeAg-negative CHB patients infected with HBV genotypes B or C from the REVEAL-HBV cohort, the combination of HBsAg <1000 IU/mL and HBV DNA <2000 IU/mL distinguished between ICs and patients with active CHB with a diagnostic accuracy of 78% [9]. Those identified as ICs and with HBsAg levels below 1000 IU/mL had a very low risk of developing HCC or liver cirrhosis and a higher likelihood of HBsAg seroclearance. In another study, 200 HBeAg-negative ICs were prospectively followed, and 15 (5%) experienced HBsAg seroclearance after 24 months. HBsAg levels below 1000 IU/mL predicted spontaneous HBsAg clearance in this cohort [10].

These findings suggest that HBsAg determination at a single time point in HBeAg-negative chronic HBV patients with low HBV DNA levels can help to identify ICs and accurately predict spontaneous HBsAg seroclearance at 24 months as well as the risk of developing HCC. Nonetheless, a few studies have pointed out that HBsAg levels are influenced by HBV genotype; hence, the usefulness of the HBsAg <1000 IU/mL cut-off can vary according to the genotype [8,11,12].

Hepatitis B core-related antigen

Hepatitis B core-related antigen (HBcrAg) has been suggested as an additional biomarker of HBV infection. HBcrAg combines the antigenic reactivity resulting from denatured HBeAg, HBV core antigen, and a core-related protein (p22cr), all products of the precore/core gene that share an identical 149 amino acid sequence. HBcrAg levels vary significantly during the different phases of HBV infection, being higher in patients with HBeAg-positive infection and CHB, lower in HBeAg-negative CHB, and very low in ICs (2.00 log U/mL). These findings suggest that HBcrAg may help to distinguish between IC state and active CHB in HBeAg-negative patients [13].

In a study including 202 consecutive HBeAg-negative patients chronically infected by HBV (135 ICs and 67 with HBV activity), serum HBcrAg was more accurate than HBsAg in identifying ICs, regardless of the HBV genotype [7]. HBsAg levels differed across the different HBV genotypes, whereas HBcrAg was stable. Although HBsAg at a cut-off of <3 log IU/mL showed good performance only for identifying genotype D inactive carriers, the combination of a single HBcrAg measurement ≤3 logU/mL plus HBV DNA ≤2000 IU/mL yielded a positive predictive value and diagnostic accuracy of more than 85% in all HBV genotypes [7].

In a multicenter European study including 1584 samples from HBeAg-negative patients, including ICs and patients with CHB, HBcrAg quantification was superior to HBsAg, suggesting a high diagnostic value to discriminate between CHB and ICs. The optimal cut-off for HBcrAg was 3.14 log U/mL, which yielded a negative predictive value of 0.91 and positive predictive value of 0.94. Addition of HBsAg determination did not improve the diagnostic performance of HBcrAg alone. Along with HBV DNA and ALT, serum HBcrAg is a better marker than HBsAg for differentiating between chronic HBV infection and CHB in HBeAg-negative patients and may be a useful biomarker for faster identification of ICs, independently of HBV genotype. Further studies including Asian patients are needed to validate the diagnostic role of HBcrAg in the HBV-infected population.

Fibrosis evaluation and noninvasive markers

Hepatitis B virus guidelines recommend histologic assessment to determine treatment candidacy, in particular when HBV-DNA and ALT levels are near the threshold for starting therapy. The role of noninvasive markers, such as the AST to platelet ratio index (APRI), Fibrosis-4 score (FIB-4), and transient elastography, has been less extensively studied in patients with CHB than in those with chronic hepatitis C [13].

Small-scale studies have suggested that the APRI and FIB-4 scores are higher in CHB patients with significant fibrosis, but a clear cut-off to distinguish between mild-to-moderate and severe fibrosis requires validation. A recent metaanalysis of 39 studies that focused on APRI and/or FIB-4 concluded that these scoring systems identify CHB-related fibrosis with only moderate sensitivity and accuracy, and are not an ideal replacement for liver biopsy [13].

Transient elastography (TE) has also been evaluated in HBV ICs. TE values ≤6.2 kPa combined with HBV DNA ≤2000 IU/mL and HBsAg ≤1000 IU/L at a single time point enabled identification of a considerable number of ICs [13]. In general, TE values in ICs are very similar to those observed in healthy controls. In a longitudinal assessment of 329 consecutive HBeAg-negative patients (201 inactive carriers), TE (median 4.8 vs 6.8 kPa, p<0.0001), Fibrotest (0.16 vs 0.35, p<0.0001), and APRI values (0.28 vs 0.43, p<0.0001) were significantly lower in ICs than in the remaining patients, but showed no differences according to HBV DNA levels. In the same study, 82 ICs underwent repeated examinations and TE values did not differ significantly over time. Conversely, significant fluctuations were observed for the Fibrotest and APRI. In addition to HBV DNA and ALT determinations, noninvasive tools such as TE could be useful to follow up HBV ICs, and improve selection of patients requiring liver biopsy [14].

Natural history

HBeAg-negative ICs are considered to have a good prognosis because of immunologic control of HBV infection. This notion is based on the results of long-term longitudinal studies performed in adult inactive carriers during the 1980s, reporting that 15–24% of patients developed HBeAg-negative CHB and very few patients developed HCC [1]. It is estimated that the incidence of HBeAg-negative CHB in ICs ranges from 1 to 3 per 100 person-years. More recent studies performed in the last 10 years have shown similar results. HCC rates, only reported in some of the studies, ranged from 0% to 1.6%, and HBsAg loss occurred in 0.7% annually [5,15,16]. In another recent study, the risk of developing HCC was null in 338 HBeAg-negative Japanese ICs followed up for 1035 days [17].

In a study carried out in 1932 HBeAg-negative ICs followed for a mean of 13 years, the annual HCC rates and liver-related deaths were 0.06% and 0.04%, respectively, in HBV ICs, and 0.02% and 0.02% in controls. These results provide evidence that ICs are at higher risk of developing HCC and liver-related complications than uninfected individuals. Older age and alcohol intake were independent predictors of HCC development [18].

Other studies have focused on the risk of meeting antiviral therapy criteria during follow-up. Wong et al. analyzed 361 HBeAg-negative patients with HBV DNA levels <20 000 IU/mL, normal ALT, and mean TE at 5.4 kPa [5]. After an interval of 44 ± 7 months, liver fibrosis progression, defined as a TE increase of 30% or higher, was observed in 10 (2.8%) patients, and 49 (13.6%) started antiviral therapy. Patient sex and age, and ALT, HBV DNA, and HBsAg levels were not associated with progression of liver fibrosis. In addition, in 244 patients with baseline HBV DNA <2000 IU/mL, 2.9% had liver fibrosis progression, 8.2% started antiviral therapy, and 4.1% had HBV DNA ≥20 000 IU/mL during follow-up.

In another study, 153 HBeAg-negative patients with normal ALT and HBV DNA ≤20 000 IU/mL were prospectively followed for 57.2 months [15]. During follow-up, none of the 87 ICs reactivated and 19 (21.8%) cleared HBsAg, particularly those who were older (p=0.004), had lower HBsAg values (p<0.001), or a higher yearly HBsAg decline (p<0.001). Twenty-five of 46 (54.3%) HBeAg-negative patients with low viremia (HBV DNA ≤20 000 IU/mL) remained stable, 20 (43.5%) became ICs, and one (2.2%) developed CHB. Viremia persistently ≤20 000 IU/mL predicted a benign clinical outcome, being associated with transition to ICs in 43%. Nevertheless, 13.1% of those with low viremia at presentation developed CHB within one year. These studies support the EASL's recommendation of regular monitoring of these patients [1].

Inactive HBsAg carriers are at risk of HBV reactivation if they receive chemotherapy or immunosuppressive therapy, including the established and emerging new biological response modifiers [19]. The risk of HBV reactivation can be high, particularly in patients receiving rituximab alone or in combination with steroids. Therefore, all CHB patients, including ICs, should receive a nucleos(t)ide analog (NA) such as lamivudine, entecavir or tenofovir disoproxil to prevent HBV reactivation. In contrast, the optimal management of patients with chronic HBV infection (without CHB) remains controversial.

Therapy

Currently, the various HBV guidelines do not recommend therapy for ICs [1,3,20]. It has been estimated that every year 1–3% of ICs lose HBsAg spontaneously, which represents clinical cure of the infection [1].

A recent study conducted in China evaluated pegylated-interferon alpha-2a (PEG-IFN-alpha-2a) as a therapeutic option for ICs [21]. In total, 144 inactive HBsAg carriers were divided into a therapy group receiving either PEG-IFN-alpha-2a or PEG-IFN-alpha-2a combined with adefovir dipivoxil for no more than 96 weeks (102 individuals) versus an untreated control group (42 individuals). HBsAg clearance and seroconversion rates in the treated patients were 29.8% and 20.2% at week 48, which increased to 44.7% and 38.3% at week 96, respectively. In the control group, HBsAg clearance was 2.4% at weeks 48 and 96, and none achieved seroconversion. Despite limitations such as a lack of randomization, an inability to evaluate the effect of HBV DNA level on treatment, and a short posttreatment follow-up, this is the first proof of concept that interferon can increase HBsAg clearance in HBV ICs [21].

Nucleoside analogs are the treatment of choice for HBeAg-negative CHB. High viral suppression rates have been achieved, with very low rates of HBsAg clearance. NAs have not been evaluated in ICs because most of these patients have low HBV DNA levels and minimal or no liver disease. However, several novel antivirals for CHB patients are now being tested in phase 1 and 2 clinical trials. These include capsid inhibitors, miRNA, and immunomodulatory compounds, whose aim is to achieve a functional cure of chronic HBV infection. Depending on the results of these clinical studies, the management of ICs may completely change in the future.

References

1. EASL. 2017 Clinical Practice Guidelines on the management of hepatitis B virus infection. *Journal of Hepatology* 2017;67: 370–398.
2. Di Bisceglie AM, Lombardero M, Teckman J et al. Determination of hepatitis B phenotype using biochemical and serological markers. *Journal of Viral Hepatitis* 2017;24:320–329.
3. Terrault NA, Lok ASF, McMahon BJ et al. Update on prevention, diagnosis, and treatment of chronic hepatitis B: AASLD 2018 hepatitis B guidance. *Hepatology* 2018;67:1560–1599.
4. Ruhl CE, Everhart JE. Upper limits of normal for alanine aminotransferase activity in the United States population. *Hepatology* 2012;55:447–454.
5. Wong GL, Chan HL, Yu Z, Chan HY, Tse CH, Wong VW. Liver fibrosis progression is uncommon in patients with inactive chronic hepatitis B: a prospective cohort study with paired transient elastography examination. *Journal of Gastroenterology and Hepatology* 2013;28:1842–1848.
6. Brunetto MR, Oliveri F, Colombatto P et al. Hepatitis B surface antigen serum levels help to distinguish active from inactive hepatitis B virus genotype D carriers. *Gastroenterology* 2010;139:483–490.
7. Riveiro-Barciela M, Bes M, Rodriguez-Frias F et al. Serum hepatitis B core-related antigen is more accurate than hepatitis B surface antigen to identify inactive carriers, regardless of hepatitis B virus genotype. *Clinical Microbiology and Infection* 2017;23:860–867.
8. Jaroszewicz J, Calle Serrano B, Wursthorn K et al. Hepatitis B surface antigen (HBsAg) levels in the natural history of hepatitis B virus (HBV)-infection: a European perspective. *Journal of Hepatology* 2010;52:514–522.
9. Liu J, Yang HI, Lee MH et al. Serum levels of hepatitis B surface antigen and DNA can predict inactive carriers with low risk of disease progression. *Hepatology* 2016;64:381–389.
10. Ungtrakul T, Sriprayoon T, Kusuman P et al. Role of quantitative hepatitis B surface antigen in predicting inactive carriers and HBsAg seroclearance in HBeAg-negative chronic hepatitis B patients. *Medicine* 2017;96:e6554.
11. Peiffer KH, Kuhnhenn L, Jiang B et al. Divergent preS sequences in virion-associated hepatitis B virus genomes and subviral HBV surface antigen particles from HBV e antigen-negative patients. *Journal of Infectious Diseases* 2018;218: 114–123.
12. Brunetto MR, Marcellin P, Cherubini B et al. Response to peginterferon alfa-2a (40KD) in HBeAg-negative CHB: on-treatment kinetics of HBsAg serum levels vary by HBV genotype. *Journal of Hepatology* 2013;59:1153–1159.
13. Maimone S, Caccamo G, Squadrito G et al. A combination of different diagnostic tools allows identification of inactive hepatitis B virus carriers at a single time point evaluation. *Liver International* 2017;37:362–368.
14. Castera L, Bernard PH, Le Bail B et al. Transient elastography and biomarkers for liver fibrosis assessment and follow-up of inactive hepatitis B carriers. *Alimentary Pharmacology and Therapeutics* 2011;33:455–465.
15. Oliveri F, Surace L, Cavallone D et al. Long-term outcome of inactive and active, low viraemic HBeAg-negative-hepatitis B virus infection: benign course towards HBsAg clearance. *Liver International* 2017;37:1622–1631.
16. Habersetzer F, Moenne-Loccoz R, Meyer N et al. Loss of hepatitis B surface antigen in a real-life clinical cohort of patients with chronic hepatitis B virus infection. *Liver International* 2015;35:130–139.
17. Taida T, Arai M, Kanda T et al. The prognosis of hepatitis B inactive carriers in Japan: a multicenter prospective study. *Journal of Gastroenterology* 2017;52:113–122.
18. Chen JD, Yang HI, Iloeje UH et al. Carriers of inactive hepatitis B virus are still at risk for hepatocellular carcinoma and liver-related death. *Gastroenterology* 2010;138:1747–1754.

19. Perrillo RP, Gish R, Falck-Ytter YT. American Gastroenterological Association Institute technical review on prevention and treatment of hepatitis B virus reactivation during immunosuppressive drug therapy. *Gastroenterology* 2015;148: 221–244.e223.

20. Sarin SK, Kumar M, Lau GK et al. Asian-Pacific clinical practice guidelines on the management of hepatitis B: a 2015 update. *Hepatology International* 2016;10:1–98.

21. Cao Z, Liu Y, Ma L et al. A potent hepatitis B surface antigen response in subjects with inactive hepatitis B surface antigen carrier treated with pegylated-interferon alpha. *Hepatology* 2017;66:1058–1066.

22. Tong MJ, Trieu J. Hepatitis B inactive carriers: clinical course and outcomes. *Journal of Digestive Diseases* 2013;14:311–317.

23. Magalhaes MJ, Pedroto I. Hepatitis B virus inactive carriers: which follow-up strategy? *Portuguese Journal of Gastroenterology* 2015;22:47–51.

27 Hepatitis B e antigen-positive chronic hepatitis B infection with minimal changes on liver biopsy: what to do next

Apostolos Koffas and Patrick T. Kennedy

Barts Liver Centre, The Blizard Institute, Queen Mary University of London, London, UK

LEARNING POINTS

- HBeAg-positive chronic infection is not benign and events associated with hepatocarcinogenesis appear to be already under way at this early stage of the disease.

- Virus-specific T-cell responses appear to be preserved in those formerly referred to as "immune tolerant" and these responses are no different from those seen in the HBeAg-positive "immune active" disease phase.

- Early initiation of antiviral treatment in HBeAg-positive chronic infection can reduce the risk of HCC development, in addition to reducing the pool of HBV infection and the risk of transmission in young individuals.

An estimated 240 million people worldwide are chronic carriers of hepatitis B surface antigen (HBsAg), the hallmark of chronic infection [1]. Chronic hepatitis B (CHB) mortality is consequent to the development of cirrhosis and/or primary liver cancer, accounting for 850 000 deaths in 2015, which represents the leading cause of hepatocellular carcinoma (HCC) worldwide [2]. The World Health Organization (WHO) published global targets to combat the burden of hepatitis B and C by reducing new chronic infections by 90% and relevant mortality by 65% by the year 2030 [3].

The primary goal in the treatment of CHB is the prevention of all-cause morbidity and mortality associated with hepatitis B virus (HBV)-related cirrhosis and/or HCC development. Currently, the backbone of CHB treatment is nucleos(t)ide analogs (NAs); in particular, tenofovir disoproxil (TDF), entecavir (ETV), and tenofovir alafenamide (TAF) are the preferred treatment options, owing to their favorable profiles, once-daily administration, and high genetic barriers to resistance. A second therapeutic option is pegylated interferon-alpha (peg-IFN-alpha) for a finite treatment duration (48 weeks); however, peg-IFN-alpha is effective only in a small proportion of patients and even with careful patient selection, its efficacy remains suboptimal in addition to its unfavorable systemic effects [4].

Chronic hepatitis B has traditionally been divided into four disease phases – immune tolerant (IT), immune active (IA), inactive carrier, and immune escape – taking into account the presence or absence of hepatitis B e antigen (HBeAg), HBV DNA levels, serum alanine aminotransferase (ALT) values, and the presence or absence of inflammations/fibrosis. Additionally, HBsAg-negative, hepatitis B core antibody (anti-HBc)-positive individuals are considered to have "occult" hepatitis B, being at risk of hepatitis B reactivation when immunosuppressed. More recently, the European Association for the Study of the Liver (EASL), proposed a change in the nomenclature, as shown in Table 27.1, based primarily on the presence or absence of HBeAg [5].

HBeAg-positive chronic infection, formerly referred to as the IT phase, is classically characterized by high-titer viremia, normal ALT levels, and absence or minimal inflammation/fibrosis on liver biopsy (or other, noninvasive modalities). Patients can remain in this disease phase for several decades. Historically, this early disease phase has been perceived as a

Clinical Dilemmas in Viral Liver Disease, Second Edition. Edited by Graham R. Foster and K. Rajender Reddy.
© 2020 John Wiley & Sons Ltd. Published 2020 by John Wiley & Sons Ltd.

Table 27.1 Clinical parameters during disease phases of chronic hepatitis B

	Immune tolerant (IT)	Immune active (IA)	Inactive carrier	Immune escape	HBsAg negative, anti-HBc positive
	HBeAg positive		HBeAg negative		
	Chronic infection	Chronic hepatitis	Chronic infection	Chronic hepatitis	
Duration	20–30 years	Can be protracted	Many years	Variable if occurs	HBsAg clearance usually sustained except in context of immune suppression
Anti-HBe	Negative	Negative	Positive	Positive	Positive
HBV DNA (IU/mL)	>1 000 000	>20 000	<2000	2000–20 000	Usually undetectable
Liver enzymes	Normal	Elevated (fluctuating)	Normal	Elevated	Normal
Liver histology	No/minimal fibrosis and inflammation	Moderate/severe fibrosis and inflammation	No fibrosis and inflammation	Moderate fibrosis and inflammation	No/minimal fibrosis and inflammation
HBsAg level	High	High/moderate	Low	Low/moderate	Undetectable

anti-HBe, hepatitis B e antibody; HBeAg, hepatitis B e antigen; HBsAg, hepatitis B surface antigen; HBV DNA, hepatitis B viral load; IU/mL, international units/milliliter.

"benign", disease-free phase, so these patients were excluded from therapy. HBeAg-positive chronic infection/IT phase is often followed by a period of immune activity (HBeAg-positive chronic hepatitis), when patients are considered antiviral treatment candidates. The current debate in the field is whether patients should be started on antiviral treatment earlier, irrespective of serum ALT values [6].

The perception that this is a benign disease phase devoid of disease progression, including HCC initiation, has been challenged by recent data. Kennedy et al. challenged the concept of immunologic tolerance in young patients by demonstrating HBV-specific T-cell responses in young individuals, which were no different to their peers considered IA. In particular, T-cells from young patients with CHB demonstrated a superior ability to produce Th1 cytokines (IFN-gamma and tumor necrosis factor [TNF]-alpha) in comparison to healthy subjects. It was also observed that PD-1+ CD8 T-cells, a surrogate of immune activity, were no different between HBeAg-positive chronic infection/IT and HBeAg-positive chronic hepatitis/IA, in age-matched peers under the age of 30. Additionally, the observation that PD-1+ CD 127 low CD8 T-cells increase with age in patients with CHB indicates that HBV infection over time induces a progressive state of T-cell exhaustion [7]. The above findings highlight the inadequacy of serum

ALT levels in reflecting the presence/absence of antiviral T-cell responses in these patients, and challenge the classic dogma that treatment should be withheld until there is a persistent elevation in serum ALT [8].

Mason et al. demonstrated that HBV DNA integration and clonal hepatocyte expansion, both considered initiating events for HCC development, were similar between patients in HBeAg-positive chronic infection/IT phase and HBeAg-positive chronic hepatitis/IA phase. In particular, HBV DNA integration was shown to be prevalent in both the early and late stages of CHB. It was demonstrated that at least $\sim 5 \times 10^6$ distinct integration sites were present in a liver of 5×10^{11} hepatocytes in each patient group, including those characterized as IT, irrespective of the presence or absence of advanced liver disease. It was also shown that clonal hepatocyte expansion, a risk factor for development of HCC, is present across all the disease phases. The principle is that clonal hepatocyte expansion in mutated hepatocytes could contribute to tumorigenesis. The average hepatocyte clone sizes in both the "IT" and "IA" phases were beyond those predicted for normal liver turnover, reflecting ongoing immune-mediated liver injury, a key driver in the development of HCC [9]. The above results indicate that the risk of HCC may already be present in the HBeAg-positive chronic infection phase, hence necessitating a reevaluation of early treatment in young patients with CHB [6,10].

Additionally, the REVEAL study showed a correlation between high viral load and the risk of HCC, independent of cirrhosis [5]. Subsequently, Kim et al. studied whether administration of antiviral therapy in the "IT phase," which as previously described is characterized by significant viremia, would reduce HCC risk and overall mortality. The 10-year estimated cumulative incidences of HCC (12.7% vs 6.1%; p=0.001) and death/transplantation (9.7% vs 3.4%; p<0.001) were significantly higher in HBeAg-positive chronic infection/IT phase than in treated HBeAg-positive chronic hepatitis/IA phase [11].

Considering the growing body of evidence indicating that events associated with hepatocarcinogenesis appear to be already present in this early phase of CHB, the EASL updated its 2017 guidance to broaden treatment consideration for individuals with HBeAg-positive chronic infection/IT phase, provided they are 30 years or older, or they have a family history of HCC or cirrhosis, or there is evidence of extrahepatic disease, regardless of ALT level and the presence or absence of underlying inflammation or fibrosis [12]. The American Association for the Study of Liver Disease (AASLD) and the Asian Pacific Association for the Study of the Liver (APASL) also released their 2018 and 2016 recommendations respectively. The AASLD rec-

ommends 3–6-monthly follow-up for these patients. Treatment should be considered in cases where HBV DNA levels are greater than 20 000 IU/mL, with elevated serum ALT levels (greater than twice the upper normal limit), and remain elevated for more than 3–6 months. In patients whose ALT levels remains borderline normal or slightly elevated, especially in those over age 40 who acquired the infection at a young age, antiviral therapy should be considered provided that a liver biopsy or a noninvasive modality is performed and either moderate-to-severe inflammation and/or fibrosis (F2 or higher) is demonstrated [12]. Similarly, the APASL recommends that HBeAg-positive viremic patients older than 35–40 years, with high normal or minimally raised ALT levels or family history of HCC or cirrhosis, should undergo assessment of fibrosis with noninvasive modalities and should be considered for a liver biopsy, aiming to identify patients with significant fibrosis or moderate/severe inflammation requiring treatment. In HBeAg-positive patients under 30 years of age with persistently normal ALT level, high-titer viremia, no evidence of underlying liver disease and no family history of HCC or cirrhosis, the APASL generally does not recommend antiviral therapy, but favors noninvasive assessment of liver fibrosis and follow-up at regular intervals [13]. Table 27.2 summarizes treatment recommendations from the EASL, AASLD, and APASL.

Table 27.2 Guidance for management of noncirrhotic HBeAg-positive chronic infection/immune tolerant

	Definition	Treatment recommendation
[tb]EASL (2017)	HBsAg high ALT normal HBV DNA >10⁷ IU/mL None/minimal liver disease	Monitor every 3–6 months May treat if >30 years even if ALT and biopsy normal Consider treatment if patient has extrahepatic manifestations of HBV or a family history of HCC/ cirrhosis
AASLD (2018)	HBsAg present for ≥6 months Normal or minimally elevated ALT and/or AST HBV DNA levels are very high (typically >1 million IU/mL) Liver biopsy or noninvasive test results show no fibrosis and minimal inflammation	Monitor every 3–6 months May treat if HBV DNA >20 000 IU/mL and ALT persistently higher than 2 times the upper normal limit Consider treatment if >40 years and biopsy shows moderate-to-severe necroinflammation/fibrosis even if ALT persistently borderline/normal
APASL (2016)	ALT persistently normal Elevated HBV DNA Absence of significant inflammation or fibrosis on biopsy	Monitor every 3–6 months Exclude other causes if elevated ALT Assess fibrosis noninvasively Individualize liver biopsy Treat if evidence of significant inflammation or fibrosis on biopsy

ALT, alanine aminotransferase; HBeAg, hepatitis B e Antigen; HBsAg, bepatitis B surface antigen; HBV DNA, hepatitis B viral load; IU/mL, international units/milliliter.

Nucleoside analogs and peg-IFN-alpha represent the mainstay of treatment in CHB, although there is a paucity of data regarding antiviral treatment in HBeAg chronic infection. Overall, treatment with NAs remains the first-line treatment option, owing to good tolerability, favorable side effect profile, once-daily administration, high genetic barrier to resistance, and potential reduction of HCC risk [4]. Recent studies have explored the use of combination or sequential therapies with NAs and peg-IFN-alpha to potentially improve treatment outcomes. However, in spite of some promising findings, further studies are needed to better define the immunologic effects of these combination or sequential treatment strategies. Furthermore, recent advances with *in vitro* and *in vivo* models of HBV infection indicate that multiple therapeutic strategies both targeting the viral life cycle and restoring the host immune response are likely to be required in combination with existing licensed treatment options to achieve HBV functional cure [1].

Conclusion

In essence, recent data suggest that HBeAg-positive chronic infection, formerly known as the IT disease phase, is not a benign state devoid of disease progression but that events associated with tumorigenesis may already be present. In contrast to the historic perception, virus-specific T-cell responses appear to be preserved at this early stage of CHB. These recent findings challenge the historical dogma that patients in this disease phase should be excluded from antiviral treatment, primarily owing to drug costs and potential toxicity associated with long-term therapy, but more importantly due to the misperception of the absence of disease activity in this phase. Guidance from international governing bodies has been updated to consider the above reinterpretation of disease phase in CHB; for instance, the EASL now recommends treatment consideration for HBeAg-positive patients who do not fulfill the traditional treatment criteria. With the widespread availability of potent NAs and the emergence of novel pipeline therapies, careful consideration should now be given to treatment candidacy. The initiation of antiviral treatment in such patients and the broadening of treatment candidacy has the potential to prevent disease progression, reduce the risk of HCC

development, and reduce the pool of HBV-infected patients, not to mention the potential to achieve HBsAg loss and functional cure with the employment of novel agents.

References

1. Collier J, Sherman M. Screening for hepatocellular carcinoma. *Hepatology* 1998;27(1):273–278.
2. El-Serag HB, Rudolph KL. Hepatocellular carcinoma: epidemiology and molecular carcinogenesis. *Gastroenterology* 2007;132(7):2557–2576.
3. Bruix J, Sherman M. Management of hepatocellular carcinoma. *Hepatology* 2005;42(5):1208–1236.
4. Singal A, Volk ML, Waljee A et al. Meta analysis: surveillance with ultrasound for early stage hepatocellular carcinoma in patients with cirrhosis. *Alimentary Pharmacology and Therapeutics* 2009;307–47.
5. Gebo KA, Chander G, Jenckes MW et al. Screening tests for hepatocellular carcinoma in patients with chronic hepatitis C: a systematic review. *Hepatology* 2002;36(5 Suppl 1):S84–92.
6. Colli A, Fraquelli M, Casazza G et al. Accuracy of ultrasonography, spiral CT, magnetic resonance, and alpha-fetoprotein in diagnosing hepatocellular carcinoma: a systematic review. *American Journal of Gastroenterology* 2006;101(3):513–523.
7. Kennedy PTF, Sandalova E, Jo J et al. Preserved T-cell function in children and young adults with immune-tolerant chronic hepatitis B. *Gastroenterology* 2012;143(3):637–645.
8. Chen JG, Parkin DM, Chen QG et al. Screening for liver cancer: results of a randomised controlled trial in Qidong, China. *Journal of Medical Screening* 2003;10(4):204–209.
9. Mason WS, Gill US, Litwin S et al. HBV DNA integration and clonal hepatocyte expansion in chronic hepatitis B patients considered immune tolerant. *Gastroenterology* 2016;151(5):986–998.
10. Gupta S, Bent S, Kohlwes J. Test characteristics of alpha-fetoprotein for detecting hepatocellular carcinoma in patients with hepatitis C. A systematic review and critical analysis. *Annals of Internal Medicine* 2003;139(1):46–50.
11. Kim GA, Lim YS, Han S et al. High risk of hepatocellular carcinoma and death in patients with immune-tolerant-phase chronic hepatitis B Gut. 2018;67(5):945–952.
12. Pepe MS, Etzioni R, Feng Z et al. Phases of biomarker development for early detection of cancer. *Journal of the National Cancer Institute* 2001;93(14):1054–1061.
13. Marrero JA. Screening tests for hepatocellular carcinoma. *Clinical Liver Disease* 2005;9(2):235–251, vi.

28 The management of hepatitis B virus in pregnancy

Henry L.Y. Chan

Department of Medicine and Therapeutics, The Chinese University of Hong Kong, Hong Kong SAR, China

---

LEARNING POINTS

- Risk of maternal-to-infant HBV transmission persists despite vaccination of the newborn when maternal viral load exceeds 6 log IU/mL.

- Use of tenofovir disoproxil fumarate in the third trimester of gestation for mothers with high viral load can greatly reduce the risk of HBV transmission to infants.

- Close monitoring of HBV DNA and ALT for six months postpartum is recommended after cessation of tenofovir disoproxil fumarate.

- Tenofovir disoproxil fumarate is generally safe for both mothers and infants, and breastfeeding is not contraindicated for mothers on tenofovir disoproxil fumarate.

Prevention of hepatitis B virus transmission by vaccination

Before the introduction of hepatitis B virus (HBV) vaccination, mother-to-baby transmission was a key route of HBV acquisition, particularly in Asian countries. After acquisition of HBV at birth, 95% of infants will develop chronic HBV infection. A standard three-dose universal HBV vaccination with first dose started within 24 hours after birth is recommended by the World Health Organization to prevent mother-to-baby transmission of HBV. For HBV-infected mothers, coadministration of hepatitis B immunoglobulin with birth dose vaccine can offer additional protection to the newborn to prevent perinatal transmission.

Universal vaccination was first introduced in Taiwan in 1984. By the end of 2016, hepatitis B vaccine had been introduced in 186 countries and global coverage with three doses of HBV vaccine was estimated at 84%. The United Kingdom is one of the last European countries to introduce universal vaccination for newborns; all babies born after August 2017 are eligible for HBV vaccine. Five European countries (Denmark, Finland, Iceland, Norway, and Sweden) have not yet introduced universal HBV vaccination policy due to the low local prevalence of HBV infection.

Introduction of universal vaccination has led to a dramatic reduction in the global prevalence of HBV infection. In Taiwan, where maternal HBV infection is prevalent, among freshmen aged 15 years who have received vaccination at birth, protective anti-HBs level ($\geq 10\,\mathrm{IU/mL}$) was found in 48.3% and amnestic response in 72% of the remaining subjects [1]. Approximately 0.5% of Taiwanese children aged <15 years still have positive hepatitis B surface antigen (HBsAg), and a few subjects with occult HBV infection (negative HBsAg, positive anti-HBc, and detectable HBV DNA) were also identified 25 years after the launch of the universal vaccination program [2]. Various reports from China and Taiwan have shown that positive maternal hepatitis B e antigen (HBeAg) status and high maternal viral load are the key factors associated with risk of HBV transmission despite vaccination of newborns [3]. In general, the risk of HBV transmission to newborn starts to increase when maternal HBV DNA is higher than 6 log IU/mL, and the risk increases exponentially with each

Clinical Dilemmas in Viral Liver Disease, Second Edition. Edited by Graham R. Foster and K. Rajender Reddy.
© 2020 John Wiley & Sons Ltd. Published 2020 by John Wiley & Sons Ltd.

logarithmic increase in maternal viral load. As serum HBsAg has good correlation with HBV DNA level in HBeAg-positive mothers, serum HBsAg >4 log IU/mL is also found to associate with increased risk of maternal-to-infant HBV transmission.

Antiviral prophylaxis for high viral load mothers

As recommended by the US Food and Drug Administration, telbivudine and tenofovir disoproxil fumarate are category B anti-HBV drugs for pregnant women. Based on data from antiretroviral registries, lamivudine appears to have similar safety to tenofovir disoproxil fumarate in pregnancy [4].

To further reduce the risk of HBV transmission to newborns by HBV carrier mothers with high viral load, many centers studied the use of antiviral agents in the third trimester at week 28–32 of gestation in addition to vaccination of the newborn [5]. In general, HBV transmission was reduced by a relative risk of 70% by antiviral treatment. A randomized controlled trial was conducted in China comparing tenofovir disoproxil fumarate started at 30–32 weeks of gestation versus no antiviral treatment for mothers with HBV DNA >200 000 IU/mL [6]. All infants received a combination of three-dose HBV vaccine and hepatitis B immunoglobulin at birth. On per protocol analysis, 7% of babies born from 88 deliveries without tenofovir disoproxil fumarate versus 0% babies from 97 deliveries with tenofovir disoproxil fumarate treatment had HBV infection (p=0.01). Another randomized placebo-controlled trial in Thailand showed only 2% infant HBV infection rate with an intensive five-dose HBV vaccine regime with birth dose started 1.2 hours after birth, which is not significantly different from that of the tenofovir disoproxil fumarate arm (0%) [7]. However, isolated cases of HBV infection have been reported among infants born to HBV-infected mothers who received tenofovir disoproxil fumarate since the third trimester and the maternal viral load at delivery was about 4–5 log IU/mL [8,9].

As the use of lamivudine or telbivudine may induce drug resistance, particularly among high viral load carrier mothers, tenofovir disoproxil fumarate should be the preferred antiviral drug to use during pregnancy. The American Association for the Study of Liver Diseases (AASLD) and the European Association for the Study of the Liver (EASL) recommend tenofovir disoproxil fumarate

treatment for all pregnant women with high HBV DNA load (>200 000 IU/mL) [10,11]. There is some controversy on the threshold of maternal HBV DNA for commencement of tenofovir disoproxil fumarate, as most carriers had HBV DNA >6–7 log IU/mL in the randomized controlled trials in China and Thailand [6,7]. The AASLD recommends treatment commencement at week 28–32 of gestation, whereas the EASL recommends an earlier start at week 24–28. There are insufficient data to recommend the commencement of tenofovir disoproxil fumarate at an earlier phase of pregnancy, although some experts suggest starting it in the second trimester for mothers with HBV DNA >9 log IU/mL. Nonetheless, with the safety data of tenofovir disoproxil fumarate during pregnancy from antiretroviral registries, pregnant women on this drug should be continued, and those on other antiviral drugs should be switched to tenofovir disoproxil fumarate throughout their pregnancy.

Hepatitis flare after stopping antiviral therapy

Pregnancy is a special stage of life when cell-mediated immunity is suppressed to tolerate paternally derived fetal antigens, while the immunology changes are reversed back to normal postpartum. As a result, elevation of alanine aminotransferase (ALT) may develop in the postpartum period in HBV carrier mothers. Approximately 10–25% of HBV-infected women develop elevation of ALT after delivery; most ALT flares are <5 times the upper limit of normal and self-limiting, and rarely lead to hepatic decompensation [12–14]. Mothers with positive HBeAg and higher HBV DNA seem to have a higher risk of postpartum ALT flare.

For mothers who are in the phase of HBeAg-positive chronic infection (or immune-tolerant phase), which is characterized by very high viral load but absence of significant hepatic necroinflammation or fibrosis, long-term antiviral treatment may not be desirable or indicated [10,11]. In a clinical trial using tenofovir disoproxil fumarate among patients in the immune-tolerant phase, only 45% had HBV DNA <29 IU/mL and 5% had HBeAg seroconversion at the end of four years of treatment [15]. the AASLD and EASL recommend that discontinuation of tenofovir disoproxil fumarate can be considered within 12 weeks after delivery [10,11]. As antiviral drugs can only suppress HBV DNA replication but cannot eliminate HBV in the liver, viral relapse after stopping antiviral drugs after pregnancy should be expected. Based on the randomized controlled trial conducted in China, the risk of any ALT elevation postpartum was slightly higher among HBV carrier mothers who stopped tenofovir disoproxil fumarate (46%) versus those who were untreated (30%) [6]. Only 1% of mothers developed ALT level >10 times upper limit of normal after stopping tenofovir disoproxil fumarate, and ALT was normalized after reinitiation of antiviral therapy. In the randomized trial in Thailand, postpartum ALT flare to >300 IU/mL was similar between mothers who stopped tenofovir disoproxil fumarate (9%) and placebo (6%) [7]. Nonetheless, among mothers with indications for antiviral treatment, for example those who have evidence of significant liver fibrosis, antiviral treatment should not be stopped after delivery and long-term antiviral treatment should be offered.

Regardless of the use of antiviral therapy, ALT elevation may occur postpartum in HBV carrier mothers. Most ALT elevation develops within the first six months postpartum in both untreated mothers and those who have stopped antiviral treatment. A large-scale follow-up study in China revealed two bursts of hepatic flare at one month (19.8%) and three months (17.1%) after delivery, and the time pattern was similar among mothers with and without antiviral therapy [16]. Hence, close monitoring for HBV DNA and ALT at four-weekly intervals is recommended in the initial six months postpartum. Mild ALT elevation can be observed without antiviral therapy as it is usually self-limiting. Reinitiation of antiviral therapy should be considered if ALT is elevated to >10 times the upper limit of normal.

Safety of antiviral drugs during pregnancy and breastfeeding

The use of antiviral therapy (lamivudine, telbivudine, tenofovir disoproxil fumarate) is safe for both the mother and the fetus [5]. Based on reports from observational studies, there was no increase in congenital malformation and prematurity for infants or increase in postpartum hemorrhage, cesarean section rate or elevated creatine kinase rate for mothers who received antiviral therapy. According to the label of tenofovir disoproxil fumarate, breastfeeding is not recommended.

However, available data from animal and human in current literature suggest that the concentration of tenofovir disoproxil fumarate in breast milk is low and should not be harmful to the infant [17]. Balancing the risk and benefit of tenofovir disoproxil fumarate for HBV-infected mothers and infants, the AASLD and EASL recommend no contraindication to breastfeeding in HBsAg-positive women treated with tenofovir disoproxil fumarate [10,11].

References

1. Wu TW, Lin HH, Wang LY. Chronic hepatitis B infection in adolescents who received primary infantile vaccination. *Hepatology* 2013;57:38–45.
2. Ni YH, Chang MH, Wu JF, Hsu HY, Chen HL, Chan DS. Minimization of hepatitis B infection by 25-year universal vaccination program. *Journal of Hepatology* 2012;57:730–735.
3. Wen WH, Huang CW, Chie WC et al. Quantitative maternal hepatitis B surface antigen predicts maternally transmitted hepatitis B virus infection. *Hepatology* 2016;64:1451–1461.
4. Bzowej NH. Hepatitis B therapy in pregnancy. *Current Hepatitis Reports* 2010;9:197–204.
5. Brown Jr RS, McMahon BJ, Lok AS et al. Antiviral therapy in chronic hepatitis B viral infection during pregnancy: a systemic review and meta-analysis. *Hepatology* 2016;63:319–333.
6. Pan CQ, Duan Z, Dai E et al. Tenofovir to prevent hepatitis B transmission in mothers with high viral load. *New England Journal of Medicine* 2016;374:2324–2334.
7. Jourdain G, Ngo-Giang-Huong N, Harrison L et al. Tenofovir versus placebo to prevent perinatal transmission of hepatitis B. *New England Journal of Medicine* 2018;378:911–923.
8. Chen HL, Lee CN, Chang CH, Ni YH, Shyu MK, Chen SM. Efficacy of maternal tenofovir disoproxil fumarate in interrupting mother-to-infant transmission of hepatitis B virus. *Hepatology* 2015;62:375–386.
9. Greenup AJ, Tan PK, Nguyen V et al. Efficacy and safety of tenofovir disoproxil fumarate in pregnancy to prevent perinatal transmission of hepatitis B virus. *Journal of Hepatology* 2014;61:502–507.
10. European Association for the Study of the Liver. EASL 2017 clinical practice guideline on the management of hepatitis B virus infection. *Journal of Hepatology* 2017;67:370–398.
11. Terrault NA, Lok ASF, McMahon BJ et al. Update on prevention, diagnosis, and treatment of chronic hepatitis B: AASLD 2018 hepatitis B guidance. *Hepatology* 2018;67:1560–1599.
12. Giles M, Visvanathan K, Lewin S et al. Clinical and virological predictors of hepatic flares in pregnant women with chronic hepatitis B. *Gut* 2015;64:1810–1815.

13. Chang CY, Aziz N, Poongkunran M et al. Serum alanine aminotransferase and hepatitis B DNA flares in pregnant and postpartum women with chronic hepatitis B. *American Journal of Gastroenterology* 2016;111:1410–1415.

14. Kushner T, Shaw PA, Kalra A et al. Incidence, determinants and outcomes of pregnancy-associated hepatitis B flares: a regional hospital-based cohort study. *Liver International* 2017;38:813–820.

15. Chan HLY, Chan CK, Hui AJ et al. Effects of tenofovir disoproxil fumarate in hepatitis B e antigen-positive patients with normal levels of alanine aminotransferase and high levels of hepatitis B virus DNA. *Gastroenterology* 2014;146: 1240–1248.

16. Liu J, Wang J, Qi C et al. Baseline hepatitis B virus titer predicts initial postpartum hepatic flare. *Journal of Clinical Gastroenterology* 2018;52:902–907.

17. Ehrhardt S, Xie C, Guo N, Nelson K, Thio CL. Breastfeeding while taking lamivudine or tenofovir disoproxil fumarate: a review of the evidence. *Clinical Infectious Disease* 2015; 60:275–278.

29 Treatment of hepatitis B in children

Maureen M. Jonas

Children's Hospital Boston, Division of Gastroenterology, Boston, MA, USA

LEARNING POINTS

- Most individuals with chronic hepatitis B virus (HBV) acquired infection either perinatally or during childhood. Chronic HBV acquired during childhood may be associated with significant morbidity later in life, such as cirrhosis and hepatocellular carcinoma (HCC).

- Most children with chronic HBV are in the immune-tolerant stage. Treatment is not helpful or indicated during this stage, and indiscriminate use of nucleotide/nucleoside analogs may elicit resistance, with serious negative ramifications for later treatment.

- Some children with chronic HBV may be candidates for treatment. This includes those primarily in the immune active phase, with persistently abnormal ALT values and histologic chronic hepatitis.

- There are now several therapeutic options for chronic HBV during childhood.

When making treatment decisions, it is important to remember that the natural history of chronic HBV infection in children is variable, depending upon age, mode of acquisition, and ethnicity. These differences are likely due to the immune tolerance that is known to develop when infection occurs at an early age, although the exact mechanisms are unknown. Children from endemic countries in whom HBV is acquired perinatally are usually HBeAg positive with high levels of viral replication [1]. Rates of spontaneous seroconversion are less than 2% per year in children younger than 3 years of age, and 4–5% after age 3. By contrast, children in nonendemic countries are less likely to have acquired the disease perinatally. In this case, they frequently clear HBeAg and IIBV DNA from serum during the first two decades of life [2]. In a 29-year longitudinal study of Italian children with chronic HBV who underwent HBeAg seroconversion, 95% of those without cirrhosis had inactive HBV infection at most recent follow-up and 15% cleared HBsAg [3]. Children who seroconvert spontaneously tend to have higher alanine aminotransferase (ALT) levels early in life.

Although inflammatory changes are often mild in liver biopsies from children with chronic hepatitis B, fibrosis may be significant. In a study of 76 children with chronic HBeAg-positive HBV and elevated ALT (mean age 9.8 years), at least half had moderate-to-severe fibrosis, with 35% having either bridging fibrosis with lobular distortion or cirrhosis [4]. Cirrhosis is an infrequent complication of HBV infection during childhood, although precise incidence is uncertain. One of the largest studies included 292 consecutive children who were HBsAg positive and had an elevated serum ALT level [5]. Cirrhosis was found in 10 patients (3%) at a mean age 4.0 ± 3.3 years. No child developed cirrhosis during follow-up (ranging from 1 to 10 years).

There are no data regarding treatment of acute HBV infection in children. Most children infected perinatally are asymptomatic, and the small percentage in whom acute, even fulminant, hepatitis develops rapidly clear HBsAg and viremia.

Some children with chronic HBV infection require treatment in order to prevent serious sequelae, such as cirrhosis and HCC, in young adult life. Management of children with chronic HBV infection involves education and

Clinical Dilemmas in Viral Liver Disease, Second Edition. Edited by Graham R. Foster and K. Rajender Reddy.
© 2020 John Wiley & Sons Ltd. Published 2020 by John Wiley & Sons Ltd.

counseling, surveillance for hepatocellular carcinoma, and antiviral therapies in some cases.

There are some large trials in children to guide treatment decisions. Treatment is generally considered in patients who are in the immune active phase, usually defined as ALT more than 1.5–2 times upper limit of normal (ULN) and HBV DNA >20 000 IU/mL for at least six months [6]. Almost all children with chronic HBV are HBeAg positive, but therapy can also be considered for the few in whom HBeAg is negative, provided that viremia >10^4 IU/mL is documented and other diseases are excluded. The choice of whether to treat depends on patient-specific characteristics that predict the efficacy of treatment, including persistently abnormal ALT levels, and active disease on liver biopsy, as well as considerations regarding the likelihood of achieving appropriate therapeutic goals.

The likelihood of response to some of the available therapies depends upon the degree of elevation of the serum aminotransferases [7–9]. ALT levels less than 1.5–2 times ULN generally indicate that the patient is in the immune-tolerant phase of HBV infection. Such children are not typically candidates for treatment, because treatment with any of the currently available drugs does not result in higher rates of HBeAg seroconversion compared with no treatment. Prolonged treatment with nucleoside/nucleotide analogs at this stage is associated with little benefit, but imposes the important risk of viral resistance, both to the agent chosen and similar drugs. An exception may be those immune-tolerant children who will be undergoing immunosuppression, such as those who will have chemotherapy, or stem cell or solid organ transplantation. Just as in adults, HBV suppression should be considered during these critical periods to avoid activation of hepatitis.

Children with ALT values greater than 10 times ULN may be in the process of spontaneous HBeAg seroconversion, and should be observed for several months before treatment is begun. There may be several other considerations in deciding upon treatment in individual patients, such as coinfection with hepatitis C (HCV), hepatitis D, human immunodeficiency virus, or other comorbidities.

Interferon (IFN)-alpha, PEG-IFN-alpha, lamivudine, and entecavir are licensed for use in children as young as 2–3 years of age, and tenofovir disoproxil fumarate is also available for use in those over 12 years of age [8].

A large multinational randomized controlled trial of IFN-alpha was performed in 144 children with chronic HBeAg-positive infection and ALT greater than twice ULN [9]. Serum HBeAg and HBV DNA became negative in 26% of treated children in comparison to 11% of untreated controls. In addition, 10% of treated children lost HBsAg compared to 1% of controls. In a recently published trial, children with immune-active HBeAg+ chronic hepatitis B without cirrhosis were randomized to receive either pegylated interferon-alpha or no treatment for 48 weeks [10]. HBeAg seroconversion rates at 24 weeks post treatment were significantly higher in treated children (25.7% vs 6%; p=0.0043), as were the rates of hepatitis B surface antigen (HBsAg) clearance (8.9% vs 0%; p=0.03), hepatitis B virus (HBV) DNA <2000 IU/mL (28.7% vs 2.0%; p<0.001) or undetectable (16.8% vs 2.0%; p=0.0069), and ALT normalization (51.5% vs 12%; p<0.001). Overall, PEG-IFN alpha-2a treatment was efficacious and well tolerated, and associated with higher incidence of HBsAg clearance than in adults. This treatment has now been approved for children 2 years of age and older.

Interferon-alpha leads to a beneficial response in 30–40% of patients. Success rates of IFN-alpha treatment in children have varied significantly in different regions of the world. Response rates have been highest in Western countries, where treatment with IFN-alpha results in loss of HBV DNA or HBeAg seroconversion in 20–58% compared to 8–17% in untreated controls. In contrast, only 3–17% of children treated with IFN-alpha in Asian countries clear HBV DNA or seroconvert from HBeAg to anti-HBe. However, if aminotransferases are elevated, there may be no difference in response rates between children born in Asian countries (22%) and those from Europe and North America (26%) [11]. Children most likely to respond to IFN-alpha, regardless of ethnicity, are of younger age with elevated aminotransferases and low HBV DNA levels.

An advantage of IFN is that it has a finite duration of treatment and is not associated with the development of resistant HBV mutants. For children with HBeAg-positive chronic HBV infection, standard IFN-alpha is given at a dose of 6 million units (MU) per m^2 (maximum 10 MU) three times a week for 24 weeks, followed by an observation period of 6–12 months. A year of treatment may be preferable in those with HBeAg-negative chronic HBV infection, based upon data in adults. PEG-IFN is given at 180 μg/1.73 m^2 weekly for 48 weeks. IFN treatment may be accompanied by frequent and unpleasant side effects such as neutropenia, anorexia, fever, and transient growth delay.

In addition, IFN is not a good option in children with an underlying autoimmune disorder, organ transplant, cirrhosis, or serious neuropsychiatric disease. Patients should be monitored regularly for hepatitis flares during the first few months after the drug is discontinued.

Lamivudine was the first oral nucleoside analog approved in the United States for treatment of children younger than 12 years with chronic HBV. In 2002, a multicenter randomized, double-blind, placebo-controlled trial in HBeAg-positive children with ALT greater than 1.3 times ULN demonstrated clearance of HBeAg and HBV DNA at 52 weeks in 23% of treated children in comparison to 13% of controls [7]. In children whose baseline ALT was at least twice normal, this response rate increased to 35%. Subsequently, open-label lamivudine given to nonresponders showed a cumulative three-year virologic response rate of 35%. HBsAg loss occurred in 3% of patients. HBeAg seroconversion from the first year was durable in 88% of patients at three years [12]. However, viral resistance developed in 64% of children who received lamivudine for three years. Lamivudine is safe for children with hepatitis B, and is well tolerated. Serious side effects were not reported after three years of continuous treatment. In comparison to treatment with IFN-alpha, decreased height velocity and weight loss were not observed [13]. However, lamivudine has been largely displaced by entecavir as the first-line oral agent, since resistance to entecavir is very uncommon, particularly in individuals who have never been exposed to lamivudine.

Entecavir was studied in a multinational, randomized, double-blind, placebo-controlled trial of HBeAg-positive children aged 2 to <17 years of age [14]. The children were treated with either entecavir 0.015 mg/kg, up to a maximum of 0.5 mg/day, or placebo for 48 weeks. The primary endpoint was defined as HBeAg seroconversion and HBV DNA <50 IU/mL at week 48; this was met in 24.2% of those who received entecavir compared to 3.3% of those who received placebo (p=0.0008), and the rate increased with longer duration of treatment. Compared to subjects who received placebo, treated patients had higher rates of ALT normalization (relative risk [RR] 2.9), HBV DNA suppression (RR 14.8), and HBeAg seroconversion (RR 2.4). Entecavir was well tolerated, with no observed differences in adverse events or change in growth between the two groups.

A double-blind, placebo-controlled trial of the adult formulation adefovir dipivoxil was reported in 2008 [15], and the drug was subsequently approved for that age group,

but it has been virtually completely replaced with either entecavir or tenofovir disoproxil fumarate in the treatment of chronic hepatitis B in adolescents. In a randomized, double-blind study, either the adult formulation of tenofovir disoproxil fumarate or placebo was given to adolescents 12 to < 18 years of age with immune-active chronic hepatitis B, 91% of whom were HBeAg positive [16]. The primary study endpoint of HBV DNA <400 copies/mL was achieved in 89% of tenofovir disoproxil fumarate-treated and 0% of placebo-treated patients. Among patients with an ALT level greater than ULN at baseline, normalization of ALT occurred in 74% of patients receiving tenofovir disoproxil fumarate and 31% of patients receiving placebo (p<0.001). However, among patients who were HBeAg positive at baseline, 21% (10/48) in the tenofovir disoproxil fumarate group and 15% (7/48) in the placebo group experienced HBeAg loss by week 72, a difference that was not statistically significant. Although there was some baseline concern about bone mineralization in patients treated with tenofovir disoproxil fumarate, no patients met the safety endpoint of a 6% decrease in spine bone mineral density at week 72. The rate of grade 3 or 4 adverse events, primarily ALT flares, was higher in the placebo group.

A study of tenofovir disoproxil fumarate in younger children with chronic hepatitis B has recently been completed, and publication of results is expected soon. Tenofovir alafenamide is currently being evaluated in adolescents.

Although entecavir and tenofovir are very effective in reducing HBV DNA levels, there remains no rationale for treating children and adolescents whose HBV infection is in the immune-tolerant stage with persistently normal ALT values [17]. The results of a trial of entecavir with PEG-IFN-alpha-2a in 60 immune-tolerant children demonstrated no beneficial effect [18]. The primary endpoint of HBeAg loss and HBVDNA ≤1000 IU/mL 48 weeks after the end of treatment was met by only two patients (3%) but adverse events were noted in 37 of the 60 children. For these reasons, initiation of treatment should be reserved for those children with persistently abnormal ALT and histologic evidence of chronic hepatitis or fibrosis [17].

At this time, there are no recommendations regarding the best treatment of children with coinfections such as hepatitis C or HIV, since these are rare in pediatric patients.

Children with chronic HBV in the immune-tolerant stage (normal ALT, HBeAg positive) need to be monitored carefully for activation. ALT should be determined twice yearly, and HBeAg and anti-HBe yearly. Patients who are in the inactive phase of hepatitis B infection (HBeAg negative, anti HBe positive, persistently normal ALT, serum HBV DNA $<10^4$ copies/mL) should undergo monitoring of ALT every 6–12 months. The infection may reactivate even after years of quiescence; 4–20% of inactive "carriers" have one or more reversions back to HBeAg, and approximately 20–25% will develop HBeAg-negative chronic HBV. Periodic measurement of serum alpha-fetoprotein levels and hepatic ultrasound for hepatocellular cancer surveillance have been recommended in adults based upon observational data and expert opinion, even after HBeAg seroconversion, either spontaneous or after treatment. The risk of HCC increases with increasing age, but childhood cases have been described. Currently, there are no guidelines as to when this surveillance should be initiated, and how often testing should be done.

Children with HBV should be allowed to participate in all the regular activities of childhood. There is no need to exclude infected children from regular school and sports participation [19]. HBV-infected children should receive hepatitis A vaccine. Household contacts should receive HBV immunization and be tested to ensure vaccine efficacy. They should be counseled not to share items that may be contaminated with blood and to carefully dispose of such items. Adolescents need to be informed of the risks of HBV transmission by sexual activity and needle sharing.

Optimal treatment for children with chronic HBV should be individualized, depending on clinical and histologic status, comorbid conditions, ability to take medications, contraindications, and family concerns. The goal of treatment should be suppression of HBV DNA and durable HBeAg seroconversion, indicating cessation of active viral replication, to prevent the long-term consequences. Appropriate patient selection and understanding of the strengths and limitations of each of the therapeutic options are key to successful treatment.

References

1. Lok ASF, Lai CL. A longitudinal follow-up of asymptomatic hepatitis B surface antigen-positive Chinese children. *Hepatology* 1988;8:1130–1133.
2. Bortolotti F, Cadrobbi P, Crivellaro C et al. Long-term outcome of chronic type B hepatitis in patients who acquire hepatitis B virus infection in childhood. *Gastroenterology* 1990;99:805–810.
3. Bortolotti F, Guido M, Bartolacci S et al. Chronic hepatitis B in children after e antigen seroclearance: final report of a 29-year longitudinal study. *Hepatology* 2006;43:556–562.
4. Godra A, Perez-Atayde AR, Jonas MM. Histologic features of chronic hepatitis B in children (abstract). *Hepatology* 2005; 42:478A.
5. Bortolotti F, Calzia R, Cadrobbi P et al. Liver cirrhosis associated with chronic hepatitis B virus infection in childhood. *Journal of Pediatrics* 1986;108:224–227.
6. Shah U, Kelly D, Chang M-H et al. Management of chronic hepatitis B in children. *Journal of Pediatric Gastroenterology and Nutrition* 2009;48:399–404.
7. Jonas MM, Kelly DA, Mizerski J et al. Clinical trial of lamivudine in children with chronic hepatitis B. *New England Journal of Medicine* 2002;346:1706–1713.
8. Jonas MM, Lok A, McMahon BJ et al. Antiviral therapy in management of chronic hepatitis B viral infection in children: a systemic review and meta-analysis. *Hepatology* 2016; 63307–318.
9. Sokal EM, Conjeevaram HS, Roberts EA et al. Interferon alpha therapy for chronic hepatitis B in children: a multinational randomized controlled trial. *Gastroenterology* 1998; 114:988–995.
10. Wirth S, Zhang H, Hardikar W et al. Efficacy and safety of peginterferon-alpha-2a (40KD) in children with chronic hepatitis B: the PEG-B-ACTIVE study. *Hepatology* 2018; 68:1681–1694.
11. Narkewicz MR, Smith D, Silverman A, Vierling J, Sokol RJ. Clearance of chronic hepatitis B virus infection in young children after alpha interferon treatment. *Journal of Pediatrics* 1995;127:815–818.
12. Sokal EM, Kelly DA, Mizerski J et al. Long-term lamivudine therapy for children with HBeAg-positive chronic hepatitis B. *Hepatology* 2006;43:225–232.
13. Jonas MM, Little NR, Gardner SD. Long-term lamivudine treatment of children with chronic hepatitis B: durability of therapeutic responses and safety. *Journal of Viral Hepatology* 2007;15(1):20–27.
14. Jonas MM, Chang M-H, Sokal E et al. Randomized controlled trial of entecavir versus placebo in children with HBeAg-positive chronic hepatitis B. *Hepatology* 2016;63: 377–387.
15. Jonas MM, Kelly D, Pollack H et al. Safety, efficacy, and pharmacokinetics of adefovir dipivoxil in children and adolescents (age 2 to < 18 years) with chronic hepatitis B. *Hepatology* 2008;47(6):1863–1871.
16. Murray KF, Szenborn L, Wysocki J et al. Randomized, placebo-controlled trial of tenofovir disoproxil fumarate in adolescents with chronic hepatitis B. *Hepatology* 2012;56: 2018–2026.

17. Terrault NA, Bzowej NH, Chang KM, Hwang JP, Jonas MM, Murad MH. AASLD guidelines for treatment of chronic hepatitis B. *Hepatology* 2016;63(10):261–283.

18. Rosenthal P, Ling SC, Belle SH et al. Combination of entecavir/peginterferon alpha-2a in children with Hepatitis B e antigen-positive immune tolerant chronic hepatitis B virus infection. *Hepatology* 2019;69:2326–2337.

19. American Academy of Pediatrics. Red Book Online 2018. Section 2: Recommendations for care of children in special circumstances. https://redbook.solutions.aap.org/chapter.aspx?sectionid=88187019&bookid=1484

30 Hepatitis B vaccine failures: how do we handle them?

Daniel Shouval

Liver Unit, Hadassah-Hebrew University Hospital, Jerusalem, Israel

LEARNING POINTS

- Risk factors for nonresponse to vaccination include overweight, male gender, immune suppression, older age, chronic inflammatory conditions, malnutrition, and genetic predisposition.

- Risk groups for nonresponse to conventional vaccination against HBV include patients with renal failure, HIV, immune-suppressed patients such as organ transplant recipients, patients with non-HBV chronic liver disease, celiac disease, PWID, sex partners of HBsAg carriers including MSM, and healthcare workers engaged in exposure-prone procedures.

- Nonresponse to vaccination against HBV should be confirmed through anti-HBs and anti-HBc testing in defined risk groups following conventional immunization with three vaccine doses

- Strategies for circumventing vaccine nonresponse include:

  - administration of a second series of three vaccine doses using the conventional dose or double dose per injection

  - intradermal vaccination with more than three doses

  - use of vaccines with enhanced immunogenicity including vaccines formulated with new adjuvants other than aluminum hydroxide, and immunization with a PreS/S HBV vaccine (only available in a few countries).

Introduction

About 2 billion people have contracted hepatitis B virus (HBV) during their lifetime worldwide and approximately 240 million remained HBV carriers. Following the recommendation of the World Health Organization (WHO), so far, 184 countries have introduced universal vaccination of newborns with a stunning impact on reduced incidence of acute and chronic hepatitis B, cirrhosis of the liver, and liver cancer worldwide. Further to universal vaccination of newborns (UV), HBV immunization is also recommended for a large number of risk groups including, among others, healthcare workers (especially those involved in exposure-prone procedures), patients with non-HBV chronic liver disease (i.e., chronic hepatitis C), patients with chronic renal failure on dialysis, immune-suppressed patients (i.e., transplant recipients, HIV) or multitransfused patients, men who have sex with men (MSM) as well as people who inject drugs (PWID). Yet, in contrast to immunization against hepatitis A, which is highly successful in almost 100% of vaccinees and with a very low rate of nonresponders, immunization failures against HBV affect a relatively high number of vaccinees worldwide. The present review provides the background and the currently available information regarding the reported but not always available means to cope with vaccination failures against HBV infection.

History

Since 1979, three generations of efficacious, safe, and well-tolerated HBV vaccines have been developed for intramuscular (IM) injections. These include the first-generation, plasma-derived vaccines containing mainly the small S

Clinical Dilemmas in Viral Liver Disease, Second Edition. Edited by Graham R. Foster and K. Rajender Reddy.
© 2020 John Wiley & Sons Ltd. Published 2020 by John Wiley & Sons Ltd.

envelope protein, the second-generation yeast-derived recombinant vaccines containing exclusively the small S antigen, which are currently the mostly used vaccines globally, and various third-generation recombinant vaccines produced in mammalian cells (Chinese hamster ovary [CHO] or mouse cell lines), expressing the small S, middle Pre-S2, and large Pre-S1 envelope antigens [1–3]. In contrast to yeasts, HBV-transfected CHO cells secrete one or more glycosylated envelope protein(s) while glycosylation apparently contributes to an enhanced immunogenicity. Such vaccines have been developed in France, Germany, the UK, China, and Israel. Only one CHO-derived PreS1/PreS2/S vaccine, Sci B vac™, is currently licensed in Israel and available in a few countries in East Asia [2].

As recommended by the World Health Organization (WHO) and the United States Centers for Disease Control, three IM doses of licensed recombinant HBV vaccines formulated in aluminum hydroxide (alum), given in the deltoid muscle (in adults) or the anterolateral thigh (in newborns and children) at month 0, 1, and 6, lead to anti-HBs seroconversion in 90–100% of immune-competent recipients. These seroprotection rates drop to 50–60% in various risk groups mentioned above. Vaccine-induced seroprotection against HBV infection is defined by a minimal anti-HBs antibody titer of ≥10 mIU/mL. Measurement of anti-HBs levels about four weeks after the third dose in vaccinees belonging to specific risk groups is recommended. Fading (waning) anti-HBs seropositivity over time, (eventually down to undetectable levels by conventional assays) may occur within months to years post completion of immunization. Yet, most such vaccinees remain protected, retain an immune memory against HBV, and will respond with anamnestic anti-HBs production following exposure to HBV or booster immunization (which is currently not recommended in initially seroprotected vaccinees).

Definition of nonresponse to immunization

Vaccine-acquired seroprotection is considered a surrogate of clinical protection. In situations when anti-HBs levels after the third vaccine dose are <10 mIU/mL, it is important to distinguish between the following conditions post immunization.

- Primary nonresponse to three HBV vaccine doses followed by another set of three vaccine doses.

- Fading (waning) anti-HBs seropositivity over time in vaccinees who achieved an adequate protective anti-HBs titer following a conventional three-dose immunization protocol.
- Conventional immunoassays cannot distinguish between neutralizing and nonneutralizing anti-HBs antibodies. Thus, some anti-HBs antibodies detected by commercial immunoassays may not be fully protective against wild-type HBV, envelope protein mutants or distinct genotypes/subtypes of the surface antigen.

The definition of response and nonresponse to HBV immunization varies. In general, nonresponse to primary immunization is defined as an inability of the vaccinee to generate protective anti-HBs antibody levels following the recommended three-dose protocol. True primary nonresponse is confirmed when anti-HBs levels remain <10 mIU/mL after administration of an additional series of an HBV vaccine. Most countries accept an anti-HBs threshold of 10 mIU/mL as proof for protection. Yet, an anti-HBs level of 10–100 mIU/mL is sometimes considered as a "gray zone" for protection with an unknown fraction of nonneutralizing antibodies, occasionally also present in overt or occult HBV carriers. Thus, vaccinees who develop anti-HBs levels of 10–100 mIU/mL following three vaccine doses are sometimes categorized as "low or hypo responders." Consequently, some regulatory authorities require an anti-HBs threshold of 100 mIU/mL as proof for protection, for example for healthcare workers engaged in exposure-prone procedures.

Immunization against HBV is expected in the majority of vaccinees to generate a protective antibody response to the a epitope on the envelope protein loop, present in all genotypes and subtypes. However, although nonresponse to conventional vaccination occurs in a minority of vaccinees, a solution is still required for those nonresponders at risk of contracting HBV. The mechanism(s) of HBV neutralization by anti-HBs antibodies acquired through "natural" infection or immunization are only partially understood [4,5]. There are apparently two classes of anti-HBs neutralizing antibodies. The first class comprises a fraction of antibodies targeting specific sites in the antigenic loop of HBsAg and neutralizing viral entry, blocking the interaction with the prereceptor heparan sulfate proteoglycan (HSPG). The second class comprises antibodies targeting the receptor binding "site" of the

Pre-S1 domain and blocking the interaction of virions with the sodium taurocholate cotransporting polypeptide (NTCP) receptor on hepatocytes. An additional antiviral mechanism described for antibodies directed to the antigenic loop of HBsAg involves FcRn-mediated endocytosis and the consequent intracellular blocking of HBV and HBsAg subviral particle release from infected hepatocytes [4].

Risk factors for nonresponse to vaccination

Although currently used yeast-derived vaccines are sufficiently immunogenic, safe, and efficacious, immunization failures do occur. In assessment of the risk factors associated with vaccine nonresponse, one has to distinguish between vaccine-related and host-related risk factors [6].

Vaccine-related risk factors for nonresponse include break in the cold chain and improper storage (i.e., freezing), intragluteal injection, inadequate dosing or sequence of administration as well as rare breakdowns in manufacturing.

Host-related risk factors for non-response were recently reviewed in a metaanalysis of 37 reports including >20 000 vaccinees [7]. These include, among others, various systemic diseases, immune suppression, nutrition and body weight (BMI >25–30), smoking, male gender, age >40 years (immune senescence) as well as distinct genetic determinants specifically and nonspecifically controlling the immune response to various antigens present in a particular vaccine (Box 30.1) [6,7]. An impaired response to vaccination (three IM doses given at month 0, 1, and 6) has been observed in cancer patients (57%), chronic liver disease (50%), chronic renal failure (34–81%), HIV (30%), celiac disease, Crohn disease, diabetes, PWID, and Down syndrome.

Breakthrough HBV infections following successful immunization are rare but may occur, for example in newborns to highly viremic HBsAg+ mothers despite passive and active immunization [8]. Vaccine breakthrough events (which seem to be rare) have been linked, among other factors, to a mismatch of HBV genotype between the infecting virus and the vaccine genotype used for immunization [9].

For those who respond favorably to immunization, vaccine-induced immunity against HBV infection and/or

---

Box 30.1 Host-related factors determining nonresponse to immunization against HBV

Male gender
Older age (> 40 years) – immunosenescence
Overweight (BMI ≥25)
Malnutrition; vitamin D deficiency
Lifestyle
  Heavy smoking
  Drug abuse
Genetic: distinct HLA class II haplotypes (HLA-DRB1, HLA-DQB1); specific nucleotide polymorphism in cytokine or cytokine receptor genes and Toll-like receptors
Systemic diseases:
  Chronic renal failure and dialysis
  Diabetes mellitus
  HIV
  Hematopoietic bone marrow and stem cell recipients
  Chronic, non-HBV liver disease
  Organ transplant recipients
  Immune-suppressed patients

Source: Modified from references [7,10].

---

clinical disease lasts for several decades post administration of the third dose and may be lifelong. Moreover, immune memory to envelope antigen(s) may persist for decades even in vaccinees who serorevert and in whom anti-HBs become undetectable. This condition may be verified through a vaccine booster dose which should lead to an anamnestic anti-HBs response. However, means for protection of true nonresponders to conventional vaccination against HBV are limited [5].

Ways to approach nonresponse to conventional immunization against HBV

Several methods have been suggested to bypass nonresponse to conventional vaccination and improve seroprotection in HBV vaccine non-responders (Table 30.1).

Repeated immunization and doubling vaccine dose

The easiest and most available measure to cope with HBV vaccine failure is to repeat the three-dose vaccination series with an alum adjuvanted yeast-derived vaccine. The licensed vaccines for adults contain 10–20 μg/dose of the small S antigen. In immune-suppressed patients, including those with renal failure, a double dose of the vaccine is justified

Table 30.1 Potential strategies and means to improve protection of nonresponders to conventional HBV vaccination

Strategy	Product name and manufacturer	Comments
Repeat HBV immunization series	Any licensed vaccine	Following the primary three-dose protocol
Double antigen dose	Any licensed vaccine	Three doses
Intradermal HBV immunization [11,12]	Several vaccine manufacturers	Metaanalysis of 14 trials in renal failure patients and in five trials in nonresponders receiving up to 16 doses at variable intervals.
		Data available on seroprotection rates post completion of immunization series but limited follow-up
Nasal HBV vaccine	Experimental – Cuba and Japan	Contains rHBsAg with or without rHBcAg
New adjuvants and immune stimulants [10]	ASO4 Fendrix, GSK ISS 1018 [13] (in renal failure)	Contains immunostimulatory Toll-like receptor (TLR) 4 agonist monophosphoryl lipid A with aluminum salt (use in >15y and older given IM at months 0, 1, 2, and 6). Higher local reactogenicity and more fatigue and headaches compared to aluminum salt adjuvanted vaccine
	Heplisav, Dynavax®, CpG immuno-stimulatory DNA [14]	TLR agonist 9, 2 doses given at month 0 and 1. Higher local reactogenicity compared to control vaccine
Pre-S/S HBV vaccines	Pre-S1/Pre-S2/S:	
	Hepacare® [15]	Germany, UK –discontinued
	Sci B Vac® [16]	Licensed in Israel and in several East Asian countries
	Pre-S2/S:	
	Gene Hevac B® [17]	France, discontinued

[18]. The second three-dose course is successful in 50–70% of vaccinees who do not reach the protective 10 mIU/mL threshold following primary immunization. The reported seroprotection rates in patients on hemodialysis receiving a three-dose vaccine regimen may be improved to 70% by doubling the vaccine dose. Available experience suggests that IM administration of additional vaccine doses to nonresponders to two series of vaccine is futile.

Intradermal injection (ID) [11,12]

The rationale of this strategy is based on the presence of dendritic cells in the dermis capable of presenting antigens and stimulating the innate and adaptive immune response [12]. In a comparative randomized trial, this ID strategy was tested in vaccine nonresponders with chronic kidney disease who received biweekly up to 6 doses of 5 µgHBsAg ID. Seroprotection rates have markedly improved, reaching 100% in ID recipients compared to 48% in the control group vaccinated by the conventional route [11]. Although intradermal injection requires training, this strategy is accessible and frequently successful in vaccine nonresponders. New devices for ID injection have been designed to bypass

the technical difficulty involved in ID injection. Metaanalysis of several clinical trials supports the use of this approach in nonresponders to 3 + 3 HBV vaccine doses [11,12]. The dose used for ID administration varies according to the vaccine brand and volume used for injection but is usually 50% of the recommended dose/volume in adults. The interval in follow-up of anti-HBs response in such vaccinees is flexible and dependent on clinical judgment.

Vaccine adjuvants and immune stimulators

Aluminum hydroxide (alum)

This is an adjuvant which triggers the innate immune system and enhances the humoral response to the small envelope antigen (HBsAg) in vaccine recipients. It is also an important component in many vaccine formulations, including first- and second-generation HBV vaccines [19]. Since its first recognition in 1926 and introduction into clinical vaccination practice in the 1940s, alum has had an excellent profile of safety and tolerability. Thus, absorption of small recombinant HBsAg particles to alum enables improved uptake by antigen-presenting cells. There are a number of hypotheses regarding the mechanism of action of alum reviewed in reference [19]. Aluminum salts trigger endogenous danger signals which lead to activation of multiple genes that promote antigen uptake, presentation, cytokine release, and adaptive immune responses [10]. Yet, although currently licensed second-generation HBV vaccines have a very good record of immunogenicity (and safety) in healthy immunocompetent recipients, the reduced performance of HBV vaccines in distinct risk groups and in the elderly required exploration of new means to circumvent nonresponse. Consequently, this was the rationale for developing more potent adjuvants.

ASO4

ASO4 is a combination of an aluminum salt and *Salmonella*-derived 3-o-desacyl-4'-monophophoryl lipid A(MPL). The poor immunogenicity of HBV vaccines in patients with end-stage kidney disease and on dialysis lead to development of a more immunogenic HBV vaccine, FENDrix®, which contains 20 µg rHBsAg formulated with ASO4. In controlled randomized trials, primary immunization with FENDRrix was shown to induce faster seroconversion, higher seroprotection rates, higer anti-HBs titers and prolonged anti-HBs seropositivity compared to a conventional aluminum adjuvanted HBV vaccine [10]. The inclusion of ASO4 elicits a stronger local but transient reactogenicity and more fatigue and headaches compared to the control vaccine containing only aluminum hydroxide as an adjuvant. FENDrix is approved in Europe and recommended for patients 15 years and older before or on dialysis, given in four doses at 0, 1, 2, and 6 months. Booster doses are permitted in originally seroconverted patients with fading anti-HBs titers <10 mIU/mL. FENDrix was also tested in HIV patients and patients with end-stage liver disease pending liver transplantation.

Immunostimulatory DNA sequences (ISS)

The US FDA has recently approved a new recombinant HBV vaccine, Heplisav B®, which contains 20 µg yeast-derived small S antigen formulated with a new, bacterial DNA-derived adjuvant CpG, a synthetic cytosine phosphoguanosine [10,20,21]. CpG stimulates the immune system via Toll-like receptor 9, leading to faster and higher seroprotection rates against HBV compared to an alum adjuvanted yeast-derived control vaccine, as demonstrated

by several randomized trials. These revealed a 100% seroprotection rate at age 18–29 years compared to 93.9% in recipients of Engerix B®,declining to 91.6% and 72.6% respectively in 60–70-year-old vaccinees. Local and systemic adverse events (AE) were comparable between the two vaccines. The FDA's initial concerns regarding serious systemic AEs (i.e., autoimmune manifestations, ischemic heart disease) were discarded and Heplisav was approved for healthy recipients 18 years old and older. The enhanced immunogenicity afforded by CpG enables reduction of the number of vaccine doses from three to two injections within a four-week interval. Data on immunogenicity in special risk groups of nonresponders (i.e., patients with renal failure, transplant patients, and nonresponders to conventional vaccination) are pending.

Pre-S1/Pre-S2/S vaccine

Inclusion of pre-S1 and pre-S2 epitopes into HBV vaccines enhances protection against HBV. Sci-B-Vac® is a mammalian cell-derived recombinant Pre-S1/Pre-S2/S hepatitis B vaccine formulated with alum, which has been shown to be highly immunogenic, inducing faster and higher seroprotection rates against HBV with higher anti-HBs levels at lower HBsAg doses in immune-competent recipients compared to conventional yeast-derived vaccines [2]. Furthermore, one or two 20 µg doses of this vaccine were shown to induce a higher seroprotection rate at both 100 and 10 mIU/mL levels compared to documented nonresponders who previously received 4–6 doses of a conventional vaccine [16]. Moreover, results of a clinical trial in Germany indicate that Sci-B-Vac induces a robust cellular immune response to HBsAg as well as protective anti-HBs antibody titers in nonresponders and lowresponders [22].

Approach to an individual with primary vaccine failure after receiving three conventional vaccine doses

- Test anti-HBc and if positive, evaluate HBV-DNA by polymerase chain reaction to exclude occult HBV infection. If negative, proceed to one of the following options.
- *Option 1*: Repeat a three-course immunization series (double dose optional) and test anti-HBs four weeks after the last vaccine dose.
- *Option 2*: In patients with renal failure and where available, administer four doses of FENDrix at the recommended intervals and follow anti-HBs levels.

- *Option 3*: In countries where a PreS/S vaccine is available, repeat immunization with 1–2 doses at a four-week interval and follow anti-HBs levels.

References

1. Zanetti AR, van Damme P, Shouval D. The global impact of vaccination against hepatitis B: a historical overview. *Vaccine* 2008;26:6266–6273.

2. Shouval D, Roggendorf H, Roggendorf M. Enhanced immune response to hepatitis B vaccination through immunization with a Pre-S1/Pre-S2/S vaccine. *Medical Microbiology and Immunology* 2015;204:57–68.

3. Zuckerman JN. Protective efficacy, immunotherapeutic potential, and safety of hepatitis B vaccines. *Journal of Medical Virology* 2006;78:169–177.

4. Corti D, Benigni F, Shouval D. Viral envelope-specific antibodies in chronic hepatitis B virus infection. *Current Opinion in Virology* 2018;30:48–57.

5. Gerlich WH. Do we need better hepatitis B vaccines? *Indian Journal of Medical Research* 2017;145:414–419.

6. Wiedermann U, Garner-Spitzer E, Wagner A. Primary vaccine failure to routine vaccines: why and what to do? *Human Vaccines and Immunotherapeutics* 2016;12:239–243.

7. Yang S, Tian G, Cui Y et al. Factors influencing immunologic response to hepatitis B vaccine in adults. *Scientific Reports* 2016;6:27251.

8. Wang Y, Chen T, Lu LL et al. Adolescent booster with hepatitis B virus vaccines decreases HBV infection in high-risk adults. *Vaccine* 2017;35:1064–1070.

9. Cheah BC, Davies J, Singh GR et al. Sub-optimal protection against past hepatitis B virus infection where subtype mismatch exists between vaccine and circulating viral genotype in northern Australia. *Vaccine* 2018;36:3533–3540.

10. Leroux-Roels G. Old and new adjuvants for hepatitis B vaccines. *Medical Microbiology and Immunology* 2015;204:69–78.

11. Fabrizi F, Dixit V, Messa P, Martin P. Intradermal vs intramuscular vaccine against hepatitis B infection in dialysis patients: a meta-analysis of randomized trials. *Journal of Viral Hepatitis* 2011;18:730–737.

12. Filippelli M, Lionetti E, Gennaro A et al. Hepatitis B vaccine by intradermal route in non responder patients: an update. *World Journal of Gastroenterology* 2014;20:10383–10394.

13. Kundi M. New hepatitis B vaccine formulated with an improved adjuvant system. *Expert Review of Vaccines* 2007; 6:133–140.

14. Cooper C, Mackie D. Hepatitis B surface antigen-1018 ISS adjuvant-containing vaccine: a review of HEPLISAV safety and efficacy. *Expert Review of Vaccines* 2011;10:417–427.

15. Zuckerman JN, Zuckerman AJ, Symington I et al. Evaluation of a new hepatitis B triple-antigen vaccine in inadequate responders to current vaccines. *Hepatology* 2001;34:798–802.

16. Rendi-Wagner P, Shouval D, Genton B et al. Comparative immunogenicity of a PreS/S hepatitis B vaccine in non- and low responders to conventional vaccine. *Vaccine* 2006;24: 2781–2789.

17. Marescot MR, Budkowska A, Pillot J, Debre P. HLA linked immune response to S and pre-S2 gene products in hepatitis B vaccination. *Tissue Antigens* 1989;33:495–500.

18. Cardell K, Akerlind B, Sallberg M, Fryden A. Excellent response rate to a double dose of the combined hepatitis A and B vaccine in previous nonresponders to hepatitis B vaccine. *Journal of Infectious Diseases* 2008;198:299–304.

19. Wen Y, Shi Y. Alum: an old dog with new tricks. *Emerging Microbes and Infections* 2016;5:e25.

20. Schillie S, Harris A, Link-Gelles R, Romero J, Ward J, Nelson N. Recommendations of the Advisory Committee on Immunization Practices for use of a hepatitis B vaccine with a novel adjuvant. *Morbidity and Mortality Weekly Report* 2018;67:455–458.

21. Hyer R, McGuire DK, Xing B, Jackson S, Janssen R. Safety of a two-dose investigational hepatitis B vaccine, HBsAg-1018, using a toll-like receptor 9 agonist adjuvant in adults. *Vaccine* 2018;36:2604–2611.

22. Krawczyk A, Ludwig C, Jochum C et al. Induction of a robust T- and B-cell immune response in non- and low-responders to conventional vaccination against hepatitis B by using a third generation PreS/S vaccine. *Vaccine* 2014;32:5077–5082.

31 The stopping rules in hepatitis B virus therapy: can we provide any guidance?

Florian van Bömmel and Thomas Berg

Section of Hepatology, University of Leipzig, Leipzig, Germany

LEARNING POINTS

- NA treatment may be discontinued in all patients who achieve HBsAg loss.

- In patients with advanced fibrosis/cirrhosis failing to achieve HBsAg loss, NA treatment should be continued.

- Discontinuation of NA treatment may be considered in noncirrhotic HBeAg-positive patients after one year of consolidation treatment after HBeAg seroconversion with undetectable HBV DNA levels and normal ALT.

- Discontinuation of long-term NA treatment can induce durable immune control and even HBsAg loss in some HBeAg-negative patients, but close follow-up and appropriate algorithms to initiate retreatment are essential to manage HBeAg-positive and -negative patients after NA treatment discontinuation.

The dilemma: effective control but little cure in chronic hepatitis B

Currently, pegylated interferon-alpha (PEG-IFN) and six nucleos(t)ide analogs (NAs; lamivudine, telbivudine, entecavir, adefovir dipivoxil, tenofovir disoproxil fumarate, and tenofovir alafenamid) are approved for the treatment of chronic hepatitis B infection. Treatment with these NAs suppresses hepatitis B virus (HBV) replication and ameliorates hepatic inflammation and thereby leads to decreased risk of chronic liver disease, hepatic decompensation, cirrhosis, and hepatocellular carcinoma which are common consequences of chronic hepatitis B [1–3]. Steps towards immune control over HBV infections include HBeAg to anti-HBe seroconversion, which can be achieved in up to 50% of HBeAg-positive patients, and the rare event of HBsAg loss or seroconversion. Once achieved during NA treatment, these events are considered to be a valuable endpoint in patients with chronic hepatitis B [4–6]. However, even under immune control the HBV genome tends to persist in the core of infected hepatocytes in the form of closely covalent circular DNA (cccDNA).

In recent years, a consensus has been reached aiming at "functional cure" as an optimal endpoint. The definition of functional cure includes durable HBsAg loss (with or without HBsAg seroconversion), undetectable serum HBV DNA, persistence of cccDNA in a transcriptionally inactive status, and the absence of spontaneous relapse after the cessation of treatment [7].

Unfortunately, even after eight years of treatment with tenofovir disoproxil fumarate, a functional cure was observed in no more than 10% of HBeAg-positive patients and, more disappointingly, in less than 1% of HBeAg-negative patients [8]. Functional cure rates during treatment with PEG-IFN-alpha were comparably low and associated with bothersome interferon-related side effects. As a result, while HBeAg-positive patients have a low chance for achieving functional cure but at least a fair chance to achieve HBeAg seroconversion, almost all patients with HBeAg-negative chronic hepatitis B require lifelong treatment with NAs.

Clinical Dilemmas in Viral Liver Disease, Second Edition. Edited by Graham R. Foster and K. Rajender Reddy.
© 2020 John Wiley & Sons Ltd. Published 2020 by John Wiley & Sons Ltd.

How may discontinuation of antiviral treatment increase immune control?

The reason for an individual's inability to establish immunologic control over the infection is believed to be the ineffective CD8+ T-cell responses against HBV that patients with chronic hepatitis B typically exhibit. A reason for this so-called T-cell exhaustion is thought to be chronic antigen overstimulation of virus-specific CD8+ T-cells, which gradually leads to loss of antiviral effector functions [9]. There is an ongoing debate on whether long-term suppression of HBV DNA can eventually reinvigorate exhausted CD8+ T-cells and restore immune control. Stopping NA treatment and the subsequent sudden increase in HBV DNA may also be an important trigger to reinduce T-cell responses against HBV-infected hepatocytes [10]. This suggested effect of HBV DNA increase following NA discontinuation has in this context also been designated as "autovaccination." There is also the possibility that programmed cell death protein (PD)-1 expression on

functional HBV-specific T-cells may reflect an activated, nonexhausted phenotype that may mediate immune control after NA discontinuation (Figure 31.1). Thus, in recent work studying HBV-specific T-cell response as a biomarker for HBV therapy discontinuation, it was shown that in patients who did not relapse after discontinuation of NA treatment, an increased frequency of functional PD-1+ HBV-specific T-cells directed against nucleocapsid and polymerase HBV proteins was already present during antiviral treatment [10].

Stopping NA treatment after achieving serologic endpoints

It remains controversial whether NA treatment can be stopped after NA-induced HBeAg seroconversion, as relapse rates of up to 50% have been observed. Yet, the American, Asian, and European guidelines agree that treatment discontinuation may be considered in HBeAg-positive patients without cirrhosis after a 1–3-year period

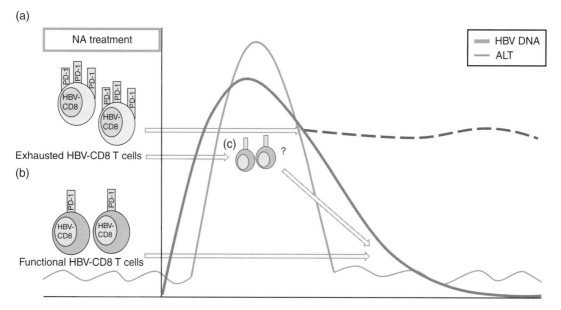

Figure 31.1 Potential role of the functional status of PD-1+ HBV-specific CD8 T-cells for the establishment of immunologic control after NA discontinuation. Exhausted HBV-specific CD8 T-cells with high PD-1 expression fail to establish a robust response and HBV DNA relapses permanently (a). HBV-specific CD8 T-cells that have reacquired their antiviral function after long-term NA therapy and have low PD-1 expression exhibit a strong response against HBV antigens and HBV DNA decreases to low or undetectable levels after an initial relapse (b). There is also discussion on whether stopping NA treatment itself may revigorate exhausted CD8 T-cells so that immune control can be established (c). HBV, hepatitis B virus; NA, nucleos(t)ide analog; PD-1, programmed cell death protein 1.

Table 31.1 Endpoints for NA treatment in noncirrhotic patients with chronic hepatitis B according to current guidelines

Treatment guidelines	EASL (2017) [4]	AASLD (2018) [6]	APASL (2015) [5]
HBeAg positive	HBeAg seroconversion after ≥12 months of consolidation treatment + undetectable HBV DNA	HBeAg seroconversion after ≥12 months of consolidation treatment + undetectable HBV DNA	HBeAg seroconversion after ≥12, better 36 months of consolidation treatment
HBeAg negative	HBeAg-negative patients who have achieved ≥3 years virologic suppression, if close post-NA monitoring can be guaranteed	Indefinite	Indefinite
After HBsAg loss[a]	NA should be discontinued	NA discontinuation can be considered	NAs can be discontinuated. After ≥12 months consolidation or if under NAs, HBV DNA was undetectable for ≥2 years

[a] Both HBeAg positive and negative.
HBV, hepatitis B virus; NA, nucleos(t)ide analog.

of consolidation (Table 31.1) [4–6]. This is supported by a systematic review that evaluated outcomes after treatment discontinuation [9]. In this report, consolidation treatment duration for patients achieving HBeAg seroconversion varied from <12 months to 12 months. The authors report that stable HBeAg seroconversion was observed in 88% of the patients 24 months after treatment discontinuation. Stable suppression of HBV DNA was observed in 53% and 51% of patients 24 and 36 months after treatment discontinuation respectively. It seems that extension of NA consolidation to up to three years after HBeAg seroconversion can increase the chance of sustainability of off-treatment response [11].

It is important to understand that the evidence in support of discontinuing NA treatment after HBeAg seroconversion is not strong as randomized trials evaluating robust clinical outcomes for this option have not yet been conducted. There is also no global consensus regarding the duration of consolidation therapy after HBeAg seroconversion and the recommended 1–3-year period was arbitrarily chosen [3–5].

Nucleoside analog treatment should not be stopped after HBeAg seroconversion in patients with liver cirrhosis. In contrast, it may be stopped in all patients with or without compensated cirrhosis who achieve HBsAg loss or seroconversion to anti-HBs, provided that close posttreatment monitoring can be provided to them [3–5].

Inducing serologic response by stopping NA treatment in HBeAg-negative patients

In 2012, Hadziyannis et al. published a small, uncontrolled single-center study of the posttreatment course of 33 patients with HBeAg-negative HBV infection who had discontinued adefovir dipivoxil after 3–5 years. Although all patients initially had a relapse of HBV DNA and most of them a subsequent biochemical relapse, at 69 months after NA withdrawal, 18 patients (55%) had achieved sustained biochemical and virologic remission. Strikingly, during the long-term follow-up, a functional cure was achieved in 39% of patients [12].

A number of studies have been inspired by this observation and researched the effect of stopping NA treatment in HBeAg-negative patients, and there is a growing body of evidence that helps to elucidate whether NA therapy cessation is safe and effective. However, there are great differences in patient selection, treatment duration before stopping, and retreatment rules across these trials. A recent metaanalysis summarizing outcomes in 25 of these studies in mainly Asian patients demonstrated that 12–36 months after NA withdrawal, 38% of 967 HBeAg-negative patients had achieved durably low HBV DNA levels and normal alanine aminotransferase (ALT) and 2% achieved HBsAg loss [13].

There are only a few prospective studies assessing the outcome of post-NA treatment in HBeAg-negative patients

(Table 31.2). The primary endpoint was the rate of HBV DNA relapse after NA discontinuation in most studies, and high HBV DNA relapse rates of 45–100% were reported. Post-NA treatment HBsAg loss rates were 8–25%. The authors of two studies assessed sustained low HBV DNA levels after NA cessation as an endpoint, and found that 8.4% and 33% of patients maintained HBV DNA ≤2000 IU/mL at one year post treatment. To date, evidence from a large, prospective and randomized trial regarding the effects of NA discontinuation in HBeAg-negative patients is missing.

How can response to NA discontinuation be predicted?

The factors shown to be associated with response to NA treatment cessation in HBeAg-negative patients were heterogeneous and partially conflicting across the available studies. They include female sex, younger age, low ALT, low HBV DNA and low HBsAg levels at baseline, the duration and the drug used for preceding NA treatment, and the immune status characterized by T-cell properties.

HBsAg is a marker believed to reflect HBV replication, and a decrease in quantitative serum HBsAg has been correlated to HBsAg clearance and highlighted as a possible predictor of sustained response and flares after NA withdrawal [14–17]. The practical value for HBsAg level seems, however, to be limited due to the low levels required for consideration of NA cessation which were found to be 100–700 IU/mL [18–21]. The predictive role of ALT, which is a classic marker for response to antiviral treatment, is controverted in the scenario of NA discontinuation. Although there is wide agreement that after NA discontinuation, ALT flares are an expression of the establishment of immune control over HBV infections, lower ALT baseline levels have been correlated with higher rates of HBsAg loss [18]. Also, it has recently been demonstrated that patients who do not flare upon treatment withdrawal are those who do not require retreatment [10]. Given the observed disparities, more research is necessary to distinguish "good" from "bad" ALT flares, and possibly it needs to be focused rather on the type of T-cell response than on the resulting ALT kinetic for a better understanding of therise of immune control. Thus, a preexisting or newly forming HBV-specific CD8 T-cell phenotype may predict acquisition of antiviral control or HBsAg loss after NA discontinuation [10,15,22].

Management of harmful ALT flares after NA discontinuation

In a metaanalysis of 25 selected studies, biochemical relapse following NA discontinuation was reported in 28/72 (39%) patients with baseline cirrhosis in three studies that provided these data [23–25]. Liver decompensation was described in 2/243 (0.8%) patients with baseline cirrhosis [13]. In the large prospective study by Seto et al., 26% of subjects had elevated ALT and 12% had ALT >2 × upper limit of normal (ULN) following virologic relapse [26]. The median ALT level in patients with elevated ALT was 97 (range 37–1058) U/L, with 88.1% (n = 37) occurring at either week 12 or 24. None of these 42 subjects had increased serum bilirubin.

To establish adequate safety measures without interrupting the trigger for immune control too early, one could refer to the following rules for retreatment initiation.

- Confirmed (i.e., two consecutive central laboratory results) increase in direct bilirubin from baseline, and ALT ULN at the confirmatory test.
- Confirmed sustained increase in prothrombin time ≥2.0 sec from baseline with appropriate vitamin K therapy and elevated ALT.
- Confirmed elevated ALT 10 × ULN with or without associated symptoms.
- ALT 2 × ULN and ≤5 × ULN persisting for ≥84 days (12 weeks) as well as a HBV DNA relapse ≥20 000 IU/mL.
- ALT 5 × ULN and ≤10 × ULN persisting for ≥28 days (4 weeks) [17].

Guidance for stopping NA treatment

The current supraregional guidelines agree that NA treatment may be stopped in all patients who achieve HBsAg loss or seroconversion to anti-HBs (see Table 31.1). For all other cases, the ideal scenario for stopping long-term treatment with NAs is a patient without advanced liver fibrosis who is compliant to close follow-up examinations and a physician experienced in the treatment of HBV infections. Considerations before stopping NA treatment in patients with chronic hepatitis B should be as follows.

For HBeAg-positive patients

- After HBeAg seroconversion and a consecutive consolidation treatment ≥12 months.
- Continuous follow-up to detect a possible HBeAg seroreversion and viral or hepatic flares.

Table 31.2 Prospective studies assessing post-NA treatment courses in HBeAg-negative patients

Study	Region	Design	Patients (n)	Endpoint	NA	Mean NA treatment duration (range) [months]	Post-NA follow-up (range) [months]	HBV DNA relapses (%)	HBsAg loss (%)	No retreatment (%)
[tb]Liu et al. [27]	China	Prospective	61	HBV DNA relapse, HBsAg loss	LMV +/- PEG-IFN	30 (24–66)	22 (1–84)	56	10	n.a.
Ha et al. [28]	China	Prospective	145	HBV DNA relapse, HBsAg loss	ADV +/- IFN-alpha	26 (24–66)[a]	16 (1–88)[a]	65.5	8.3	n.a.
Seto et al. [26]	China	Prospective	184	HBV DNA relapse, HBsAg loss, immune control	ETV	≥24	12	91.4	0	8.4[b]
Karakaya et al. [29]	Turkey	Prospective	23	HBV DNA relapse, HBsAg loss	LMV	>60	12–60	45	9	9
Cao et al. [30]	China	Prospective	22	HBV DNA relapse, HBsAg loss	ETV, ADV, LdT, LMV	47 (29–77)	n.a.	53	n.a.	n.a.
Berg, et al. [17]	Germany	Prospective, randomized	21	HBsAg loss, retreatment	TDF	33	36	100	19	43
Rivino, et al. [19]	Great Britain	Prospective	21/27	HBV DNA relapse	TDF, LMV	≥24/≥24	12/12	n.a.	0	19/51
Papatheodoridis et al. [31]	Greece	Prospective	57	HBV DNA relapse, retreatment rate	ETV, TDF	>48	18	72	25	74[b]

[a] Median;

[b] defined as continuous HBV DNA levels ≤2000 IU/mL throughout 48 weeks off-treatment.

ADV, adefovir dipivoxil; ETV, entecavir; IFN, interferon; LdT, telbivudine; LMV, lamivudine; n.a., not available; TDF, tenofovir disoproxil fumarate.

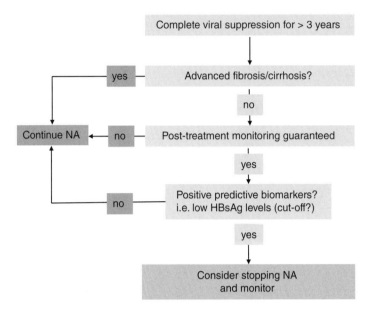

Figure 31.2 Algorithm for stopping NAs in HBeAg-negative patients.

For HBeAg-negative patients (Figure 31.2)

- Continuous suppression of HBV DNA ≥36 months during preceding NA treatment.
- Continuous *close* follow-up to monitor the anticipated viral and hepatic flares.
- Familiarity with a retreatment strategy (e.g., the one here proposed).
- Inform the patient regarding potential liver damage by biochemical flares.
- HBV biomarkers as quantitative HBsAg may help to select patients more likely to respond to NA discontinuation; however, a cut-off level has not yet been defined.

Future perspectives on the role of NA discontinuation for HBV treatment

To date, the effect of discontinuing long-term NA treatment for HBeAg-negative patients is poorly understood, but there is evidence that it leads to a higher rate of immune control and functional cure when compared to other currently available treatments. Large prospective and randomized trials are warranted to elucidate the risks and benefits of this generally safe and low-cost intervention and to help define patients likely to benefit from it. In this context, the value of HBV and immunologic biomarkers needs to be elucidated. Novel treatment options that aim at functional cure should investigate NA cessation as a possible enhancer of their efficacy.

References

1. World Health Organization. Hepatitis B. Key facts. www.who.int/mediacentre/factsheets/fs204/en/
2. Weinbaum CM, Mast EE, Ward JW. Recommendations for identification and public health management of persons with chronic hepatitis B virus infection. *Hepatology* 2009;49:535–544.
3. Liaw YF, Chu CM. Hepatitis B virus infection. *Lancet* 2009;373:582–592.
4. European Association for the Study of the Liver. EASL clinical practice guidelines: management of chronic hepatitis B virus infection. *Journal of Hepatology* 2017;67:370–398.
5. Sarin SK, Kumar M, Lau GK et al. Asia-Pacific clinical guidelines on the management of hepatitis B: a 2015 update. *Hepatology International* 2016;10:1–98.
6. Terrault NA, Lok AS, McMahon BJ et al. Update on prevention, diagnosis, and treatment of chronic hepatitis B: AASLD 2018 hepatitis B guideline. *Hepatology* 2018;67:1560–1599.
7. Zoulim F. Inhibition of hepatitis B virus gene expression: a step towards functional cure. *Journal of Hepatology* 2018;68:386–388.

8. Marcellin P, Gane EJ, Flisiak R et al. Long term treatment with tenofovir disoproxil fumarate for chronic hepatitis B infection is safe and well tolerated and associated with durable virologic response with no detectable resistance: 8 year results from two phase 3 trials. *Hepatology* 2014;60:313A.

9. Boni C, Fisicaro P, Valdatta C et al. Characterization of hepatitis B virus (HBV)-specific T-cell dysfunction in chronic HBV infection. *Journal of Virology* 2007;81:4215–4225.

10. Rivino L, Le Bert N, Gill US et al. Hepatitis B virus-specific T cells associate with viral control upon nucleos(t)ide analogue therapy discontinuation. *Journal of Clinical Investigation* 2018;128(2):668–681.

11. Chi H, Hansen BE, Yim C et al. Reduced risk of relapse after long-term nucleos(t)ide analogue consolidation therapy for chronic hepatitis B. *Alimentary and Pharmacology Therapeutics* 2015;41:867–876.

12. Hadziyannis SJ, Sevastianos V, Rapti I, Vassilopoulos D, Hadziyannis E. Sustained responses and loss of HBsAg in HBeAg-negative patients with chronic hepatitis B who stop long-term treatment with adefovir. *Gastroenterology* 2012;143:629–636.

13. Papatheodoridis G, Vlachogiannakos I, Cholongitas E et al. Discontinuation of oral antivirals in chronic hepatitis B: a systematic review. *Hepatology* 2016;63(5):1481–1492.

14. Qiu YW, Huang LH, Yang WL et al. Hepatitis B surface antigen quantification at hepatitis B e antigen seroconversion predicts virological relapse after the cessation of entecavir treatment in hepatitis B e antigen-positive patients. *International Journal of Infectious Diseases* 2016;43:43–48.

15. Höner Zu Siederdissen C, Rinker F et al. Viral and host responses after stopping long-term nucleos(t)ide analogue therapy in HBeAg-negative chronic hepatitis B. *Journal of Infectious Diseases* 2016;214:1492–1497.

16. Yao CC, Lee CM, Hung CH et al. Combining age and HBsAg level predicts post-treatment durability of nucleos(t)ide analogue induced HBeAg seroconversion. *Journal of Gastroenterology and Hepatology* 2015;30:918–924.

17. Berg T, Simon KG, Mauss S et al., FINITE CHB Study Investigators. Long-term response after stopping tenofovir disoproxil fumarate in non-cirrhotic HBeAg-negative patients – FINITE study. *Journal of Hepatology* 2017;67:918–924.

18. Chen CH, Lu SN, Hung CH et al. The role of hepatitis B surface antigen quantification in predicting HBsAg loss and HBV relapse after discontinuation of lamivudine treatment. *Journal of Hepatology* 2014;61:515–522.

19. Wang CC, Tseng KC, Hsieh TY, Tseng TC, Lin HH, Kao JH. Assessing the durability of entecavir-treated hepatitis B using quantitative HBsAg. *American Journal of Gastroenterology* 2016;111:1286–1294.

20. Hara T, Suzuki F, Kawamura Y et al. Long-term entecavir therapy results in falls in serum hepatitis B surface antigen levels and seroclearance in nucleos(t)ide-naïve chronic hepatitis B patients. *Journal of Viral Hepatology* 2014;21:802–808.

21. Hosaka T, Suzuki F, Kobayashi M et al. Clearance of hepatitis B surface antigen during long term nucleot(s)ide analog treatment in chronic hepatitis B: results from a nine-year longitudinal study. *Journal of Gastroenterology* 2013;48:930–941.

22. Tian Y, Ou JJ. HBV-specific T cells as a biomarker for discontinuation of nucleos(t)ide analogue therapy for chronic hepatitis B. *Hepatology* 2019;69:1342–1344.

23. Yeh CT, Hsu CW, Chen YC, Liaw YF. Withdrawal of lamivudine in HBeAg-positive chronic hepatitis B patients after achieving effective maintained virological suppression. *Journal of Clinical Virology* 2009;45:114–118.

24. Kuo YH, Chen CH, Wang JH et al. Extended lamivudine consolidation therapy in hepatitis B e antigen-positive chronic hepatitis B patients improves sustained hepatitis B e antigen seroconversion. *Scandinavian Journal of Gastroenterology* 2010;45:75–81.

25. Jeng WJ, Sheen IS, Chen YC et al. Off-therapy durability of response to entecavir therapy in hepatitis B e antigen-negative chronic hepatitis B patients. *Hepatology* 2013;58:1888–1896.

26. Seto WK, Hui AJ, Wong VW et al. Treatment cessation of entecavir in Asian patients with hepatitis B e antigen negative chronic hepatitis B: a multicentre prospective study. *Gut* 2015;64:667–672.

27. Liu F, Wang L, Li XY et al. Poor durability of lamivudine effectiveness despite stringent cessation criteria: a prospective clinical study in hepatitis B e antigen-negative chronic hepatitis B patients. *Journal of Gastroenterology and Hepatology* 2011;26:456–460.

28. Ha M, Zhang G, Diao S et al. A prospective clinical study in hepatitis B e antigen-negative chronic hepatitis B patients with stringent cessation criteria for adefovir. *Archives of Virology* 2012;157:285–290.

29. Karakaya F, Özer S, Kalkan Ç et al. Discontinuation of lamivudine treatment in HBeAg-negative chronic hepatitis B: a pilot study with long-term follow-up. *Antiviral Therapy* 2017;22:559–570.

30. Cao J, Chi H, Yu T et al. Off-treatment hepatitis B virus (HBV) DNA levels and the prediction of relapse after discontinuation of nucleos(t)ide analogue therapy in patients with chronic hepatitis B: a prospective stop study. *Journal of Infectious Diseases* 2017;215:581–589.

31. Papatheodoridis GV, Rigopoulou EI, Papatheodoridi M et al. DARING-B: discontinuation of effective entecavir or tenofovir disoproxil fumarate long-term therapy before HBsAg loss in non-cirrhotic HBeAg-negative chronic hepatitis B. *Antiviral Therapy* 2018;23:677–685.

32 Hepatitis C and hepatitis B coinfection

Chun-Jen Liu and Jia-Horng Kao

Graduate Institute of Clinical Medicine, National Taiwan University College of Medicine, Taipei, Taiwan
Department of Internal Medicine and Hepatitis Research Center, National Taiwan University Hospital, Taipei, Taiwan
Taiwan Liver Disease Consortium, Taipei, Taiwan

LEARNING POINTS

- HCV/HBV coinfection can be encountered in HBV- or HCV-endemic areas, and also in populations at risk of parenteral transmission.

- Value of combination therapy with PEG-interferon alpha and ribavirin in the treatment of those with HCV/HBV coinfection and positive HCV RNA has been demonstrated in previous clinical trials.

- The advent of new DAA-based anti-HCV therapy increases the rate of HCV clearance and fills the unmet need for those coinfected patients in the PEG-interferon era.

- Notably, subjects may experience HBV reactivation and related hepatitis activity while on treatment or after cure of HCV by DAA therapy. Recent trial data demonstrated that ~70% of subjects experienced a HBV reactivation event within one year after the start of DAA therapy.

- The optimal strategy to prevent HBV reactivation during and after DAA therapy for HCV/HBV coinfected patients awaits further rigorous investigation. For those not receiving prophylactic anti-HBV agent before the start of DAA therapy, close monitoring of HBV activity and prompt anti-HBV treatment on detection of clinical hepatitis activity is strongly recommended.

Introduction

Most patients with chronic hepatitis C (HCV) usually have it as a monoinfection. However, in hepatitis B virus (HBV)-endemic areas, a substantial proportion of patients are coinfected with hepatitis C and B [1–3]. Besides, HCV/HBV coinfection can be found in individuals at risk of parenteral hepatotropic viral transmission, such as people who inject drugs (PWID), and thalassemia and hemophilia patients [3]. The precise global prevalence of HCV/HBV coinfection remains unclear. Fortunately, through the worldwide launch of hepatitis B vaccination programs and the implementation of effective measures to prevent new HBV or HCV infection, it is anticipated that the prevalence of HCV/HBV coinfection will decrease dramatically in the younger populations.

In patients coinfected with HCV and HBV, disease outcomes including the development of liver cirrhosis (LC) and hepatocellular carcinoma (HCC) are usually more severe than those with HCV or HBV monoinfection [1–8]. Both cross-sectional hospital-based data and a community-based cohort study supported the combined effect of HCV/HBV coinfection on the cumulative incidence of HCC [9]. Our recent hospital-based cohort study consistently demonstrated the negative impact of HCV/HBV coinfection [10,11]. During a 10-year follow-up, patients with HCV/HBV coinfection had a higher risk of HCC and LC than those with HBV monoinfection. Therefore, coinfected patients with hepatitis C and B require timely and effective antiviral treatment.

Treatment priority in HCV/HBV coinfection can be determined by the relative viral activity of both viruses [12]. Previous clinical trials suggested that PEG-interferon (PEG-IFN)-alpha plus ribavirin (RBV) was effective in the clearance of HCV in coinfected patients with active

Clinical Dilemmas in Viral Liver Disease, Second Edition. Edited by Graham R. Foster and K. Rajender Reddy.
© 2020 John Wiley & Sons Ltd. Published 2020 by John Wiley & Sons Ltd.

hepatitis C [13–16]. Around 70% of HCV genotype 1 coinfected patients and around 90% of HCV genotype 2 coinfected achieved HCV sustained virologic response (SVR) post treatment while the SVR was durable in 97% of patients during a five-year follow-up [17]. However, the optimal treatment strategies for coinfected patients with active hepatitis B, with decompensated cirrhosis, or in other clinical situations remain largely unknown.

Long-term treatment goals in HCV/HBV coinfection are to reduce liver-related mortality and the development of HCC. Using the nationwide database from Taiwan, a recent analysis suggested that the use of PEG-IFN-alpha plus RBV in coinfected patients was associated with a lower risk of overall mortality, liver-related mortality and the development of HCC in comparison with matched untreated controls [18].

Direct-acting antiviral (DAA)-based anti-HCV therapy has markedly increased the rate of HCV clearance in monoinfected patients and would likely fill the unmet gap in such patients. Our recent multicenter trial in Taiwan demonstrated that the HCV SVR rate was high (100%) in coinfected patients with genotype 1 or 2 infection [19]. As we recognize, DAA therapy would not have any activity against HBV infection; subjects may experience HBV reactivation and even severe hepatitis activity during treatment or after cure of HCV by DAA therapy [20–27], as warned by the US FDA [21]. Our trial data demonstrated that ~70% of subjects experienced an HBV reactivation event within 48 weeks after the start of DAA therapy. Management of HBV activity and/or prevention of HBV reactivation post HCV therapy is a clinical issue that needs to be addressed in further clinical trials. Considering the lack of supportive evidence, recommendations by the EASL and AASLD differ regarding the prevention of HBV reactivation in coinfected patients [28,29].

Clinical impact of HCV/HBV coinfection

A long-term community-based study clearly demonstrated the combined effect of HCV/HBV coinfection on the cumulative incidence of HCC [9]. Our recent hospital-based cohort study consistently demonstrated the adverse impact of HCV/HBV coinfection on liver disease progression [10,11]. During a 10-year follow-up, 111 coinfected patients had a higher risk of HCC and cirrhosis than 111 patients with HBV monoinfection (hazard ratio [95% confidence interval[of 3.59 [1.56–8.22] and 2.52 [1.37–4.61], respectively). Of note, coinfected patients with alanine

aminotransferase (ALT) level >80 U/L had an increased incidence of HBsAg seroclearance and risk of HCC or cirrhosis compared to those with ALT level ≤80 U/L or matched controls with HBV monoinfection. These data clearly indicated that both higher ALT level and coexisting HBV infection were associated with increased risks of cirrhosis and HCC development. We further demonstrated the predictive value of FIB-4 index in the outcomes of coinfected patients where FIB-4 index decreased only in the treated group who achieved SVR; high baseline FIB-4 index (per 1-point increase) in the treated groups independently correlated with a higher risk of developing LC (p=0.011) and HCC (p=0.025). Based on these findings, patients coinfected with hepatitis C and B are at higher risk of liver disease progression, particularly when their serum ALT level or baseline FIB-4 value is elevated.

Evaluation and treatment of HCV and HBV coinfection (Table 32.1)

Baseline evaluation and goals of therapy

In clinical practice, risks and benefits of active treatment, dominance or evolution of hepatic inflammatory activity, severity of liver disease, concomitant delta virus (HDV) or human immunodeficiency virus (HIV) infection, and the presence of comorbidities should be taken into consideration before the selection of treatment candidates and start of antiviral therapy.

The short-term and long-term treatment goals in patients with HCV/HBV coinfection are basically similar to those with HBV or HCV monoinfection, including persistent suppression of viral replication, reduction of hepatic necroinflammation and fibrosis formation, prevention of progression to liver cirrhosis and the development of HCC, and ultimately the improvement of overall as well as liver-related survival [30,31].

Ideally, these goals can be achieved through the eradication of both viruses with effective antiviral therapy. However, if a virus cannot be eradicated, such as HBV, effective suppression is likely to provide benefit by mitigating hepatic inflammation and reducing downstream consequences of untreated infection of progressive liver disease culminating in liver failure and HCC.

Identification of target virus to be treated

A previous study noted that active hepatitis C can be found in more than 50% of coinfected patients [12]. Previous

Table 32.1 Proposed strategies for the treatment of patients with HCV/HBV coinfection

HCV RNA	HBV DNA level	Treatment goals	Proposed strategies	Remarks	Potential benefit of DAA-based therapy
Detectable	<2000 IU/mL	Cure of HCV infection	DAA[a] or PEG-IFN/RBV[a]	DAA cannot control HBV replication; HBV reactivation is a concern. AASLD and EASL have different recommendations about prophylactic NUC [28,29]	DAA increases rate of HCV SVR; avoids IFN-related adverse events. DAA regimen may replace PEG-IFN/RBV therapy for CHC
Detectable	≥2000 IU/mL	Cure of HCV infection; control of HBV infection	DAA[a] or DAA + NUC Or PEG-IFN/RBV[a] or PEG-IFN/RBV + NUC	DAA cannot control HBV replication; HBV reactivation is a concern. AASLD and EASL have different recommendations about prophylactic NUC [28,29]	DAA increases rate of HCV SVR; avoids IFN-related adverse events. DAA regimen may replace PEG-IFN/RBV therapy for CHC
Undetectable	≥2000 IU/mL	Control of HBV infection	NUC	Only small case series	No
Undetectable	<2000 IU/mL	Not necessary	Clinical observation	Expert opinion	No

[a] Data from large multicenter clinical trial.

CHB, chronic hepatitis B; CHC, chronic hepatitis C; DAA, direct-acting antiviral; NUC, nucleos(t)ide analog; RBV, ribavirin; PEG-IFN, PEG-interferon.

experiences noted that HCV could be successfully eradicated in about 70% of subjects with chronic HCV monoinfection using PEG-IFN plus RBV combination therapy [30,31]. Recent trials and real-world data demonstrated that HCV SVR rate can be higher than 95% using DAA-based therapy for HCV monoinfected patients [32–37]. Accordingly, HCV infection seems to be the ideal priority target in dually infected patients with active hepatitis C.

Treatment of subjects with HCV/HBV coinfection using PEG-IFN and RBV

The efficacy of PEG-IFN plus RBV in the treatment of coinfected subjects with active hepatitis C has been well reported [13,17,36–38]. The durability of hepatitis C clearance in HCV/HBV coinfected patients was further demonstrated by a five-year prospective follow-up study [17]. We also noted that HCV SVR was durable by using PEG-IFN-alpha and ribavirin therapy and that it was not influenced by HBV coinfection. In addition to the cure of HCV infection, PEG-IFN-based therapy may also help the control of chronic HBV infection in those with HCV/HBV coinfection. During five-year posttreatment follow-up, the rate of HBsAg seroclearance was 5.4% per year [17].

Notably, reactivation of HBV activity is an important clinical concern in coinfected subjects receiving anti-HCV therapy [39]. In our previous PEG-IFN trial, we found that reactivation of HBV DNA occurred in 47 (61.8%) of 76 patients with pretreatment serum HBV DNA <200 IU/mL. The reactivation may occur during the course of treatment (38%) or during the posttreatment follow-up period (62%) [17].

Treatment of HBV and HCV coinfection in the era of DAA

Rationale of DAA-based therapy

The new anti-HCV DAAs have revolutionized the care of HCV by offering simple regimens, providing high rates of SVR with shortened treatment duration and have great tolerability (Figure 32.1) [40]. However, the following issues need to be clarified before DAAs can be recommended for the treatment of coinfected patients

- Whether DAA-based therapy is similarly effective (as in HCV monoinfected patients) in the seroclearance of HCV RNA.
- Whether coexisting HBV infection influences the response to DAA-based therapy.

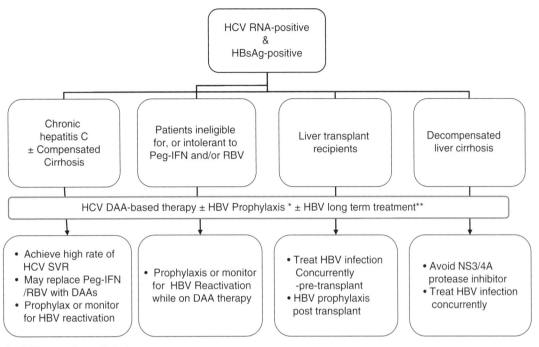

Figure 32.1 Potential benefits of DAA-based therapy in different clinical scenarios.

- What are the effects of IFN-free DAA regimens in the treatment of IFN-refractory or -ineligible subjects?

Since HCV DAAs would not affect the replication cycle of HBV or modulate immune responses to HBV infection, it would also be very interesting to examine whether HBV would reactivate after the seroclearance of HCV RNA.

HCV SVR rate using DAAs to treat coinfected subjects

To address all these issues, we conducted a multicenter study in Taiwan using sofosbuvir/ledipasvir to treat HCV/HBV coinfected patients [19]. One hundred and eleven patients were enrolled (61% HCV genotype 1 and 39% genotype 2; 16% compensated cirrhosis) and all achieved HCV SVR. Of the 37 patients with baseline HBV DNA <20 IU/mL, 31 (84%) had at least one episode of quantifiable HBV DNA through posttreatment week 12. Of the 74 patients with baseline HBV DNA ≥20 IU/mL, 39 (53%) had increases of HBV DNA by >1 $\log^{10}$ IU/mL through posttreatment week 12. Overall, five patients had an elevation in HBV DNA concomitant with an increase in ALT >2 × upper limit of normal (ULN). Of these, two started HBV treatment. No patient experienced clinical signs and symptoms of HBV reactivation. Our findings suggested that a DAA regimen such as 12-week ledipasvir/sofosbuvir was highly effective in those with HCV coinfected with HBV. The risk of HBV reactivation was high but the incidence of severe hepatitis activity was minimized through regular monitoring of serum HBV DNA and prompt administration of anti-HBV nucleotide analog therapy upon HBV reactivation.

The hidden menace of HBV reactivation: in comparison with PEG-IFN/RBV treatment

After the introduction of DAA for the treatment of chronic hepatitis C, there has been an increased awareness of HBV reactivation in coinfected chronic hepatitis C [CHC]/HBV which has been treated with DAAs. An earlier systematic review and metaanalysis was performed to compare the rate of HBV reactivation in CHC patients coinfected with HBV and treated with IFN-based therapy versus those treated with DAAs [20]. Overall, the pooled incidence rate of HBV reactivation among CHC subjects with HBV coinfection (n = 779) was similar between those treated with IFN-based therapy (14.5%, p<0.001) and DAAs (12.2%, p=0.03; p=0.91 for heterogeneity between subgroups). Interestingly, the time to HBV reactivation seems to be earlier in those treated with DAAs (4–12 weeks during treatment) than in those treated with IFN-based therapies (most at the end of treatment and some during follow-up). Also, studies with DAA-based therapies were more likely to be associated with an increased incidence of hepatitis due to HBV reactivation (12.2% in DAAs vs 0% in IFN; p=0.009 for heterogeneity between subgroups). Fortunately, HCV SVR was not affected by HBV reactivation (p=0.27).

Improvement in clinical outcomes

In patients with HCV monoinfection, successful anti-HCV therapy has demonstrated a decrease in the incidence of newly developed HCC and liver-related mortality [41]. Whether anti-HCV therapy using PEG-IFN plus ribavirin combination could obtain similar effects in HCV/HBV coinfected patients was investigated by a large population-based survey in Taiwan [18]. Using the National Health Insurance Database of Taiwan, we found that in comparison to the untreated dually infected cohort, the risk of HCC development, all-cause mortality, and liver-related mortality decreased by 35%, 62%, and 59%, respectively after anti-HCV therapy [18].

Despite the control or eradication of hepatitis virus after PEG-IFN/RBV treatment, patients may still be at risk of developing advanced liver disease, including HCC. Therefore, regular surveillance for the occurrence of HCC is advised in these dually infected patients even after achieving HCV SVR.

Regarding the long-term outcomes of subjects receiving DAA therapy and achieving SVR, usually the risk of HCC development has been noted to decrease even in those with cirrhosis and the risk of HCC recurrence has not increased after curative therapy for HCC [42]. Nevertheless, the long-term benefits post HCV cure by DAA in coinfected subjects await further investigation.

Updated international guidance on the treatment of patients with HCV and HBV coinfection

Recent EASL guidelines [28] recommend that:

- patients with HCV/HBV coinfection should be treated with the same anti-HCV regimens, following the same rules as in HCV monoinfected patients (B1)
- patients coinfected with HCV and HBV fulfilling the standard criteria for HBV treatment should receive nucleoside/nucleotide analog treatment according to the EASL 2017 guidelines on HBV (A1)
- patients who are HBsAg positive should receive nucleoside/nucleotide analog prophylaxis at least until week 12 post anti-HCV therapy and be monitored monthly if HBV treatment is stopped (B1).

In contrast, AASLD practice guidance [29] suggests that all HBsAg-positive patients should be tested for HCV infection using the anti-HCV test. HCV treatment is indicated for patients with HCV viremia. HBV treatment is determined by HBV DNA and ALT levels as per the AASLD HBV guidelines for monoinfected patients. HBsAg-positive patients are at risk of HBV DNA and ALT flares with HCV DAA therapy and monitoring of HBV DNA levels every 4–8 weeks during treatment and for three months post treatment is indicated in those who do not meet treatment criteria for monoinfected patients. HBsAg-negative, anti-HBc-positive patients with HCV are at very low risk of reactivation with HCV DAA therapy. ALT levels should be monitored at baseline, at the end of treatment, and during follow-up, with HBV DNA and HBsAg testing reserved for those whose ALT levels increase or those who fail to normalize during treatment or post treatment.

Both guidelines agree that the status of HBV infection should be monitored closely if IFN-free regimens are used since HCV DAA is anticipated to have no direct or immunomodulatory effect on the replication of HBV. Anti-HBV therapy should be implemented in timely fashion if clinically indicated.

Conclusion and Future Directions

HCV/HBV coinfection is not uncommon in endemic areas and among those at risk of parenterally transmissible infections. How two viruses interact with each other in the liver is only partly understood. Apart from academic interest, these data will help develop more effective antiviral therapy and efficient strategies to prevent HBV reactivation post HCV cure by DAA.

For HCV/HBV coinfected patients with active hepatitis C, the same genotype-dependent treatment recommendations as for single chronic hepatitis C can be applied. The effectiveness of DAA-based therapy in coinfected patients has been demonstrated in a recent clinical trial [19]. The long-term benefits of curing HCV by DAAs, in those with HCV/HBV coinfection, await further follow-up studies. HBV reactivation in those treated with DAAs for HCV remains of some concern. Last but not least, for patients with active hepatitis B and C, more studies are needed to determine the optimal regimen to treat both viruses at the same time.

Acknowledgments

The work was supported by grants from the Taiwan Liver Disease Consortium, Ministry of Science and Technology, Taiwan.

Financial support

The work was supported by grants from the Taiwan Liver Disease Consortium, Ministry of Science and Technology, Taiwan.

References

1. Liu CJ, Liou JM, Chen DS, Chen PJ. Natural course and treatment of dual hepatitis B virus and hepatitis C virus infections. *Journal of the Formosan Medical Association* 2005;104:783–791.

2. Chen DS, Kuo GC, Sung JL et al. Hepatitis C virus infection in an area hyperendemic for hepatitis B and chronic liver disease: the Taiwan experience. *Journal of Infectious Diseases* 1990;162:817–822.

3. Liu CJ, Chen PJ, Chen DS, Tseng TC, Kao JH. Perspectives on dual hepatitis B and C infection in Taiwan. *Journal of the Formosan Medical Association* 2016;115:298–305.

4. D'Amelio R, Matricardi PM, Biselli R et al. Changing epidemiology of hepatitis B in Italy: public health implications. *American Journal of Epidemiology* 1992;135:1012–1018.

5. Crespo J, Lozano JL, de la Cruz F et al. Prevalence and significance of hepatitis C viremia in chronic active hepatitis B. *American Journal of Gastroenterology* 1994;89:1147–1151.

6. Treitinger A, Spada C, Ferreira LA et al. Hepatitis B and hepatitis C prevalence among blood donors and HIV-1 infected patients in Florianopolis, Brazil. *Brazilian Journal of Infectious Diseases* 2000;4:192–196.

7. Liaw YF, Chen YC, Sheen IS, Chien RN, Yeh CT, Chu CM. Impact of acute hepatitis C virus superinfection in patients with chronic hepatitis B virus infection. *Gastroenterology* 2004;126:1024–1029.

8 . Donato F, Boffetta P, Puoti M. A meta-analysis of epidemiological studies on the combined effect of hepatitis B and C virus infections in causing hepatocellular carcinoma. *International Journal of Cancer* 1998;75:347–354.

9. Huang YT, Jen CL, Yang HI et al. Lifetime risk and sex difference of hepatocellular carcinoma among patients with chronic hepatitis B and C. *Journal of Clinical Oncology* 2011;29:3643–3650.

10. Liu CJ, Tseng TC, Yang WT et al. Profile and value of FIB-4 in patients with dual chronic hepatitis C and B. *Journal of Gastroenterology and Hepatology* 2019;34:410–417.

11. Yang WT, Wu LW, Tseng TC et al. Hepatitis B surface antigen loss and hepatocellular carcinoma development in patients with dual hepatitis B and C infection. *Medicine* 2016;95(10):e2995.

12. Raimondo G, Brunetto MR, Pontisso P et al. Longitudinal evaluation reveals a complex spectrum of virological profiles in hepatitis B virus/hepatitis C virus-co-infected patients. *Hepatology* 2006;43:100–107.

13. Liu CJ, Chuang WL, Lee CM et al. An open label, comparative, multicenter study of peginterferon alpha-2a plus ribavirin in the treatment of patients with chronic hepatitis C/hepatitis B co-infection versus those with chronic hepatitis C monoinfection. *Gastroenterology* 2009;136:496–504.

14. Uyanikoglu A, Akyuz F, Baran B et al. Co-infection with hepatitis B does not alter treatment response in chronic hepatitis C. *Clinics and Research in Hepatology and Gastroenterology* 2013;37:485–490.

15. Kim YJ, Lee JW, Kim YS et al. Clinical features and treatment efficacy of peginterferon alpha plus ribavirin in chronic hepatitis C patients coinfected with hepatitis B virus. *Korean Journal of Hepatology* 2011;17:199–205.

16. Potthoff A, Wedemeyer H, Boecher WO et al. The HEP-NET B/C co-infection trial: a prospective multicenter study to investigate the efficacy of pegylated interferon-alpha2b and ribavirin in patients with HBV/HCV co-infection. *Journal of Hepatology* 2008;49:688–694.

17. Yu ML, Lee CM, Chen CL et al. Sustained HCV clearance and increased HBsAg seroclearance in patients with dual chronic hepatitis C and B during post-treatment follow-up. *Hepatology* 2013;57:2135–2142.

18. Liu CJ, Chu YT, Shau WY, Kuo RNC, Chen PJ, Lai MS. Treatment of patients with dual hepatitis C and B by

peginterferon alpha and ribavirin reduced risk of hepatocellular carcinoma and mortality. *Gut* 2014;63:506–514.

19. Liu CJ, Chuang WL, Sheen IS et al. Efficacy of ledipasvir and sofosbuvir treatment of HCV infection in patients coinfected with HBV. *Gastroenterology* 2018;154:989–997.

20. Chen G, Wang C, Chen J et al. Hepatitis B reactivation in hepatitis B and C coinfected patients treated with antiviral agents: a systematic review and meta-analysis. *Hepatology* 2017;66:13–26.

21. Bersoff-Matcha SJ, Cao K, Jason M et al. Hepatitis B virus reactivation associated with direct-acting antiviral therapy for chronic hepatitis C virus: a review of cases reported to the U.S. Food and Drug Administration adverse event reporting system. *Annals of Internal Medicine* 2017;166:792–798.

22. Collins JM, Raphael KL, Terry C et al. Hepatitis B virus reactivation during successful treatment of hepatitis C virus with sofosbuvir and simeprevir. *Clinical Infectious Diseases* 2015;61:1304–1306.

23. Takayama H, Sato T, Ikeda F, Fujiki S. Reactivation of hepatitis B virus during interferon-free therapy with daclatasvir and asunaprevir in patient with hepatitis B virus/hepatitis C virus co-infection. *Hepatology Research* 2016;46:489–491.

24. De Monte A, Courjon J, Anty R et al. Direct-acting antiviral treatment in adults infected with hepatitis C virus: reactivation of hepatitis B virus coinfection as a further challenge. *Journal of Clinical Virology* 2016;78:27–30.

25. Wang C, Ji D, Chen J et al. Hepatitis due to reactivation of hepatitis B virus in endemic areas among patients with hepatitis C treated with direct-acting antiviral agents. *Clinical Gastroenterology and Hepatology* 2017;15:132–136.

26. Londoño MC, Lens S, Mariño Z et al. Hepatitis B reactivation in patients with chronic hepatitis C undergoing antiviral therapy with an interferon-free regimen. *Alimentary Pharmacology and Therapeutics* 2017;45:1156–1161.

27. Liu CH, Liu CJ, Su TH et al. Hepatitis B virus reactivation in patients receiving interferon-free direct-acting antiviral agents for chronic hepatitis C virus infection. *Open Forum Infectious Diseases* 2017;4:ofx028.

28. European Association for the Study of the Liver. EASL recommendations on treatment of hepatitis C 2018. *Journal of Hepatology* 2018;69:461–511.

29. Terrault NA, Lok ASF, McMahon BJ et al. Update on prevention, diagnosis, and treatment of chronic hepatitis B: AASLD 2018 hepatitis B guidance. *Hepatology* 2018;(4):1560–1599.

30. Liu CJ, Chen PJ, Chen DS. Dual chronic hepatitis B virus and hepatitis C virus infection. *Hepatology International* 2009;3:517–525.

31. Chen DS. Fighting against viral hepatitis: lessons from Taiwan. *Hepatology* 2011;54:381–392.

32. Lok AS, Gardiner DF, Lawitz E et al. Preliminary study of two antiviral agents for hepatitis C genotype 1. *New England Journal of Medicine* 2012;366:216–224.

33. Kumada H, Suzuki Y, Ikeda K et al. Daclatasvir plus asunaprevir for chronic HCV genotype 1b infection. *Hepatology* 2014;59:2083–2091.

34. European Association for the Study of the Liver. EASL recommendations on treatment of hepatitis C 2015. *Journal of Hepatology* 2015;63:199–236.

35. Kayali Z, Schmidt WN. Finally sofosbuvir: an oral anti-HCV drug with wide performance capability. *Pharmgenomics and Personalized Medicine* 2014;7:387–398.

36. Liu CJ, Chen PJ, Lai MY, Kao JH, Jeng YM, Chen DS. Ribavirin and interferon is effective for hepatitis C virus clearance in hepatitis B and C dually infected patients. *Hepatology* 2003;37:568–576.

37. Hung CH, Lee CM, Lu SN et al. Combination therapy with interferon-alpha and ribavirin in patients with dual hepatitis B and hepatitis C virus infection. *Journal of Gastroenterology and Hepatology* 2005;20:727–732.

38. Chuang WL, Dai CY, Chang WY et al. Viral interaction and responses in chronic hepatitis C and B co-infected patients with interferon-alpha plus ribavirin combination therapy. *Antiviral Therapy* 2005;10:125–131.

39. Gordon SC, Sherman KE. Treatment of HBV/HCV coinfection: releasing the enemy within. *Gastroenterology* 2009;136:393–396.

40. Cortez KJ, Kottilil S. Beyond interferon: rationale and prospects for newer treatment paradigms for chronic hepatitis C. *Therapeutic Advances in Chronic Disease* 2015;6:4–14.

41. Yu ML, Lin SM, Chuang WL et al. A sustained virological response to interferon or interferon/ribavirin reduces hepatocellular carcinoma and improves survival in chronic hepatitis C: a nationwide, multicentre study in Taiwan. *Antiviral Therapy* 2006;11:985–994.

42. Waziry R, Hajarizadeh B, Grebely J et al. Hepatocellular carcinoma risk following direct-acting antiviral HCV therapy: a systematic review, meta-analyses, and meta-regression. *Journal of Hepatology* 2017;67:1204–1212.

Chronic hepatitis E virus infection: is it reality or hype and where does it matter?

Nassim Kamar[1] and Jacques Izopet[2]

[1] Department of Nephrology, Dialysis and Organ Transplantation, CHU Rangueil, University Paul Sabatier, Toulouse, France

[2] Department of Virology, University Paul Sabatier, Toulouse, France

LEARNING POINTS

- Hepatitis E virus (HEV) infection is probably the most prevalent viral hepatitis worldwide.

- In most cases, HEV infection is asymptomatic. HEV genotype 1–4 infections can be incriminated in cases of acute liver failure and acute-on-chronic hepatitis. However, only genotypes 3 and 4 can induce chronic HEV infection, defined by the persistence of HEV replication for at least three months.

- Chronic HEV infection can lead to cirrhosis. It is observed only in immunosuppressed patients, that is, organ and stem cell transplant patients, human immunodeficiency virus patients, and patients given immunotherapy or chemotherapy.

- Ribavirin is the main treatment for chronic HEV infection.

Introduction

Hepatitis E virus (HEV) infection is probably the most prevalent viral hepatitis worldwide (Table 33.1) [1]. HEV is a RNA virus. There is one serotype and four main genotypes. Genotypes 1 and 2 (HEV1 and HEV2) are more prevalent in developing countries and are transmitted via the fecal–oral route. It is a human-to-human transmission. Genotypes 3 and 4 are mainly prevalent in high-income countries, including China. They are mainly transmitted from animals to humans. The main reservoirs for genotypes 3 and 4 (HEV3 and HEV4) are wild boars, pigs, deer, and rabbits. In this setting, HEV infection is a zoonosis.

Eating undercooked meat or shellfish and crops irrigated by water contaminated by animal feces transmits HEV3 and HEV4. It has also been clearly shown that HEV3 and HEV4 can be transmitted by the transfusion of contaminated blood products. Currently, HEV is not assessed systematically in blood donors. Finally, a couple of cases of HEV transmission by organ transplant were reported, after liver and kidney transplantations [2].

The estimated number of symptomatic HEV1 cases is 3.4 million per year. Nearly 20% of patients infected by HEV1 are symptomatic. The overall mortality is 1–2% of symptomatic cases. With respect to HEV3 and HEV4 infections, the global burden and the overall mortality are unknown. Very few cases are symptomatic (less than 5%). The high seroprevalence of HEV in several developing and developed countries highlights that in the large majority of cases, HEV infection is asymptomatic and it resolves spontaneously [2].

However, all four main genotypes can be responsible for hepatic and extrahepatic manifestations such as neurologic manifestations (neuralgic amyotrophy and Guillain–Barré syndrome) and kidney injuries (membranoproliferative glomerulonephritis with or without cryoglobulinemia and membranous nephritis) [3,4].

With respect to hepatic manifestations, HEV1, HEV3, and HEV4 can induce a severe hepatitis and liver failure. In pregnant women, infection with HEV1, but not HEV3, can lead to fulminant hepatitis, acute liver failure, and mother and child mortality in up to 25% of cases. The prevalence of HEV3 and HEV4 infection among patients presenting with

Clinical Dilemmas in Viral Liver Disease, Second Edition. Edited by Graham R. Foster and K. Rajender Reddy.
© 2020 John Wiley & Sons Ltd. Published 2020 by John Wiley & Sons Ltd.

Table 33.1 Characteristics of chronic hepatitis E virus infection

	Remarks
Target population	Immunosuppressed patients: transplant, HIV, patients given chemotherapy or immunotherapy
HEV genotype	Genotype 3 +++ Genotype 4 +
Prevalence	Unkown
Incidence	Two-thirds of organ transplant patients infected by HEV Unknown in other immunosuppressed populations
Symptoms	Mostly asymptomatic
Liver function tests	Can be normal or subnormal
Outcome	Progression of liver fibrosis that can lead to cirrhosis
Extrahepatic manifestations	Neurologic symptoms and kidney injury can occur
Treatment	Reduction of immunosuppression Ribavirin monotherapy

HEV, hepatitis E virus; HIV, human immunodeficiency virus.

acute liver failure ranges from 2.5% to 10%. Acute-on-chronic liver failure induced by all HEV genotypes was also reported and can lead to up to 70% mortality in the absence of liver transplantation [1].

Until 2008, no cases of chronic HEV infections were reported. Initially, chronic HEV infection was defined as HEV replication persisting in the blood for at least six months after infection. However, in a cohort of solid organ transplant patients followed prospectively, no spontaneous HEV clearance was observed between three and six months after infection. Hence, it has been suggested to define chronic HEV infection as persistence of HEV replication for three months.

Chronic HEV infection has mainly been described in solid organ transplant patients receiving immunosuppressive therapy [5]. However, it has also been reported in human immunodeficiency virus (HIV)-positive patients [6], stem cell transplant patients [7], hematologic patients receiving chemotherapy, and rheumatologic patients given immunotherapy. In other words, chronic HEV infection can occur in immunosuppressed patients. Scarce case reports suggested the possibility of persistent HEV infection in nonimmunosuppressed patients. However, careful analysis shows that these patients had previously received immunosuppressive drugs. Most chronic HEV cases have been observed in patients infected with HEV3. Very few cases of chronic HEV4 infections have been reported. In immunosuppressed patients infected by HEV1, no case of chronic hepatitis was reported. Hence, although HEV has a single serotype, HEV1 and 2 and HEV3 and 4 behave differently [8].

Chronic HEV infection among solid organ transplant patients

Retrospective studies have shown that among solid organ transplant patients infected by HEV, only one-third spontaneously cleared HEV, while the remainder developed a chronic hepatitis [9]. Strikingly, eight out of 85 patients developed cirrhosis relatively soon after HEV infection [9]. Indeed, liver fibrosis progression was very rapid, and cirrhosis occurred 3–4 years after infection. Some patients died from decompensated cirrhosis and portal hypertension. No case of hepatocellular carcinoma was reported. Chronic HEV infection has also been reported in pediatric transplant patients [10].

Low total lymphocyte count and low anti-HEV-specific T-cells were associated with an increased risk of developing chronic hepatitis [5,11]. In a large retrospective European multicenter study, a low platelet count at diagnosis and the use of tacrolimus rather than ciclosporin A as a main immunosuppressant were identified as independent predictive factors for chronic hepatitis [9]. Tacrolimus is a more potent immunosuppressive drug than ciclosporin A. *In vitro*, calcineurin inhibitors (tacrolimus and ciclosporin A) and mammalian target of rapamycin inhibitors increased HEV replication in culture models. Conversely, mycophenolic acid, an inosine monophosphate inhibitor, inhibits HEV replication *in vitro*.

Interestingly, it has been observed that patients who evolve to chronic infection have lower liver function tests at diagnosis compared to those who have resolving hepatitis, suggesting a lower immune response in patients who develop chronic hepatitis. HEV RNA concentration did not differ between acute and chronic phase, and between patients with chronic HEV infection with or without fibrosis progression. However, a greater HEV quasispecies heterogeneity was observed in patients with persistent HEV infection.

No cases of HEV reactivation have been reported after HEV clearance. Conversely, HEV reinfection was described in solid organ transplant patients [12]. In some cases, it led to chronic hepatitis in patients who were HEV seropositive at transplantation. In these patients, anti-HEV antibody concentration was low, at below 7 WHO IU/mL [12].

Chronic HEV infection among HIV-positive patients

Few cases of chronic HEV infection that led to cirrhosis have been reported in HIV-positive patients [6]. However, all of them had a low CD4+ T-cell count. A HEV strain obtained from an HIV-positive patient with chronic hepatitis allowed identification of a recombinant human hepatitis E virus [13].

Management of chronic HEV infection

In transplant patients, a decrease in immunosuppressive therapy, when feasible, is considered as a first-line therapeutic option [9]. Indeed, it has been shown that decreasing immunosuppressants targeting T-cells, such as calcineurin inhibitors, allows clearance of the virus in one-third of transplant patients with chronic hepatitis [9]. In patients with persisting HEV replication despite the reduction of immunosuppression and in those in whom it is not feasible, the use of ribavirin monotherapy is recommended [14,15]. In a cohort of organ transplant patients, ribavirin given at a median dose of 600 mg/day for a median period of three months promoted a sustained virologic response in nearly 80% of patients [14]. In patients who relapsed, retreatment with ribavirin for a longer period lead to a sustained virologic response of around

95% [14]. Ribavirin was also successfully used in cases of chronic HEV cases that occurred in HIV-positive stem cell transplant patients, and hematologic patients [2].

The mechanism of action of ribavirin is unknown. It has been suggested that it depletes guanosine triphosphate dehydrogenase. Mutations in HEV RNA polymerase were reported in patients who failed to respond to ribavirin or in cases of relapse after ribavirin cessation. However, on one hand these mutations increase the replication capacity of HEV and on the other, they increase the antiviral effect of ribavirin. Hence, their role is uncertain, but does not seem to be correlated with the sustained virologic response.

Pegylated interferon has also been used to treat chronic HEV infection. However, it is contraindicated in organ transplant patients, except liver transplant patients, because it increases the risk of acute rejection. Sofosbuvir combined with ribavirin was tested to treat refractory chronic HEV infection. The data are not convincing [2].

Conclusion

Hepatitis E virus infection is the leading cause of viral hepatitis worldwide. In most cases, it is asymptomatic and resolves spontaneously. It can be responsible for acute liver failure and acute-on-chronic hepatitis. In immunosuppressed patients infected with HEV3 or HEV4, HEV replication can persist, leading to chronic hepatitis. Therefore, assessment for HEV infection should be part of the work-up in patients with increased liver function tests and/or some specific extrahepatic manifestations.

References

1. Kamar N, Bendall R, Legrand-Abravanel F et al. Hepatitis E. *Lancet* 2012;379:2477–2488.
2. Kamar N, Izopet J, Pavio N et al. Hepatitis E virus infection. *Nature Review Disease Primers* 2017;3:17086.
3. Dalton HR, Kamar N, van Eijk JJ et al. Hepatitis E virus and neurological injury. *Nature Reviews Neurology* 2016;12(2):77–85.
4. Kamar N, Marion O, Abravanel F, Izopet J, Dalton HR. Extrahepatic manifestations of hepatitis E virus. *Liver International* 2016;36(4):467–472.
5. Kamar N, Selves J, Mansuy JM et al. Hepatitis E virus and chronic hepatitis in organ-transplant recipients. *New England Journal of Medicine* 2008;358(8):811–817.

6. Dalton HR, Bendall R, Keane F, Tedder R, Ijaz S. Persistent carriage of hepatitis E virus in patients with HIV infection. *New England Journal of Medicine* 2009;361(10):1025–1027.

7. Tavitian S, Peron JM, Huynh A et al. Hepatitis E virus excretion can be prolonged in patients with hematological malignancies. *Journal of Clinical Virology* 2010;49(2):141–144.

8. Kamar N, Dalton HR, Abravanel F, Izopet J. Hepatitis E virus infection. *Clinical Microbiology Reviews* 2014;27(1):116–138.

9. Kamar N, Garrouste C, Haagsma EB et al. Factors associated with chronic hepatitis in patients with hepatitis E virus infection who have received solid organ transplants. *Gastroenterology* 2011;140(5):1481–1489.

10. Halac U, Béland K, Lapierre P et al. Chronic Hepatitis E infection in children with liver transplantation. *Gut* 2012;64(4):597–603.

11. Suneetha PV, Pischke S, Schlaphoff V et al. HEV-specific T-cell responses are associated with control of HEV infection. *Hepatology* 2012;55(3):695–708.

12. Abravanel F, Lhomme S, Chapuy-Regaud S et al. Hepatitis E virus reinfections in solid-organ-transplant recipients can evolve into chronic infections. *Journal of Infectious Diseases* 2014;209(12):1900–1906.

13. Shukla P, Nguyen HT, Torian U et al. Cross-species infections of cultured cells by hepatitis *E virus and discovery of an infectious virus-host recombinant. Proceedings of the National Academy of Sciences USA* 2011;108(6):2438–2443.

14. Kamar N, Izopet J, Tripon S et al. Ribavirin for chronic hepatitis E virus infection in transplant recipients. *New England Journal of Medicine* 2014;370(12):1111–1120.

15. European Association for the Study of the Liver. EASL clinical practice guidelines on hepatitis E virus infection. *Journal of Hepatology* 2018;68(6):1256–1271.

Amit Goel[1] and Rakesh Aggarwal[2]

[1] Department of Gastroenterology, Sanjay Gandhi Postgraduate Institute of Medical Sciences, Lucknow, India
[2] Jawaharlal Institute of Postgraduate Medical Education & Research, Puducherry, India

LEARNING POINTS

- A recombinant subunit vaccine against hepatitis E virus infection has been developed.

- When administered as three intramuscular doses (30 µg each, at 0, 1, and 6 months), it is quite safe, highly immunogenic, and highly efficacious in preventing hepatitis E for at least 4.5 years.

- This vaccine is approved and marketed (Hecolin®) in China, but is not yet available elsewhere; even in China, its use has been quite limited.

- Hepatitis E virus vaccine should be useful in several settings; however, such use needs additional studies to provide certain key bridging data.

Introduction

Hepatitis E virus (HEV), a member of the genus *Hepevirus* and family Hepeviridae, is a hepatotropic virus. HEV infection in humans is caused primarily by isolates belonging to four genotypes (1–4) and has two distinct patterns.

The dominant pattern is that observed in Asia and Africa, where human-to-human transmission of genotype 1 or 2 HEV, through the fecal–oral route, most often via contamination of drinking water supplies, causes outbreaks and sporadic cases of acute viral hepatitis. The cases, mostly in young and immunocompetent persons, usually have a self-limiting disease with spontaneous recovery over a few days to weeks; a few cases develop acute liver failure, which may be fatal. Severe disease and mortality are more common when HEV infection affects pregnant women or persons with limited hepatic reserve. It is estimated that HEV genotypes 1 and 2 cause 20.1 million human infections, 3.4 million symptomatic cases, 70 000 deaths, and 3000 stillbirths annually in Asia and Africa.

The other pattern is observed in North America, Europe, and developed countries in the Asia-Pacific region, where zoonotic transmission of HEV genotype 3 or 4 through eating undercooked meat or close contact with animals causes occasional clinical cases, mostly among elderly or immunocompromised persons. In the latter group, persistent HEV infection (chronic hepatitis E) and progression to cirrhosis can occur. With either pattern, asymptomatic infection is common.

Hepatitis E virus disease can be largely prevented through simple measures, namely attention to sanitation, drinking water supplies, and adequate cooking of meat. Prevention using vaccination is another option. This chapter reviews the current status of HEV vaccines, including safety, immunogenicity, efficacy, duration of protection, availability, and indications.

Principles underlying HEV vaccines

HEV does not grow well in cell culture, precluding development of live attenuated or inactivated vaccines. The virus has a single-stranded RNA genome with three open reading frames: *orf1*, *orf2*, and *orf3*. The *orf2* encodes a 660 amino acid protein, which forms the viral capsid and plays a key role in virus assembly and its attachment to host cells.

Clinical Dilemmas in Viral Liver Disease, Second Edition. Edited by Graham R. Foster and K. Rajender Reddy.
© 2020 John Wiley & Sons Ltd. Published 2020 by John Wiley & Sons Ltd.

The protein is also highly immunogenic and contains neutralization epitopes, antibodies to which can neutralize the virus. Hence, attempts at development of HEV vaccines have focused on this protein, and several recombinant HEV ORF2 proteins expressed in different prokaryotic or eukaryotic systems have been evaluated in animal models.

Human studies with HEV vaccines: efficacy and safety

To date, two candidate vaccines have undergone clinical trials, and one has been approved and marketed, as described below.

Recombinant 56 kDa vaccine

This vaccine contains a purified 56 kDa polypeptide, produced in cultured insect (*Spodoptera frugiperda*) cells infected with a recombinant baculovirus that contains a partial genomic sequence from a genotype 1 HEV isolate from Pakistan. This protein, corresponding to amino acids 112–607 of *orf2*, is highly immunogenic. Each dose (0.5 mL) contains 20 µg of rHEV antigen in buffered saline, adsorbed to 0.5 mg of aluminum hydroxide, which acts as an adjuvant.

In a phase 2 trial among ~2000 HEV-seronegative Nepalese soldiers, who received three intramuscular doses (at 0, 1, and 6 months) of this vaccine or a matched placebo, the vaccine had 95.5% and 85.5% protective efficacy on per-protocol and intention-to-treat analysis, respectively, against clinical hepatitis during a median follow-up of 804 days [1]. The vaccine was safe, except for minor local adverse events. However, no further clinical trials or commercial development have taken place in the last decade.

HEV 239 vaccine

This vaccine uses a purified 239-amino acid long recombinant peptide, produced in *Escherichia coli*, corresponding to amino acids 368-606 of *orf2* protein of a genotype 1 Chinese HEV strain. This protein also forms virus-like particles, albeit smaller than those for the 56 kDa vaccine. Three intramuscular doses (at 0, 1 and 6 months) are recommended. It is currently approved and marketed in China, but not elsewhere, as prefilled, 0.5 mL, single-dose syringes, each containing 30 µg of purified protein along with buffers and thiomersal.

Data on HEV239 vaccine are available from animal studies, a phase 1 study, a phase 2 study, and a large randomized double-blind phase 3 field trial. In the phase 1 trial, 44 adults received two 20 µg intramuscular doses each, with no serious adverse events. The phase 2 study compared the effect of different vaccine doses (10, 20, 30 or 40 µg) and schedules (two-dose [0, 6 months] or three-dose [0, 1, 6 months]), and found similar (98–100%) seroconversion rates with various doses and higher antibody titers after the three-dose schedule. Mild injection site discomfort and occasional fever were the only adverse events observed.

The phase 3, double-blind, placebo (hepatitis B vaccine) controlled field trial included 112 604 healthy adults aged 16–65 years of either sex, nearly half of whom had detectable anti-HEV at enrolment (Table 34.1). In this trial, 98.7% of vaccinated subjects had at least a fourfold rise in anti-HEV antibody titer at one month after the third vaccine dose, compared to only 2.1% of controls; the latter increase was possibly related to subclinical HEV infection. The vaccine-induced antibody remained detectable for over 4.5 years after primary vaccination [2].

Clinical efficacy was assessed by active surveillance for 19 months from the first vaccine dose. The primary endpoint was frequency of acute hepatitis E (defined as constitutional symptoms for ≥3 days, serum alanine aminotransferase [ALT] ≥2.5-fold upper limit of normal, and evidence of HEV infection in the form of positive anti-HEV IgM and HEV RNA, ≥4-fold increase in anti-HEV IgG in paired sera collected 2–6 weeks apart, or both) during the 12 months beginning one month after the third vaccine dose. Per-protocol and intention-to-treat analyses showed 100% (95% confidence interval [CI] 72.1–100%) and 95.5% (95% CI 66.3–99.4%) proportionate reduction, respectively, in cases with acute hepatitis E in the vaccinated group. A protective effect was also observed in those who had received only two doses (a reduction of 100%; 95% CI 9.1–100%). The vaccine was extremely safe with only minor and infrequent adverse events.

Of the 23 placebo recipients with HEV infection, viral genotype could be identified in 13; of these, 12 had genotype 4 and one had genotype 1, indicating that the vaccine-induced protection was primarily due to prevention of genotype 4 infection.

The subjects in this trial underwent an extended follow-up for assessment of efficacy, immunogenicity, and safety for up to 4.5 years after vaccination. Of the 60 cases of

Table 34.1 Summary of data on safety, immunogenicity, and efficacy of HEV 239 vaccine in phase 3 human study

Authors, year	Study design	Participants (n)	Outcomes
Zhu et al. 2010	Double-blind, randomized, placebo-controlled field trial	• Overall clinical efficacy: healthy adults (n = 112 604) aged 16–65 years; either gender (vaccine group: 56 302; control group: 56 302) • Safety subset (vaccine group: 1316; control group: 1329) • Immunogenicity subset (vaccine group: 5567; control group: 5598)	• Efficacy of a three-dose schedule in preventing acute hepatitis E over 19 months (till one year beginning 28 days after dose 3: 95.5% [95% CI 66.3–99.4%] protection in intention-to-treat analysis and 100% in per-protocol analysis • In a safety subset, local adverse events during first 28 days after administration were more frequent following vaccine than a placebo (13.5% versus 7.1%; p<0.0001). However, severe adverse events (grade 3 or more) were infrequent and equally frequent in the two groups • Fourfold or higher rise in anti-HEV antibody titer at one month after the third dose was observed in 98.7% of subjects in the vaccine group and 2.1% of those in the control group
Zhang et al. 2015	Extended follow-up of participants in the above trial (Zhu et al. 2010)	Participants in vaccine and placebo groups remained unaware of their group assignment and were followed for up to 4.5 years	During a 4.5-year follow-up • 87% of those who had received three doses of vaccine maintained detectable anti-HEV antibody • In a modified intention-to-treat analysis, the vaccine had a protective efficacy of 86.8% (95% CI 71–94%)
Wu et al. 2012	Retrospective cohort study of a subset of pregnant women who received the vaccine during the efficacy trial by Zhu et al. 2010	Pregnant women who inadvertently received vaccine, or women who became pregnant during the trial and received one or more doses (vaccine group: 37; placebo group: 31)	• 37 women received 53 vaccine doses (one dose each: 22; two doses each: 14; 3 doses: 1) • Pregnant women tolerated the vaccine as well as the nonpregnant, with no adverse events • Birth weights and gestational ages of babies born to vaccinated and unvaccinated mothers were comparable • None of the babies had any congenital abnormality
Wu et al. 2013	Retrospective analysis of a cohort of HBsAg-positive persons included in the study by Zhu et al. 2010	14 065 participants whose HBsAg status was known before or after dose of vaccine (including 406 HBsAg positive and 6629 HBsAg negative) or placebo (including 424 HBsAg positive and 6606 HBsAg negative)	Participants with HBsAg-positive or HBsAg-negative status at baseline had: • comparable adverse event rates • similar antibody seroconversion rates (98.38% vs 98.69%) • similar antibody titers (19.32 versus 19.00 WHO U/mL) • similar antibody dynamics over a two-year follow-up

HEV, hepatitis E virus; WHO, World Health Organization.

hepatitis E identified during this period, 7 and 53 (0.3 versus 2.1 cases per 10 000 person-years, respectively) were in the vaccine and control group, respectively, with a vaccine efficacy of 86.8% (95% CI 71–94) in a modified intention-to-treat analysis [3]. In the immunogenicity subset, anti-HEV antibodies were detectable at the end of the 4.5-year period in 87% of subjects who were seronegative at baseline and had received three doses. No excess of adverse events was observed.

Further analysis of data from this trial has shown that the vaccine was equally immunogenic in some selected subject subgroups, namely in a few pregnant women who inadvertently received the vaccine and in persons with chronic hepatitis B virus infection (see Table 34.1) [4,5].

Subsequent to, and based on the results of this trial, this vaccine was approved by the China Food and Drug Administration in 2011. It has since been marketed in that country as Hecolin®, but has not yet received approval in any other country or a WHO prequalification – conditions usually considered mandatory for its use outside the country of origin.

The vaccine is supplied as ready-to-use, single-dose pre-loaded syringes that need refrigeration. There are no data on the safety and efficacy of the vaccine in those aged <16 years or >65 years, pregnant women, those with coexisting diseases, such as chronic liver disease, immunosuppression, etc.

Indications for use of HEV vaccine

Availability of a safe and effective vaccine led to the World Health Organization's Strategic Advisory Group of Experts on Immunization (SAGE) setting up a Hepatitis E Vaccine Working Group in 2013 to define the role of this vaccine (Table 34.2). Based on the available knowledge about HEV epidemiology and HEV vaccine [6], and the report of this group and the consequent recommendations of SAGE [7], the role of HEV vaccine in various settings and populations is summarized below.

General population in high-endemicity regions

In several resource-constrained countries with limited access to safe drinking water, HEV infection causes significant preventable morbidity among young adults in the form of hepatitis E outbreaks and cases of sporadic acute viral hepatitis E. This burden is believed to be comparable to that of measles and pertussis, diseases for which vaccination is routinely practiced. However, these estimates are based on several broad assumptions and robust data on the absolute morbidity or mortality due to HEV infection in high-endemicity countries are lacking. This makes it impossible to assess the cost-effectiveness of HEV vaccine in this setting. Since most of the HEV disease occurs in young adults, any population-based vaccination program would need to target adolescents, an age group currently not targeted by any large health or vaccination programs in these areas. Further, since the disease occurs over a wide age range and the available data on duration of protection following HEV vaccine extend only to 4.5 years, periodic boosters may be necessary, adding to cost as well as logistic challenges.

Pregnant women or those of child-bearing age

Pregnant women with HEV infection are at particularly high risk of severe disease, acute liver failure and death, as compared to similarly placed men and nonpregnant women. In addition, hepatitis E during pregnancy is associated with increased risk of stillbirth, premature delivery, neonatal complications, and mother-to-infant transmission of HEV.

Data on safety of HEV vaccine during pregnancy are extremely limited and the vaccine is currently not approved for use in pregnant women. Thus, to ameliorate the burden of pregnancy-related hepatitis E, one would need to vaccinate young women of child-bearing age before they become pregnant – a hard-to-reach group in most countries. Another problem relates to the data on duration of vaccine-induced protection compared to the length of the reproductive age period, suggesting the need for periodic boosters. Further, data on absolute burden of HEV disease among pregnant women are not available for any country with high endemicity of this infection, making it difficult to assess the cost-effectiveness of this intervention.

Vaccination of patients with preexisting chronic liver disease

Acute liver damage due to any cause can be expected to lead to clinical deterioration in patients with chronic liver disease. HEV infection in such patients can lead to a further reduction in functional capacity of their residual liver mass, tilting the balance and resulting in clinical decompensation.

Table 34.2 Current status of application of HEV vaccine in various settings or population subgroups, important issues involved in each situation, and World Health Organization (WHO) recommendations

Population group	Explanations and comments	WHO recommendation*
General population residing in high-endemicity regions	• Limited data on HEV-related morbidity and mortality in high endemic regions, making it impossible to calculate absolute effectiveness and cost-effectiveness • No safety and efficacy data on its use in those aged <16 years or >65 years • Data on protection beyond 4.5 years are not available • Vaccine efficacy was proven primarily against genotype 4 HEV, whereas the disease in high endemic regions is caused by genotype 1 or 2 virus (however, other evidence suggests that the vaccine is likely to protect against these genotypes too) • Role of vaccine in reducing fecal viral excretion or transmission of infection is unknown • No data on vaccine efficacy from high-endemicity regions where virus inoculum may be higher than that in the area where phase 3 trial was done	No recommendation. However, national authorities may decide to use the vaccine based on the local epidemiology
Pregnant women or women of child-bearing age	• No population-based data on the incidence of or mortality related to hepatitis E among pregnant women or neonates in any region of the world • Very limited data on safety and efficacy of the vaccine during pregnancy • Not known whether the vaccine protects against severe hepatitis E seen during pregnancy • Identification and vaccination of women of child-bearing age in high-endemicity areas poses logistic challenges	The use of vaccine to mitigate consequences in high-risk groups such as pregnant women can be considered
Patients with preexisting chronic liver disease	• Data on immunogenicity (and safety) of the vaccine in such subjects are lacking • Limited data on absolute or relative risk of disease or death due to HEV infection among patients with chronic liver disease	
Organ transplant recipients and other immunosuppressed people	• Data on immunogenicity (and safety) of the vaccine in such subjects are lacking • Most such patients have genotype 3 HEV infection, and data on protective efficacy of the vaccine against that genotype are not available	

(Continued)

Table 34.2 (Continued)

Population group	Explanations and comments	WHO recommendation*
Travelers from low-endemic to high-endemic areas	• Epidemiologic data suggest a low absolute burden of hepatitis E among travellers • Usual precautions related to water and food prevent most of the travel-associated HEV infections • Current vaccination schedule (0–1–6 months) is too prolonged for a traveler's vaccine	Not recommended routinely. May be recommended for travelers at a higher risk of HEV infection (such as humanitarian relief workers traveling to an outbreak area) or of serious disease following HEV infection (e.g., pregnant women)
Prevention and control of HEV outbreaks	• No data on the efficacy of the vaccine when administered post exposure • No data on whether vaccination reduces fecal shedding or transmission of HEV • Current vaccination schedule is too prolonged (0–1–6 months) Data for efficacy following two doses (0 and 1 month) are extremely limited • Efficacy data are primarily against genotype 4 HEV, whereas outbreaks are usually due to genotype 1 or 2 HEV	The use of vaccine to mitigate or prevent outbreaks of hepatitis E should be considered

*Based on recommendations of the Strategic Advisory Group of Experts on Immunization [7].
HEV, hepatitis E virus.

This risk is particularly high in HEV-endemic regions, and should be preventable through vaccination. However, patients with chronic liver disease have a suboptimal response to several vaccines. No data are yet available on the immunogenicity or efficacy of the HEV vaccine in this group, though it appears to be safe and immunogenic in persons with chronic hepatitis B virus infection without significant liver disease. The absence of these data makes it difficult to currently recommend the routine administration of HEV vaccine in this group.

HEV vaccine for organ transplant recipients and other immunosuppressed groups

Immunocompromised persons, particularly those with prior solid organ transplantation, in several countries have been shown to be at risk of acute and chronic HEV infection. Chronic HEV infection can progress to liver cirrhosis and, in those with prior liver transplantation, may result in loss of the transplanted organ. These chronic HEV infections occur primarily in areas where genotypes 3 and/or 4 HEV occur, and genotypes 1 and 2 HEV appear not to cause chronic infection.

Unfortunately, no direct data are available on the role of HEV vaccine to prevent HEV infection or chronic hepatitis E, or even for generation of of anti-HEV antibodies, among

immunosuppressed persons. Also, the HEV infection in this setting is primarily caused by genotype 3. The available HEV vaccine is based on genotype 1 virus, and showed protection against genotype 4 HEV in the large field trial; no direct evidence is available to show that it can prevent genotype 3 HEV infection.

Vaccine for international travelers from low- to high-endemic regions

Travelers can acquire HEV infection through consumption of unsafe water and food. Travel-associated acute hepatitis E cases have mostly been reported following travel to the Indian subcontinent. However, the frequency of HEV disease following such travel is very low, partly because travelers frequently take precautions, albeit of varying degrees, to avoid food/water-borne infections. The long duration of the currently recommended schedule for HEV vaccine also poses a challenge to its use as a travelers' vaccine, since travelers do not often consult a clinic 6–7 months before departure.

Prevention and control of HEV outbreaks

Large water-borne outbreaks of HEV infection have been reported from several developing countries in Asia and Africa. The outbreaks in Africa have in particular been related to humanitarian emergencies such as war, large-scale migration, etc., and have tended to be prolonged. Theoretically, HEV vaccination could be expected to prevent further transmission and hence interrupt such outbreaks. However, since the incubation period of HEV ranges from two to 10 weeks, by the time an outbreak is identified, the period of water contamination is already over and many people may already be infected and be in the late incubation phase. Whether administration of HEV vaccine at this time (postexposure administration) has any protective efficacy remains unknown. Further, most of the outbreaks of HEV disease are rapidly controlled once water supplies are improved – a measure which is likely to be much cheaper, besides having additional advantage of protecting against other water-borne infections. Whether vaccination can provide an additive effect remains unclear.

Further, there are no data to show whether the use of HEV vaccine is associated with reduction in viral excretion, an effect which could help reduce disease transmission. Also, the vaccine is currently not approved for those aged below 16 years or above 65 years, and the failure to vaccinate such members of the population could allow the outbreak to proceed uninterrupted. Finally, it is possible that the large outbreaks are caused by intense contamination of water supplies, and the vaccine may not prevent disease following infection with a large inoculum as effectively as observed in the trial in China, where contamination is likely to have been mild. A selective approach of vaccinating women in early pregnancy in such settings is particularly attractive, but is limited by the lack of safety data for administration during pregnancy.

Conclusion

From the above, it is clear that the available HEV vaccine is a major advance. It is safe and appears to have good protective efficacy. However, based on the information currently available, it is difficult to unambiguously recommend its use in various clinical and epidemiologic situations. The WHO Position Paper on this vaccine has identified a number of issues where it would help bridge the existing gap between the successful development of an effective vaccine and the population deriving benefit from it [7]. Hopefully, the manufacturer and academic researchers will collaborate in the next few years to answer these questions.

References

1. Shrestha MP, Scott RM, Joshi DM et al. Safety and efficacy of a recombinant hepatitis E vaccine. *New England Journal of Medicine* 2007;356:895–903.
2. Zhu FC, Zhang J, Zhang XF et al. Efficacy and safety of a recombinant hepatitis E vaccine in healthy adults: a large-scale, randomised, double-blind placebo-controlled, phase 3 trial. *Lancet* 2010;376:895–902.
3. Zhang J, Zhang XF, Huang SJ et al. Long-term efficacy of a hepatitis E vaccine. *New England Journal of Medicine* 2015;372:914–922.
4. Wu T, Zhu FC, Huang SJ et al. Safety of the hepatitis E vaccine for pregnant women: a preliminary analysis. *Hepatology* 2012;55:2038.
5. Wu T, Huang SJ, Zhu FC et al. Immunogenicity and safety of hepatitis E vaccine in healthy hepatitis B surface antigen positive adults. *Human Vaccines and Immunotherapy* 2013;9:2474–2479.
6. WHO Hepatitis E Vaccine Working Group. Recommendations of HEV Working Group on the use of hepatitis E vaccine. www.who.int/immunization/sage/meetings/2014/october/3_Hep_E_vacc_WG_SAGE_Recs_final_1Oct2014.pdf?ua=1
7. WHO. Hepatitis E vaccine: WHO position paper. *Weekly Epidemiological Record* 2015;90:185–200.

PART III
Clinical Set-up and the Future

35 Do we need expert hepatitis C virus treaters or are amateur treaters good enough?

Shyamasundaran Kottilil and Poonam Mathur

Institute of Human Virology, University of Maryland School of Medicine, Baltimore, MD, USA

LEARNING POINTS

- The development of DAAs has made HCV treatment more simple and successful, with few adverse effects or safety concerns.

- Despite the advent of DAAs, the goal for HCV elimination by 2030 remains distant due to the lack of access to specialist providers who treat hepatitis C, especially in rural or resource-limited settings (RLS).

- Since HCV treatment has become more straightforward, the concept of task-shifting can be applied in underserved areas so that nonspecialist providers who have never before treated HCV can be taught how to prescribe these medications and manage hepatitis C through dedicated teaching sessions.

- Task-shifting programs have been shown to train providers successfully in the United States, Rwanda, and India, with no significant difference in the rates of sustained virologic response (SVR) among general practitioners compared to specialists.

- Transition of care to nonspecialists through task-shifting will be essential to meet WHO HCV elimination goals.

Infection with hepatitis C virus (HCV) affects an estimated 71 million people globally [1] and is associated with long-term sequelae of cirrhosis, hepatocellular carcinoma, and an increased risk of mortality [2]. Prior to 2011, the standard of care for HCV was the use of pegylated interferon-alpha (PEG-IFN-alpha) and ribavirin (RBV), although fewer than 25% of infected patients were treated with this regimen [3]. Treatment with PEG-IFN-alpha and RBV required a long course of 24–48 weeks [4] but was associated with a success rate of only 40–50% [4,5] and a number of adverse effects including depression, hemolytic anemia, and teratogenicity [6].

The advent of direct-acting antivirals (DAAs) has provided noninjectable HCV treatment options that are well tolerated with few side effects and high success rates. Despite this paradigm shift, however, the number of people successfully treated for HCV globally is estimated to be only 1.1 million, or 7% of those infected [1]. Due to this significant discrepancy, the World Health Organization (WHO) has set a goal for hepatitis C elimination by 2030. In order to achieve this goal, gaps in the HCV cascade of care must be appropriately assessed and analyzed in the context of HCV epidemiology. Eighty percent of the population infected with HCV is in low- and middle-income countries (LMICs), and the largest burden of HCV is in the eastern hemisphere, with Africa and the Asia-Pacific region representing 10 million and 24 million, respectively, of those infected worldwide [7]. Unfortunately, LMICs often lack access to resources to address not only HCV care but management for other diseases as well. For example, though Africa accounts for the largest burden of the world's infectious diseases [8], it represents only 3% of the global workforce [9]. The lack of healthcare workers also affects Asia; combined, southeast Asia and Africa have a shortage of about 11 million healthcare workers [10].

The lack of adequate healthcare workers for treatment of infectious diseases, including HCV, is one of the many obstacles to escalating HCV treatment not just in LMICs

Clinical Dilemmas in Viral Liver Disease, Second Edition. Edited by Graham R. Foster and K. Rajender Reddy.
© 2020 John Wiley & Sons Ltd. Published 2020 by John Wiley & Sons Ltd.

but also in the United States (Figures 35.1 and 35.2). In addition to the limited number of HCV treatment-competent practitioners, access to these providers is difficult for patients in rural or resource-limited areas, as they are usually based in urban settings. In a survey by McGowan et al. [11], which represented 697 physicians in 29 countries and eight global regions, most physicians stated they practiced in private, urban settings. The lack of rural-based providers was most discordant in the Asia-Pacific and Middle East/Africa regions, where 86% and 80% of providers, respectively, identified themselves as based in urban locations [9].

In order to overcome the low provider-to-patient ratio and decentralize care from urban to rural settings, task-shifting should be used to expand HCV care. Task-shifting is when nonspecialists or general providers, who are greater in number than specialists, are trained to perform tasks which are normally reserved for specialists [12]. By task-shifting, nonspecialist providers who practice in RLS can learn how to manage hepatitis C competently and serve a nonurban population.

There are two models of task-shifting: partial and complete. In a partial task-shifting model, specialists maintain constant supervision of trained general providers. Project ECHO (Extension for Community Healthcare Models) was a study designed to expand HCV care to rural areas and prisons in New Mexico, utilizing partial task-shifting [13]. One of the first analyses from Project ECHO examined the rate of SVR among primary care physicians (PCPs), compared to specialists at the University of New Mexico HCV clinic. Overall, 407 treatment-naive HCV patients were treated with interferon and ribavirin. The SVR rate among university-based specialists was 57.5%, and 58.2% among the rural and prison-based physicians (p=0.89) [14], demonstrating that partial task-shifting is an effective method for expanding the number of providers available to treat

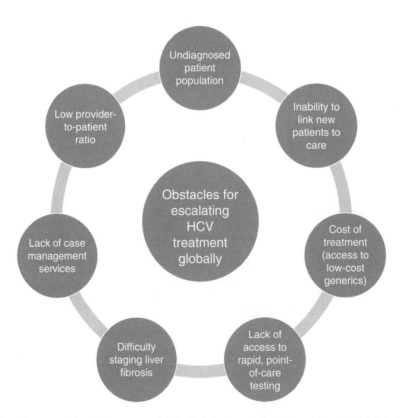

Figure 35.1 Obstacles to escalating HCV treatment globally. Each factor contributes to and is inextricably linked to the other factors that inhibit escalation of care.

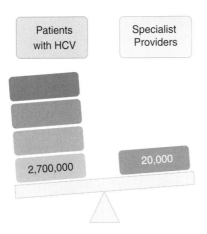

Figure 35.2 The estimated number of HCV-infected patients in the US, compared to the number of specialist providers available to treat hepatitis C in the country. The low provider-to-patient ratio is an obstacle for escalating healthcare not just globally, but in the US as well.

HCV in RLS. Since its initiation in 2003, Project ECHO has expanded to different rural sites and underserved areas using telemedicine and DAAs for HCV treatment. There are 10 sites globally that use the ECHO model, and over 30 sites in the US.

In contrast to Project ECHO, a complete task-shifting model allows for nonspecialist providers to eventually become independent from specialists after sufficient training, by demonstrating competence in the specialty treatment. A complete task-shifting model has been adopted by the government of Western Australia, since less than 1% of the population has access to treatment [15]. The Western Australian Department of Health trains providers who are geographically isolated via face-to-face didactic sessions, webinars, and videoconferences. The trainings have been developed by universities and national groups such as the School of Medicine at the University of Queensland and the Australian Association of HIV Medicine. The workforce development plan will focus on educating physicians, nurses, and Aboriginal health workers, in order to target as many diverse populations as possible. Nurses will play a critical role in the coordination of HCV programs since they serve as the first point of contact.

Complete task-shifting models have been successful in expansion of HIV programs in Africa, particularly in Rwanda, which saw a rapid increase in the incidence of HIV infections after the genocide in 1994. The Rwandan Ministry of Health implemented a complete task-shifting model for HIV, which included teaching nurses how to prescribe antiretroviral therapy. In a follow-up study assessing patients' uptake of treatment, adherence, and CD4 counts, there was no difference between physicians and trained Rwandan nurses who provided HIV care [16]. In fact, the nurses' patients showed improvement in mortality and retention in care, and decreased loss to follow-up compared to physicians. By utilizing a task-shifting model, Rwanda led African nations in escalation of HIV care [17].

A complete task-shifting model for HCV treatment has also been developed and implemented in the US. In 2015, the ASCEND study used complete task-shifting in the RLS of Washington, DC, in order to increase the number of providers competent to treat HCV, and assess the success of nonspecialists practicing independently of specialist supervision in a real-world, urban setting [18]. General practitioners in federally qualified health clinics (FQHCs), including PCPs and nurse practitioners (NPs), underwent a three-hour training session on the comprehensive care and management of patients with HCV. Six hundred patients were treated in less than a year, and had characteristics that are deemed difficult to treat, such as cirrhosis (20%), genotype 1a infection (72%), HIV (23%), and black race (96%). The overall SVR rate was 86%; the SVR rates among the three provider types – NP, PCP, and specialist – were 89.3%, 86.9%, and 83.8%, respectively, with no statistically significant difference. There was also no difference in SVR rates among the three types of providers for patients who were HIV positive or had cirrhosis. HIV-positive patients had an SVR rate of 85.4%, comparable to that of the entire study population. ASCEND corroborates the observation of several other studies which have demonstrated comparable rates of HIV- and non-HIV-infected patients (e.g., ALLY-2, ION-4, EXPEDITION-2, ASTRAL-5). Patients with cirrhosis had an SVR rate of 83.5%, comparable to another real-world study [19]. Visit adherence was higher among patients seen by a PCP or NP for HCV treatment (63.1% and 73.6%, respectively), compared to a specialist (55.9%). This demonstrated that a complete task-shifting model for HCV treatment to general practitioners was safe and effective in a real-world cohort.

The promising findings from the ASCEND study and the availability of less expensive, generic DAAs manufactured globally have prompted complete task-shifting pilot studies, with concise educational training, to be successfully implemented in Kigali, Rwanda [20], and Imphal, India [21], where a lack of trained providers to treat HCV is one of the countries' main obstacles to expanding care. Through these international pilot studies, more than 60 providers in these LMICs, who had never before treated HCV, were trained by specialist infectious disease physicians and NPs in a three-hour session on the screening, diagnosis, and treatment of HCV. Providers were also taught how to stage liver disease and evaluate for hepatocellular carcinoma.

In order to assess the efficacy of the training session, a multiple-choice assessment test was administered to the providers before and immediately after each training session. The test addressed topics including risk factors for HCV infection, screening and diagnostic modalities, treatment regimens and durations, and post-SVR follow-up for patients with cirrhosis. In both Rwanda and India, providers' test scores increased after the training.

Complete task-shifting models in RLS and LMICs have the potential to rapidly increase the number of providers available to treat HCV in a few years, as new providers (i.e., general practitioners) can be trained annually by their previously trained peers who have demonstrated competence in HCV treatment (Figure 35.3). In this fashion, complete task-shifting models are self-perpetuating, exponentially increasing the number of patients treated, while allowing communities, and even countries, to maintain independence

during healthcare escalation. By containing efforts within each nation, governments can easily track outcomes, such as the number of patients linked to care, started on treatment, and who achieve SVR. In addition, the lowered cost of and increased access to generic DAAs make successful HCV treatment in LMICs and RLS more feasible than it was a few years ago.

In order to meet the WHO's goal for worldwide HCV elimination by 2030, several barriers must be addressed and overcome through financial and administrative support from national ministries of health and community healthcare providers in each country. First, effective campaigns to increase the public's awareness on the sequelae of untreated hepatitis C are vital to educate patients about the importance of HCV screening and diagnosis. Second, with increased knowledge of hepatitis C, rapid, low-cost, point-of-care tests must be made available for efficient HCV diagnosis and linkage to care. Last, with the large number of newly diagnosed HCV cases, task-shifting must be incorporated into the global plan for hepatitis C elimination so that the number of providers available to treat HCV is sufficient to meet the need in both urban and rural settings. Compete task-shifting is possible for HCV treatment, since DAAs are simple to prescribe and use, with few adverse effects to manage. Implementing complete task-shifting projects in LMICs and RLS is essential to continuing on the path towards HCV elimination.

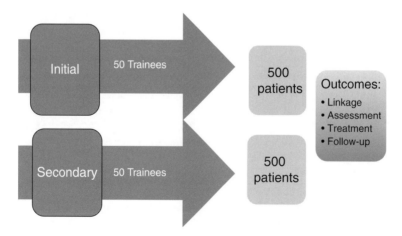

Figure 35.3 Task-shifting models are self-perpetuating in that the number of trained providers can increase each year, through the mentorship of previously trained nonspecialists who have demonstrated competence in hepatitis C treatment. By using this model, the low provider-to-patient ratio can be overcome, the number of patients treated is multiplied, and outcomes on linkage, assessment, successful treatment, and retention in care can be easily ascertained.

References

1. World Health Organization. Global Hepatitis Report 2017. www.who.int/hepatitis/publications/global-hepatitis-report2017/en/

2. Stanaway JD, Flaxman AD, Naghavi M et al. The global burden of viral hepatitis from 1990 to 2013: findings from the Global Burden of Disease Study 2013. *Lancet* 2016;388:1081–1088.

3. Vutien P, Jin M, Le MH et al. Regional differences in treatment rates for patients with chronic hepatitis C infection: systematic review and meta-analysis. *PLoS One* 2017;12:e0183851.

4. Kish T, Aziz A, Sorio M. Hepatitis C in a new era: a review of current therapies. *P T* 2017;42:316–329.

5. Nordstrom EM, Keniston A, Baouchi F, Martinez-Camacho A. Interferon-based hepatitis C therapy in a safety net hospital: access, efficacy, and safety. *European Journal of Gastroenterology and Hepatology* 2017;29:10–16.

6. Kohli A, Shaffer A, Sherman A, Kottilil S. Treatment of hepatitis C: a systematic review. *JAMA* 2014;312:631–640.

7. WHO data. www.mhahs.org.au/index.php/en/media-page/statistics/hepatitis-c-statistics

8. Umutesi J, Simmons B, Makuza JD et al. Prevalence of hepatitis B and C infection in persons living with HIV enrolled in care in Rwanda. *BMC Infectious Diseases* 2017;17:315.

9. Iwu EN, Holzemer WL. Task shifting of HIV management from doctors to nurses in Africa: clinical outcomes and evidence on nurse self-efficacy and job satisfaction. *AIDS Care* 2014;26:42–52.

10. Global Health Observatory data. www.who.int/gho/health_workforce/hrh_012.jpg?ua=1

11. McGowan CE, Monis A, Bacon BR et al. A global view of hepatitis C: physician knowledge, opinions, and perceived barriers to care. *Hepatology* 2013;57:1325–1332.

12. Jayasekera CR, Arora S, Ahmed A. Hepatitis C treatment delivery mandates optimizing available health care human resources: a case for task shifting. *JAMA* 2016;315:1947–1948.

13. Arora S, Kalishman S, Thornton K et al. Expanding access to hepatitis C virus treatment – Extension for Community Healthcare Outcomes (ECHO) project: disruptive innovation in specialty care. *Hepatology* 2010;52:1124–1133.

14. Arora S, Thornton K, Murata G et al. Outcomes of treatment for hepatitis C virus infection by primary care providers. *New England Journal of Medicine* 2011;364:2199–2207.

15. Western Australia Department of Health. Hepatitis C Virus Model of Care Health Networks Branch. Perth: Department of Health, 2009.

16. Shumbusho F, van Griensven J, Lowrance D et al. Task shifting for scale-up of HIV care: evaluation of nurse-centered antiretroviral treatment at rural health centers in Rwanda. *PLoS Medicine* 2009;6:e1000163.

17. Nsanzimana S, Ruton H, Lowrance DW et al. Cell phone-based and internet-based monitoring and evaluation of the National Antiretroviral Treatment Program during rapid scale-up in Rwanda: TRACnet, 2004–2010. *Journal of Acquired Immune Deficiency Syndrome Ac2012*;59:e17–23.

18. Kattakuzhy S, Gross C, Emmanuel B et al. Expansion of treatment for hepatitis C virus infection by task shifting to community-based nonspecialist providers: a nonrandomized clinical trial. *Annals of Internal Medicine* 2017;167:311–318.

19. Miotto N, Mendes LC, Zanaga LP et al. All-oral direct antiviral treatment for hepatitis C chronic infection in a real-life cohort: the role of cirrhosis and comorbidities in treatment response. *PLoS One* 2018;13:e0199941.

20. Mathur P, Comstock E, Makuza JD et al. Implementation of a unique hepatitis C care continuum model in Rwanda. *Journal of Public Health* 2019;41:e203–e208.

21. Mathur P, Comstock E, McSweegan E, Mercer N, Kumar NS, Kottilil S. A pilot study to expand treatment of chronic hepatitis C in resource-limited settings. *Antiviral Research* 2017;146:184–190.

36 Hepatitis C vaccines: how close are we to the promised land?

Timothy Donnison[1], Senthil Chinnakannan[1], Paola Cicconi[1,2], and Eleanor Barnes[1]

[1]Peter Medawar Building for Pathogen Research, University of Oxford, Oxford, UK
[2]Jenner Vaccine Trials, Nuffield Department of Medicine, University of Oxford, Oxford, UK

LEARNING POINTS

- HCV elimination by 2030 is highly unlikely without the implementation of a prophylactic HCV vaccination program as a part of a broader strategy.

- Results from a phase 2 clinical trial will reveal the efficacy of a prophylactic HCV vaccine in a high-risk population, with results expected shortly.

- Next-generation HCV vaccines should provide pangenotype immunity and generate an antibody and T-cell immune response.

- Overcoming major obstacles such as developing immunocompetent small animal challenge models, patient cohorts for vaccine testing, and attracting charity and government investment in vaccine research is critical to advance an HCV vaccine through human trials.

The need for an HCV vaccine

A vaccination strategy for the prevention of hepatitis C virus (HCV) remains an important goal for the global elimination of HCV. Whilst the development of highly effective directly-acting antivirals (DAAs) has revolutionized the treatment of HCV [1], these drugs remain unaffordable in many resource-limited healthcare settings and may be associated with the development of viral resistant variants that are transmitted to other people [2,3]. In addition, most HCV-infected people are asymptomatic and do not present to healthcare professionals until liver disease is advanced. These observations should drive the development of an HCV vaccine that would prevent chronic infection rather than focusing exclusively on scaling up diagnostics and therapy to identify and treat infected people once chronic disease is established. An HCV vaccine would have major benefits for people at risk of HCV infection and would be a major contributor, possibly essential for population strategies that aim to eliminate infection (Box 36.1).

Recent World Health Organization (WHO) modeling (Global Hepatitis Report 2017) showed that in 2015 alone, there were 1.75 million new HCV infections, with mean global incidence rates of 23.7/100 000 people, with higher rates (>60/100 000) in Europe and the Eastern Mediterranean regions. Although overall incidence rates declined in the latter part of the 20th century, the incidence rate in some populations has increased recently, particularly in people who inject drugs (PWID) in the USA [4,5], and in men who have sex with men in major European, American, and Australian cities. Overall, to decrease the prevalence of HCV, the number of people who are treated or who die with HCV needs to exceed the number of new infections. Notably, the recent WHO report shows that in 2015 the number of newly infected people was greater than the number of people dying of disease or receiving curative therapy.

With HCV incidence rates exceeding cure rates, the WHO has established the Global Health Sector Strategy with the aim of eliminating viral hepatitis by 2030. Central to this goal is the scaling up of global diagnosis (from 20% to >80%) and treatment rates (currently 7.4% of diagnosed cases). This will require committed political leadership and a reduction in drug costs. A limited number of "early

Clinical Dilemmas in Viral Liver Disease, Second Edition. Edited by Graham R. Foster and K. Rajender Reddy.
© 2020 John Wiley & Sons Ltd. Published 2020 by John Wiley & Sons Ltd.

adopter" countries have implemented nationwide hepatitis C action plans. However, meeting the 2030 target is an ambitious global venture, and current data suggest that without an affordable vaccine that significantly affects HCV incidence rates, this goal is unlikely to be met [6]. Clear target populations could be readily defined in Western countries including PWID, prison populations, and family members and sexual contacts of infected people, whilst population vaccination strategies could be deployed in countries where HCV is endemic. Vaccination strategies are particularly attractive in PWIDs where drug therapy delivered over many weeks is likely to limit treatment compliance and where most HCV transmission events occur in the early years after infection before any active engagement with healthcare workers [7]. Mathematical modeling suggests that introducing even a moderately efficacious vaccine would have a significant impact on reducing HCV incidence [8,9], and that this could be effectively used alongside antiviral therapy [10]. However, global research efforts to develop an HCV vaccine will need to be supported by major funding bodies and policy makers if HCV is to be eliminated by 2030.

Box 36.1 Desirable characteristics for an HCV vaccine

Delivered as one or two intramuscular or subcutaneous injections
Provides long-lasting immunity against infection
Effective against multiple HCV genotypes
Affordable
Readily manufactured, scalable, and transportable for wide distribution

HCV vaccine rationale: insights from natural infection and animal studies

In theory, the development of a vaccine for the prevention of HCV should be possible since approximately 20% of HCV-infected people spontaneously clear the virus, and these individuals are less likely to develop chronic infection when reexposed [11,12]. However, despite two decades of research, the exact correlates of immune protection in natural history studies are not completely defined. Whilst B-cell immunity generating HCV antibodies are thought to play a role in viral clearance [13], T-cell immunity (as evidenced by HLA association studies [14], genome-wide association studies [15], and chimpanzee T-cell blocking experiments) also plays a critical role in viral control [16,17]. Current vaccine efforts focus on the development of B cell vaccines that generate antibodies against the viral envelope or T-cell vaccines that target the HCV genome more widely.

To date, very few strategies have been assessed in humans [18–22], and only a single HCV vaccine has progressed to efficacy testing in humans with results expected shortly. Whilst further studies that seek to understand the mechanism of HCV persistence may inform future vaccine development, there are currently major obstacles to the downstream development of existing HCV vaccines (Table 36.1), including a lack of immune-competent animal models, a shortage of well-characterized human cohorts of "at-risk people" for vaccine testing in addition to a lack of investment by industry that should be tackled as a priority.

Table 36.1 Obstacles and solutions in vaccine development

Barrier to HCV vaccine development	Solution
Genetic variability of the HCV virus	a. Using novel immunogens that are designed to target multiple genotypes b. Targeting genotype-specific vaccines to regions where that genotype dominates c. Giving multiple or mixed genotype vaccines
No animal models of infection	a. Further development of small animal models b. Investment in phase 1/2 human studies
No human challenge models	Could be considered now
Few well-characterized cohorts of at-risk patients for phase 2/3 studies	Funding for cohort studies
No clear correlate of protection identified	Natural history studies supported by phase 2 data released in 2018 (ClinicalTrials.gov Identifier NCT01436357)
Lack of pharmaceutical investment	Research charity and government funding streams

Generating anti-HCV immunity with vaccines

Current vaccine efforts primarily utilize either the antibody response to structural HCV proteins or a T-cell response targeting the HCV genome more widely.

B-cell vaccine development

All currently licensed vaccines induce antibodies that target pathogen surface proteins that are exposed during circulation and therefore prevent pathogen entry into host cells, conferring sterilizing immunity. Unfortunately, this traditional approach to vaccine design is not universally applicable due to the high variability of surface proteins in some pathogens – including human immunodeficiency virus (HIV), dengue, malaria, and HCV – that readily escape antibody recognition and establish infection. Strikingly, HCV is highly genetically variable (10 times more than HIV) with high sequence variability focused in its surface envelope proteins E1 and E2 that are the primary targets of the host antibody response. Consequently, while anti-HCV antibodies are detected in natural infection and in vaccinated healthy volunteers, these are typically restricted to specific strains with only a small percentage of vaccinated individuals generating broadly neutralizing antibodies (bNAbs) to multiple genotypes [20,21,23]. Therefore, the generation of broadly neutralizing anti-HCV antibodies by vaccination is a significant obstacle within the field.

Several approaches to developing B cell vaccines are currently being investigated. The most advanced uses an HCV envelope protein heterodimer that has been tested in phase 1 healthy human studies [20,21,23–25]. Another approach, currently in advanced preclinical testing, seeks to generate envelope antibodies with the envelope hypervariable regions deleted in order to focus an antibody response on conserved genetic regions of the HCV envelope [26,27].

The costs of generating protein-based vaccines to GMP, without the possibility of proof-of-principle preclinical animal studies, is a major hurdle in the development of HCV B-cell vaccines. Alternative strategies that aim to develop high-titer HCV antibodies through the expression of HCV proteins using more accessible platforms (viral vectors or viral-like particles) have not yet progressed to human studies [28–30].

T-cell vaccine development

In recent years, remarkable progress has been made in the development of vaccine strategies that seek to induce viral-specific T-cells in HCV-uninfected people. T-cell vaccines do not aim to induce sterilizing immunity. Rather, infection of host cells is a requirement so that HCV epitopes can be presented in association with human leukocyte antigen (HLA) to T-cells. T-cell vaccines aim to abort acute infection and prevent the development of chronic disease.

Early efforts focused on protein, peptide or epitope string vaccines that were poorly immunogenic and which were, by design, restricted to people with a narrow range of HLA types. More recently, adenoviral (Ad) vectors encoding large HCV immunogens have been shown to be highly effective in inducing high-magnitude responses against a broad range of epitopes that are presented by individuals of all HLA types. A proof-of-principle study in chimpanzees showed that animals vaccinated with Ad vectors encoding an HCV immunogen were protected from infection with a heterologous HCV viral challenge [31]. The recent development of simian adenoviral vectors to which humans have not been exposed overcomes the issue of preexisting antivector immunity that may limit vaccine efficacy [32]. The magnitude of T-cell response can be further enhanced by the use of MVA vectors encoding the same immunogen used in a prime/boost strategy. This approach, using an HCV genotype-1b immunogen, has now progressed through phase 1 human studies [19] and is in efficacy testing with results expected shortly (ClinicalTrials.gov Identifier NCT01436357)

Universal HCV vaccines to target multiple genotypes

Hepatitis C virus exists as six major genotypes globally that are broadly distributed by geographical region [33]. These share approximately 70% sequence homology at the nucleotide level. However, a mixture of several genotypes typically circulates within any one country and even within a single host HCV exists as a swarm of closely related but distinct viruses. Therefore, it is likely that the development of a global vaccine strategy will require multiple genotype-specific vaccines to be deployed in any one region, or single vaccines with immunogens that are designed to target multiple HCV genotypes. Our own approach, currently in preclinical testing, is to utilize conserved HCV sequence segments across all genotypes combined within a single mosaic immunogen encoded in viral vector vaccines to elicit T-cell responses capable of targeting conserved epitopes across genotypes that cannot undergo mutation without a detrimental fitness cost to the virus [34].

Combining antibody and T-cell components in rational vaccine design

While the exact immune correlates of protection against HCV are not fully understood, both B-cell and T-cell immunity are associated with spontaneous resolution of HCV infection. Therefore, a combination of approaches in an HCV vaccine strategy to harness T-cell and B-cell responses may provide the best chance of successfully clearing an acute HCV infection. We are currently working on an HCV vaccine strategy that aims to induce both B- and T-cell HCV immunity in a viral vectored platform.

Remaining challenges to overcome in HCV vaccine development

Despite promising results for HCV vaccines in preclinical and human clinical trials, a number of obstacles remain if a prophylactic vaccine is to progress all the way through the clinical pipeline to be used as part of a broader strategy to eliminate HCV by 2030.

Immunologic challenges

While natural history studies and animal challenge studies have revealed, to some degree, what constitutes a host immune response to clear HCV, the exact immune correlates of protection within the 20% of those who resolve acute HCV infection are not fully understood. Complete understanding of immune-mediated HCV clearance is critical to devise vaccination strategies to overcome viral escape mechanisms, highlighting the importance of basic science to inform rational vaccine design.

Despite a diverse HCV population in infected individuals, the impact of a prophylactic vaccine may be compounded by the heterogeneity of the human population. For example, rational vaccine design should include a variety of epitopes that can be presented by heterogenic HLA molecules – the major histocompatibility complexes (MHC) – to T-cells. Furthermore, a vaccine strategy would need to account for host factors associated with high-risk

HCV populations such as ethnicity, age, liver disease status, opioid usage, HIV coinfection, and previous HCV infection or treatment.

Lack of immunocompetent animal models for vaccine testing

Humans and chimpanzees are the only two species that are permissive to HCV infection. Proof of immunogenicity of the two most clinically advanced HCV was first demonstrated in chimpanzees [31,35]. Since legislation was passed that prohibited chimpanzee use in research in the USA, the lack of a challenge model has been a significant block to HCV vaccine development. Efforts to improve suboptimal preclinical models are ongoing and the recent discovery of a rat hepacivirus represents a step towards an immunocompetent challenge model. The rat hepacivirus displays chronic infection in rat livers and mimics many of the characteristics of human HCV chronic infection [36].

Human challenge models are clinical trials by which vaccinated healthy volunteers are challenged with a pathogen, resulting in pathogen clearance or enrolment on therapeutic treatment if the vaccine is ineffective. This approach has been successfully completed with human pathogens salmonella and malaria. With the advent of anti-HCV DAA treatment with cure rates of almost 100% for genotype 1 infection and effective retreatment strategies for those in whom therapy fails, a human challenge model for HCV could now be considered as an alternative approach to expensive and logistically challenging phase 2 efficacious clinical trials.

Developing "at-risk" cohorts for vaccine efficacy testing

Due to the prohibited use of chimpanzees and the lack of small animal models permissive to HCV infection, well-characterized patient cohorts have utility in vaccine efficacy testing. However, the frequency of "at-risk" patients is limited due to the increased use of DAA treatments in these populations, therefore developing large cohorts for vaccine testing is increasingly difficult. Nevertheless, intravenous drug user (IVDU) cohorts from major US cities are enrolled in the phase 2 T-cell vaccine efficacy study. Further characterization of equivalent IVDU cohorts in the UK and Europe may provide opportunities for vaccine testing.

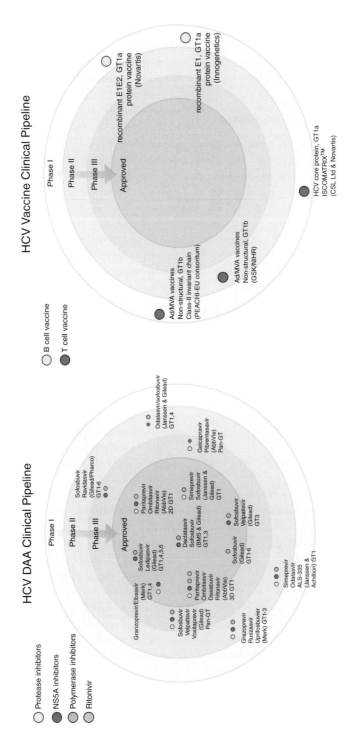

Figure 36.1 DAA versus vaccine pipeline 2019.

Overcoming HCV sequence variability

The HCV genotype 1b vaccine now in efficacy testing shows a reduction in cross-reactivity to nongenotype 1b HCV antigens *in vitro* [19]. Additional studies have shown that T-cells between genotypes 1 and 3 are largely not cross-reactive [37]. Furthermore, HCV's vast genetic diversity ensures it can readily escape immune selection pressure in these epitopes, as evidenced by a reduction in vaccine immunogenicity to HCV epitope sequence variants [38].

An ideal HCV vaccine should generate pangenotype immunity and recognize epitope variants to ensure the vaccination is efficacious in any setting regardless of infecting genotypes and to minimize immune escape under immune selection pressure. Therefore, prior to preclinical testing, vaccine design should consider the sequence variability of dominant and subdominant epitopes on the premise that mutation in highly conserved epitopes between genotypes may confer a detrimental fitness cost to the virus.

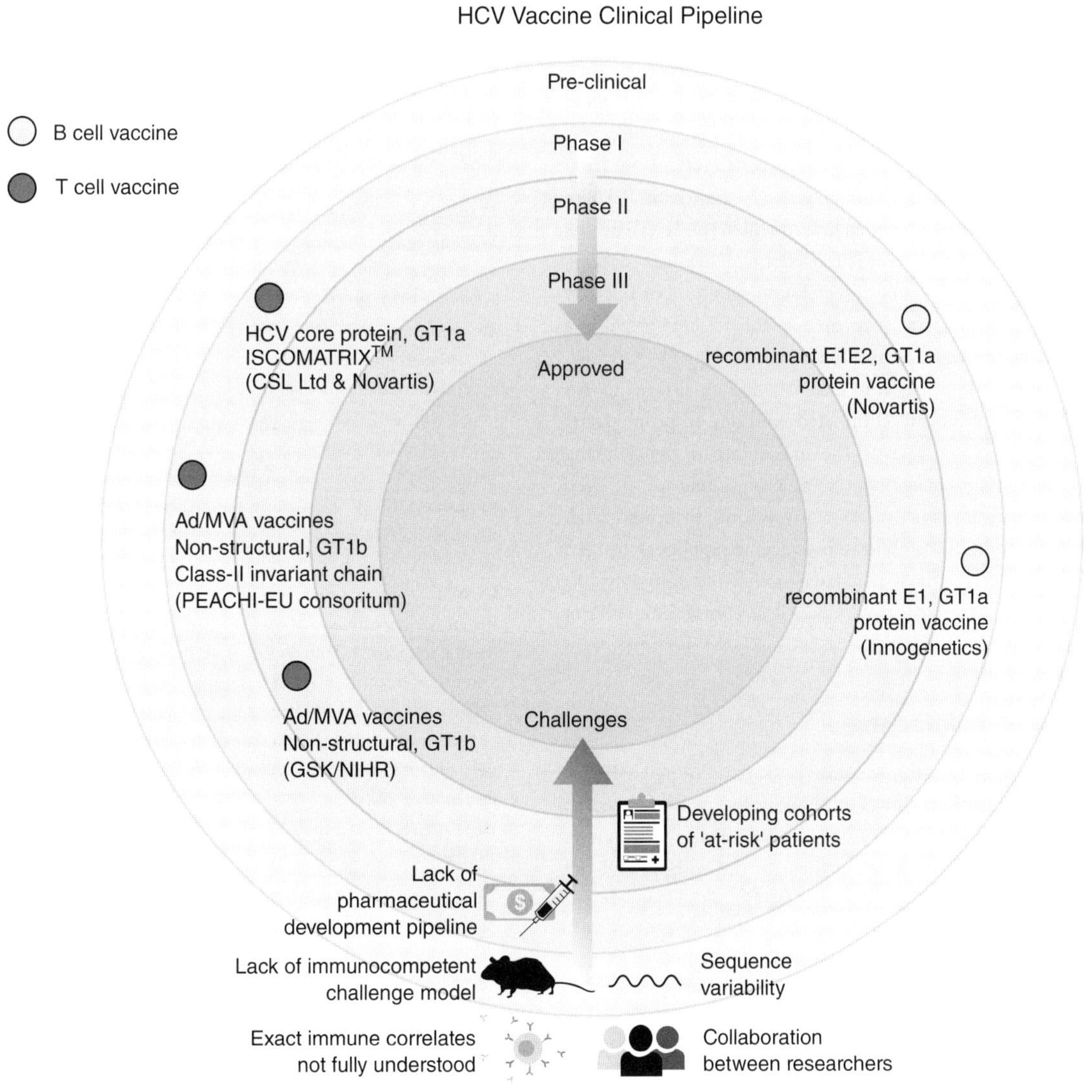

Figure 36.2 Vaccine pipeline and challenges 2019.

Promoting collaboration between researchers

A combination of a T-cell and B-cell vaccine would be an optimal vaccination strategy to confer pangenotypic anti-HCV protective immunity. As research groups have well-established T-cell and B-cell vaccine technology and expertise, efforts to collaborate between groups should be a priority. It is probable that collaborations to identify an optimal vaccine candidate will provide the best chance of securing funding for human clinical trials, particularly prudent as funds and well-characterized patient cohorts are limited.

Lack of a pharmaceutical development pipeline

Industry investment in DAAs with huge financial returns (Gilead Sciences' estimated financial return in 2015 was approximately £15 billion) has diverted attention from HCV vaccine development (Figures 36.1 and 36.2). There is minimal privately funded investment in the HCV vaccine pipeline despite the urgent need for a licensed vaccine being advocated by the research community. For publicly funded healthcare systems, an available vaccine provides a cheaper alternative to prohibitively expensive DAAs which may attract funding from charities and governments. No pathogen has been eliminated without a prophylactic vaccine and considering the major impediments facing current HCV management, there is an urgent unmet need for vaccine investment. We can reach the promised land, but only with investment in the vaccine pipeline. Our own view and that of those who have modeled the ongoing epidemic is that without a vaccine, HCV elimination will not be achieved.

Acknowledgments

TD is funded by the Medical Research Council UK. EB receives funds from the Oxford NIHR Biomedical Research Centre and is an NIHR Senior Investigator. The views expressed in this article are those of the authors and not necessarily those of the NHS, the NIHR, or the Department of Health.

References

1. Feld JJ, Jacobson IM, Hézode C et al. Sofosbuvir and velpatasvir for HCV Genotype 1, 2, 4, 5, and 6 infection. *New England Journal of Medicine* 2015;373(27):2599–2607.

2. Abravanel F, Métivier S, Chauveau M, Péron J-M, Izopet J. Transmission of HCV NS5A inhibitor-resistant variants among HIV-infected men who have sex with men. *Clinical Infectious Diseases* 2016;63(9):1271–1272.

3. Franco S, Tural C, Nevot M et al. Detection of a sexually transmitted hepatitis C virus protease inhibitor-resistance variant in a human immunodeficiency virus-infected homosexual man. *Gastroenterology* 2014;147(3):599–601.e1

4. Buckley GJ, Strom BL (eds). Eliminating the Public Health Problem of Hepatitis B and C in the United States. Washington, DC: National Academies Press, 2016.

5. Suryaprasad AG, White JZ, Xu F et al. Emerging epidemic of hepatitis C virus infections among young nonurban persons who inject drugs in the United States, 2006–2012. *Clinical Infectious Diseases* 2014;59(10):1411–1419.

6. Hill A, Khwairakpam G, Wang J et al. High sustained virological response rates using imported generic direct acting antiviral treatment for hepatitis C. *Journal of Virus Eradication* 2017;3(4):200–203.

7. Wedemeyer H, Duberg AS, Buti M et al. Strategies to manage hepatitis C virus (HCV) disease burden. *Journal of Viral Hepatitis* 2014;21:60–89.

8. Stone J, Martin NK, Hickman M et al. The potential impact of a hepatitis C vaccine for people who inject drugs: is a vaccine needed in the age of direct-acting antivirals? *PLoS One* 2016;11(5):e0156213–e0156213.

9. Major M, Gutfraind A, Shekhtman L et al. Modeling of patient virus titers suggests that availability of a vaccine could reduce hepatitis C virus transmission among injecting drug users. *Science Translation Medicine* 2018;10(449):eaao4496.

10. Scott N, McBryde E, Vickerman P et al. The role of a hepatitis C virus vaccine: modelling the benefits alongside direct-acting antiviral treatments. *BMC Medicine* 2015;13(1):198.

11. Mehta SH, Cox A, Hoover DR et al. Protection against persistence of hepatitis C. *Lancet* 2002;359(9316):1478–1483.

12. Osburn WO, Fisher BE, Dowd KA et al. Spontaneous control of primary hepatitis C virus infection and immunity against persistent reinfection. *Gastroenterology* 2010;138(1):315–324.

13. Pestka JM, Zeisel MB, Bläser E et al. Rapid induction of virus-neutralizing antibodies and viral clearance in a single-source outbreak of hepatitis C. *Proceedings of the National Academy of Sciences USA* 2007;104(14):6025–6030.

14. Neumann-Haefelin C, McKiernan S, Ward S et al. Dominant influence of an HLA-B27 restricted CD8+ T cell response in mediating HCV clearance and evolution. *Hepatology* 2006;43(3):563–572.

15. Duggal P, Thio CL, Wojcik GL et al. Genome-wide association study of spontaneous resolution of hepatitis C virus infection: data from multiple cohorts. *Annals of Internal Medicine* 2013;158(4):235.

16. Shoukry NH, Grakoui A, Houghton M et al. Memory CD8 $^+$ T cells are required for protection from persistent hepatitis C virus infection. *Journal of Experimental Medicine* 2003;197(12):1645–1655.

17. Grakoui A, Shoukry NH, Woollard DJ et al. HCV persistence and immune evasion in the absence of memory T cell help. *Science* 2003;302(5645):659–662.

18. Barnes E, Folgori A, Capone S et al. Novel adenovirus-based vaccines induce broad and sustained T cell responses to HCV in man. *Science Translational Medicine* 2012;4(115):115ra1.

19. Swadling L, Capone S, Antrobus RD et al. A human vaccine strategy based on chimpanzee adenoviral and MVA vectors that primes, boosts, and sustains functional HCV-specific T cell memory. *Science Translational Medicine* 2014;6(261):261ra153.

20. Frey SE, Houghton M, Coates S et al. Safety and immunogenicity of HCV E1E2 vaccine adjuvanted with MF59 administered to healthy adults. *Vaccine* 2010;28(38):6367–6373.

21. Law JLM, Chen C, Wong J et al. A hepatitis C virus (HCV) vaccine comprising envelope glycoproteins gpE1/gpE2 derived from a single isolate elicits broad cross-genotype neutralizing antibodies in humans. *PLoS One* 2013;8(3):e59776.

22. Houghton M, Abrignani S. Prospects for a vaccine against the hepatitis C virus. *Nature* 2005;436(7053):961–966.

23. Houghton M. Prospects for prophylactic and therapeutic vaccines against the hepatitis C viruses. *Immunological Reviews* 2011;239(1):99–108.

24. Choo QL, Kuo G, Ralston R et al. Vaccination of chimpanzees against infection by the hepatitis C virus. *Proceedings of the National Academy of Sciences USA* 1994;91(4):1294–1298.

25. Ray R, Meyer K, Banerjee A et al. Characterization of antibodies induced by vaccination with hepatitis C virus envelope glycoproteins. *Journal of Infectious Diseases* 2010;202(6):862–866.

26. McCaffrey K, Boo I, Owczarek CM et al. An optimized hepatitis C virus E2 glycoprotein core adopts a functional homodimer that efficiently blocks virus entry. *Journal of Virology* 2017;91(5):e01668-16.

27. Vietheer P, Boo I, Gu J et al. The core domain of hepatitis C virus glycoprotein E2 generates potent cross-neutralizing antibodies. *Hepatology* 2017;65:1117–1131.

28. Chmielewska AM, Naddeo M, Capone S et al. Combined adenovirus vector and hepatitis C virus envelope protein prime-boost regimen elicits T cell and neutralizing antibody immune responses. *Journal of Virology* 2014;88(10):5502–5510.

29. Bellier B, Klatzmann D. Virus-like particle-based vaccines against hepatitis C virus infection. *Expert Review of Vaccines* 2013;12(2):143–154.

30. Kumar A, Das S, Mullick R et al. Immune responses against hepatitis C virus genotype 3a virus-like particles in mice: a novel VLP prime-adenovirus boost strategy. *Vaccine* 2016;34(8):1115–1125.

31. Folgori A, Capone S, Ruggeri L et al. A T-cell HCV vaccine eliciting effective immunity against heterologous virus challenge in chimpanzees. *Nature Medicine* 2006;12(2):190–197.

32. Colloca S, Barnes E, Folgori A et al. Vaccine vectors derived from a large collection of simian adenoviruses induce potent cellular immunity across multiple species. *Science Translational Medicine* 2012;4(115):115ra2.

33. Smith DB, Bukh J, Kuiken C et al. Expanded classification of hepatitis C virus into 7 genotypes and 67 subtypes: updated criteria and genotype assignment web resource. *Hepatology* 2014;59(1):318–327.

34. von Delft A, Donnison TA, Lourenço J et al. The generation of a simian adenoviral vectored HCV vaccine encoding genetically conserved gene segments to target multiple HCV genotypes. *Vaccine* 2018;36(2):313–321.

35. Choo QL, Kuo G, Ralston R et al. Vaccination of chimpanzees against infection by the hepatitis C virus. *Proceedings of the National Academy of Sciences USA* 1994;91(4):1294–1298.

36. Trivedi S, Murthy S, Sharma H et al. Viral persistence, liver disease and host response in hepatitis C-like virus rat model. *Hepatology* 2018;68:435–448.

37. von Delft A, Humphreys IS, Brown A et al. The broad assessment of HCV genotypes 1 and 3 antigenic targets reveals limited cross-reactivity with implications for vaccine design. *Gut* 2016;65:112–123.

38. Kelly C, Swadling L, Brown A et al. Cross-reactivity of hepatitis C virus specific vaccine-induced T cells at immunodominant epitopes. *European Journal of Immunology* 2015;45(1):309–316.

37 Elimination of hepatitis C virus in high-prevalence, low-income countries: is it feasible?

Mahmoud Abdo and Hadeel Gamal Eldeen

Department of Endemic Medicine and Hepatology, Faculty of Medicine, Cairo University, Cairo, Egypt

LEARNING POINTS

- The WHO goal of global elimination of HCV by 2030 is challenging and will not be easy to achieve.

- Elimination will require both ready access to antiviral medication and improvements in infection control.

- The Egyptian model of care involving easy access to locally delivered treatment with a universal web-based registry has proven to be highly effective.

- The Egyptian experience with commitment from government and the clinical community demonstrates that, with the right support, ambitious treatment goals can be achieved.

The hope

The introduction of interferon-free all-oral, direct-acting antiviral (DAAs) regimens for the treatment of hepatitis C virus (HCV) infection has led to greatly improved chances of cure and, combined with the excellent tolerance profile, raises the possibility of eliminating HCV by 2030. This is now a World Health Organization goal [1].

The barriers

Budget limitation

This is the main challenge for HCV elimination in low-income countries. The costs of diagnosis and treatment make the HCV elimination challenge more complex. Infection is usually asymptomatic and most patients are unaware of their infected status. This translates into low HCV awareness among the general population, especially regarding modes of transmission and high-risk behaviors [2]. To achieve the 2030 disease elimination target in a low-income country like Egypt, the number of newly diagnosed patients must exceed 350 000/year together with a decrease in the incidence of new cases by >20% annually [3]. An integrated approach is needed to train health are personnel to deliver appropriate care, counseling, and therapy to patients with chronic HCV according to national and international guidelines.

Infection control

Infection control is another major limitation to HCV elimination in low-income countries. Many low-income countries lack formal infection control programs in many healthcare facilities, there are few professional healthcare workers with training or expertise in infection control, and adequate equipment sterilization, reprocessing practices, and waste management are rarely practiced. To decrease HCV transmission rates in these countries, wider application of infection control standards to all aspects of health and dental care beyond approved government facilities is required as well as a marked increase in community awareness. In Egypt, the overall WHO infection control score was 19 out of 100 in 2003. In response, the Egyptian Ministry of Health launched an infection control program to promote safe practices in hospitals and healthcare facilities and this increased the overall score to 68.9 in 2011,

Clinical Dilemmas in Viral Liver Disease, Second Edition. Edited by Graham R. Foster and K. Rajender Reddy.
© 2020 John Wiley & Sons Ltd. Published 2020 by John Wiley & Sons Ltd.

indicating that with political will, significant improvements can rapidly be achieved.

Inadequate screening

This is a major obstacle in many countires. In this contextm national health surveys need to be expanded to ensure that all infected individuals are aware of their infection status so that they can seek treatment.

Funding

It is axiomatic that lack of access to funding for antiviral therapy is a major barrier to effective elimination.

Pursuit of a model of care: the Egyptian experience

Formation and measures adopted by the National Committee for Control of Viral Hepatitis

Treatment of HCV in Egypt has been one of the top national priorities since 2006 when Egypt started a national treatment program intending to provide cure for Egyptian HCV-infected patients. With the development of highly effective DAAs for HCV, elimination of viral hepatitis has become a real possibility. Egypt, a resource-limited country with the highest HCV burden, has become a role model in HCV management. This involved establishing a novel model of care (MOC) to contain the epidemic, deliver patient care, and ensure global treatment access. The HCV MOC came into being in 2006 with the establishment of the National Committee for Control of Viral Hepatitis (NCCVH) to set up and implement a national control strategy for the disease and other causes of viral hepatitis [4,5].

The committee is divided into an advisory board and an executive working group for planning and developing the strategy and an implementation plan for monitoring progress of the MOC. Its main mission was to deliver equitable, safe, and standardized medical evaluation and treatment services to all HCV patients, without discrimination, while considering cost-effectiveness to maintain sustainability in a resource-limited country.

The strategy required a dual approach. Initially, this involved planning prevention strategies to reduce further risk of transmission through raising public awareness of modes of transmission and high-risk behaviors, providing

safe blood products, improving infection control in healthcare facilities, adopting safer injection practices, and strengthening surveillance. The second intervention involved active management through establishing approved evidence-based national guidelines for the treatment of chronic HCV, training healthcare professionals (hepatologists, infectious disease specialists, physicians, and nurses) to deliver an efficient counseling, care and treatment program for patients with chronic HCV in accordance with the updated national guidelines. Pharmacists and information technology specialists were also trained to coordinate dispensing medications and data management through a well-regulated system implemented on a nationwide basis [4].

In 2006, the NCCVH set several targets, including assessment of the disease burden, establishing an infrastructure for a national treatment program, development of a national strategy for viral hepatitis control, and management of advanced liver disease, while continuing to perform clinical and epidemiologic research activities. The initial target was to provide antiviral treatment for HCV-infected individuals either at minimum cost or totally free of charge (government sponsored) for those who do not have health insurance, and ensure that all costs are fully covered for those treated through the Health Insurance Organization (HIO). In addition, a procurement process negotiated affordable drug prices of medicines for the MOH-supported treatment program [4,5].

In 2007, the NCCVH established its first specialized centers for the treatment of viral hepatitis. Centers were planned to be geographically distributed in the most populous areas, so that eventually no patient would have to travel more than 50 km to a center. This ensured better access to care and treatment for patients everywhere. These centers are managed by a well-trained team of specialist hepatologists providing a full spectrum of care for patients, starting with initial screening for treatment elegibility up to providing standard of care management according to the national protocols. More than 24 centers were established between 2007 and 2016.

In 2014, with the availability of DAAs suitable for patients with HCV genotype 4, negotiations between the Egyptian government, represented by the NCCVH, and Gilead Sciences, the US manufacturer of sofosbuvir (Sovaldi®), led to an agreement providing the medication for patients treated through the government program at the reduced price of $300 per bottle (a reduction from $28 000 per bottle in the USA market) [4].

The deal with Gilead Sciences paved the way to similar negotiations with other manufacturers of DAAs and resulted in equivalent reduction of prices of their medications, including simeprevir (Janssen Pharmaceutica, Belgium) and daclatasvir (Bristol-Myers-Squibb, USA), at $250 for a month's supply each, paritaprevir-ombitasvir (AbbVie, USA) at $300 for a month's supply, and sofosbuvir-ledipasvir (Gilead Sciences) for the equivalent of $400 for a month's supply [4].

Meanwhile, the agreements signed with the manufacturers of the original brands of DAAs did not preclude the MOH and other official bodies from contracting with other companies to manufacture the drug locally. The local production of DAAs and the support given to generic production led to price competition with further marked reduction in the price in the Egyptian market [4].

The initial demand and anticipated numbers were beyond the capacity of the centers. This necessitated a novel administration solution that was developed for the first time in the healthcare setting of Egypt. The Ministry of State for Administrative Development developed an online registration system website (www.nccvh.org.eg) once the first DAA was registered in Egypt. The system has an appropriate bandwidth that withstands the highest possible submissions per second. This portal was designed for registration of patients with HCV and allows scheduling of appointments at the treatment centers. Inputs from the patients' registry include their national identification number, residence, and a simple question for validation. Daily workload and appointments were set according to each center's capacity. Patients' appointments were automatically set to the first time available in the treatment center nearest to their residence.

With the initial wave of patient registration, waiting times for first appointments reached six months or more in some centers (depending on prevalence in the area and the center's capacity). This eased off with the opening of new centers and with treatment of the patients on the waiting list. Eventually, by mid-2016, there was no waiting time for the first appointment in any of the centers, and patients are now evaluated in the same week of registration. By the end of November 2016, around 1 500 000 patients had registered and received appointments through the web-based system.

The Ministry of Communication provided easy access for the appointment and reservation portal and offered a mobile phone messaging service via SMS (in addition to the web-based service) for notification about appointment dates and changes when needed. Helplines are available to answer patients' queries and receive complaints, if any. This patient support service provides sufficient information to make appointments and treatment decisions that best suit patients' lifestyles, occupational and social responsibilities, personal needs, and preferences.

Almost 88% of treated patients were totally sponsored by the government (29% through the HIO and 56% through governmental support funds). The remaining 12% of patients were treated using their own resources but taking advantage of the reduced prices negotiated nationally.

Challenges faced by the NCCVH

One of the major challenges following the introduction of DAAs was the failure of a significant number of patients (approximately 40%) to return for evaluation of SVR. Patients were motivated to come back 12 weeks after therapy for clinical and laboratory results follow-up through issuing a certificate of "cure from hepatitis C" for patients who remain HCV-RNA negative at 12 weeks after the end of therapy. Patients who relapse are retreated according to the guidelines and protocols of managing treatment failures.

Another challenge was the significant discrimination against patients with HCV within the community and, sadly, also within healthcare settings. A call for legal action to prohibit discrimination against HCV-infected patients was addressed by the NCCVH in the National Council, where discussions to consider it illegal to discriminate against people on the basis of disability caused by an infectious disease were initiated. Exceptions were introduced where discrimination is necessary to protect public health.

Economic aspects of HCV screening

If HCV cure is cost-effective, then there must be a strategy to effectively screen for HCV and link infected patients to care. However, initiating a screening program is expensive and implementation can be complex. Several investigators have assessed the costs associated with effective screening programs for HCV. Although some have demonstrated that HCV screening of the entire population (in comparison to screening the at-risk population) is cost-effective, others have argued that large-scale population-based screening can only be considered in the context of a national policy and registry [6–9].

In October 2018, the MOH launched a three-phase campaign "100 Million Health". This involves a huge screening campaign for HCV over the whole country. It divides the country into three sectors, each involving 7–11 governates with around 3–11 million people per governate. All patients who test positive for HCV, using a rapid test, will complete their evaluation and receive appropriate therapy within a couple of weeks totally free of charge.

Conclusion

In order to eliminate HCV, national policies should be in place to support screening, linkage to care, and affordable treatment. More integrated international efforts are required, involving health policy makers, healthcare practitioners, public health organizations, antiviral drug manufacturers, health insurance companies, and all major stakeholders. In addition, effective prevention, comprehensive screening programs, accessibility to the new anti-HCV treatment regimens, and public education should be considered the top priorities of any health policy initiative to eliminate HCV infection. With national, regional, and global policies, the dream of HCV elimination in countries with limited resources can come true.

References

1. Younossi Z, Papatheodoridis G, Cacoub P et al. The comprehensive outcomes of hepatitis C virus infection: a multi-faceted chronic disease. *Journal of Viral Hepatitis* 2018;25 Suppl 3:6–14.
2. Central Agency for Public Mobilisation and Statistics (CAPMAS). Poverty indicators according to income, expenditure and consumption data 2012–2013. www.capmas.gov.eg
3. Waked I, Doss W, El-Sayed MH et al. The current and future disease burden of chronic hepatitis C virus infection in Egypt. *Arab Journal of Gastroenterology* 2014;15:45–52.
4. El-Akel W, El-Sayed MH, El Kassas M et al. National treatment programme of hepatitis C in Egypt: hepatitis C virus model of care. *Journal of Viral Hepatitis* 2017;24(4):262–267.
5. Omran D, Alboraie M, Zayed R et al. Towards hepatitis C virus elimination: Egyptian experience, achievements and limitations. *World Journal of Gastroenterology* 2018;24(38):4330–4340.
6. Deuffic-Burban S, Huneau A, Verleene A et al. Assessing the cost-effectiveness of hepatitis C screening strategies in France. *Journal of Hepatology* 2018;69(4):785–792.
7. Marshall AD, Pawlotsky JM, Lazarus JV, Aghemo A, Dore GJ, Grebely J. The removal of DAA restrictions in Europe – one step closer to eliminating HCV as a major public health threat. *Journal of Hepatology* 2018;69(5):1188–1196.
8. Ethgen O, Sanchez Gonzalez Y, Jeanblanc G, Duguet A, Misurski D, Juday T. Public health impact of comprehensive hepatitis C screening and treatment in the French baby-boomer population. *Journal of Medical Economics* 2017;20(2):162–170.
9. Chevaliez S, Pawlotsky JM. New virological tools for screening, diagnosis and monitoring of hepatitis B and C in resource-limited settings. *Journal of Hepatology* 2018;69(4):916–926.

38 Hepatitis B virus diagnostics: anything new?

Dina Ginzberg[1], Robert J. Wong[2], and Robert G. Gish[3]

[1] Department of Medicine, Alameda Health System – Highland Hospital, Oakland, CA, USA
[2] Division of Gastroenterology and Hepatology, Alameda Health System – Highland Hospital, Oakland, CA, USA
[3] Division of Gastroenterology and Hepatology, Stanford Health Care, Palo Alto, CA, USA

LEARNING POINTS

- Early detection of chronic HBV is critical and emphasizes the need for improved diagnostic assays with improved performance characteristics.

- While qualitative HBV surface antigen (HBsAg) has been primarily used for confirmation of chronic HBV infection, the role of quantitative HBsAg for monitoring response to antiviral therapy is evolving.

- HBV core-related antigen (HBcrAg) is also an emerging diagnostic assay, the quantification of which may have an evolving role in determining response to antiviral therapy and predicting disease progression.

- Other newer HBV diagnostic assays continue to enhance the field and provide more tools to help assess disease progression, response to therapy, and potentially discontinuation of therapy.

Introduction

Viral hepatitis is the seventh leading cause of morbidity and mortality worldwide, surpassing HIV, malaria and tuberculosis by annual death rate, and accounting for 1.45 million deaths annually. Worldwide, an estimated 292 million individuals are chronically infected with hepatitis B virus (HBV) [1] which accounts for one death every minute in the Asia-Pacific region. Chronic HBV (denoted by the seroprevalence of HBsAg for at least six months) accounts for 50% of viral hepatitis-related deaths and 21 million disability-adjusted life-years owing to progression to cirrhosis and hepatocellular carcinoma [2]. Recognizing the global burden of HBV, the 2016 World Health Assembly championed the elimination of viral hepatitis B along with hepatitis C as a global threat by 2030.

Achievement of this goal requires diagnosis, linkage to care, correct staging of disease, timely and cost-effective treatment options, and public health initiatives. Perhaps the key to elimination targets are accessible, accurate and validated diagnostic means for identifying and monitoring viral activity in infected individuals. While means of diagnosing HBV have been available since the 1970s, diagnostic rates remain suboptimal and we are a long way from the 90% target proposed by the WHO. In 2016, only 10% of infected individuals (29 million) were aware of their HBV sero-status, with estimates as low as 5% in low-income countries, where prevalence of HBV is disproportionately higher [1].

Diagnosis of HBV infection is intimately linked to determining the natural history of the virus (Figure 38.1). HBV is an enveloped DNA virus that clinically manifests as self-limited acute hepatitis, chronic hepatitis or fulminant liver failure. A sterilizing cure, defined as the eradication of detectable HBsAg, intrahepatic covalently closed circular DNA (cccDNA) and integrated HBV DNA, is the ultimate goal for HBV treatment but remains unachievable with current treatment regimens (nuceos(t)ide analogs [NAs] and PEG-interferon). A more feasible goal is functional cure, defined by a sustained loss of HBsAg with or without hepatitis B surface antibody seroconversion in patients who are DNA negative.

Clinical Dilemmas in Viral Liver Disease, Second Edition. Edited by Graham R. Foster and K. Rajender Reddy.
© 2020 John Wiley & Sons Ltd. Published 2020 by John Wiley & Sons Ltd.

Disease Phases	Phase 1 Immune Tolerant	Phase 2 Immune Active	Phase 3 Inactive/Carrier	Phase 4 Reactivation	Phase 5 Resolved/Occult
	HBeAg-positive CHBV Infection / Highly replicative / Non-inflammatory / Prolonged in perinatal infection / ↓IL-10, IL-6,IL-8 & TNF-α	HBeAg-positive chronic hepatitis / ↑ Core & precore mutations	HBeAg-negative CHBV infection / Low replicative	HBeAg-negative chronic hepatitis	Functional Cure / Risk of reactivation with immunosuppression
Current Diagnostic Tests					
qHBsAg	HBsAg				Anti-HBs
Serum HBV DNA	Elevated >20,000 IU/mL	Elevated but declining	Low <2,000–20,000 IU/mL	Elevated >2,000–20,000 IU/mL	Undetectable → low
HBeAg	HBeAg		Anti-HBe		
ALT level	Normal	High	Normal-mildly elevated	Fluctuating	Normal
Liver Inflammation	Minimal	Active	Mild	Active	Inactive
Risk for Disease Progression to cirrhosis & HCC	Minimal	Present	Minimal	Greatest	None
Future Markers					
Anti-HBc	Low	High	Low	High	Positive
HBcrAg	V. High	High	Intermediate	Low	Undetectable
HBV RNA	V. High	High	High-intermediate	Low-Intermediate	Undetectable

Figure 38.1 Hepatitis B virus disease phases.

Given the impracticality of using liver biopsies to quantify transcription of intrahepatic cccDNA, surrogate noninvasive biomarkers are necessary to diagnose HBV infection, monitor viral replication, trend disease progression, and assess therapeutic response to current and future antivirals.

Hepatitis B surface antigen

Hepatitis B surface antigen plays a vital role in characterizing acute or chronic HBV infection, and guiding treatment in chronic HBV infection (CHB) [3]. Levels of HBsAg help differentiate HBeAg-negative immune-active hepatitis from inactive carriers when measured in conjunction with ALT and HBV DNA (Table 38.1). Comprising proteins subtypes – small (SHBsAg), middle (MHBsAg) and large (LHBsAg) – HBsAg composes the envelope of secreted HBV virions and is secreted independently into serum as spherical or filamentous noninfectious subviral particles (SVPs) whose levels exceed mature virions by 100–100 000-fold. HBsAg is derived from episomal cccDNA or integrated HBV DNA and translated from preS1 and preS2/S messenger RNA in the endoplasmic reticulum (Figure 38.2). HBsAg levels (quantified in IU/mL) correlate with HBV DNA and cccDNA in HBeAg-positive patients; no such correlation exists in HBeAg-negative patients, possibly due to expression of HBsAg with increased HBV integration with later phase of HBV chronic infections [4]. HBsAg seroclearance is the current goal for functional cure, and loss of HBsAg (testing threshold is 0.05 IU/mL) remains a vital endpoint in studies of novel HBV therapies although more sensitive quantitation assays may confound this standard in the near future.

The role of HBsAg quantification in patients on NA therapy is currently evolving, with potential to identify patients with low HBsAg levels (<100 IU/mL) who may be candidates for treatment discontinuation owing to low risk of relapse after treatment discontinuation. HBsAg is detected both by immunoassays and by point-of-care (POC) tests in resource-limited settings where standard serology testing is more expensive, cumbersome or unavailable [5].

Quantitative HBV DNA testing

Hepatitis B virus is a DNA-containing enveloped virus. Infectious particles (Dane particles) circulating in the serum contain a single copy of viral DNA that serves as the template

for intrahepatic transcription of cccDNA (see Figure 38.2). Peripheral HBV DNA levels thus correlate with intrahepatic transcription. Higher levels of HBV DNA are associated with more advanced liver disease and hepatocellular carcinoma (HCC) in a dose-dependent manner (see Figure 38.1) [6]. Detection and quantification of serum HBV DNA via PCR amplification or POC nucleic acid tests are essential for diagnosing acute or chronic HBV infection, guiding treatment, and monitoring treatment response and treatment resistance (see Table 38.1). HBV DNA plays a vital role in diagnosing the phases or stages of HBV infection, helping with diagnosis during the "window period" of acute or recent infection, and helping with diagnosis of chronic infections with HBsAg escape mutants that compromise the diagnostic accuracy of serologic assays. Suppression of serum HBV DNA levels is achievable with NA therapy, and remains an important endpoint in treatment guidelines.

Covalently closed circular DNA

Contained as a minichromosome within the nucleus of infected hepatic cells, covalently closed circular DNA (cccDNA) is the transcriptional template for most of 1 HBV RNA – pregenomic RNA (pgRNA), precore-RNA, subgenomic RNA (sgRNA) (see Figure 38.2, Table 38.2) – noting that integrants of HBV can also express mRNA that is truncated. Current treatment modalities (nucleos(t)ide antagonists) do not directly target cccDNA. Interferon weakly targets cccDNA via intracellular signaling pathways [7]. For these reasons, a sterilizing cure is not yet attainable, and virologic relapse occurs occasionally in patients with HBsAg seroclearance more frequently in those on immnosuppressive therapy [7]. Quantification of cccDNA is complicated by the need for liver biopsy, and the absence of simple, efficient and standardized methods for quantification. On account of this, cccDNA is unlikely to become a routine biomarker for HBV diagnosis, yet new assays for qHBV RNA and HBcrAg may allow accurate assessment of cccDNA levels and transcriptionally active cccDNA

Hepatitis B e antigen and antibody

Hepatitis B e antigen (HBeAg) is a nonstructural protein derived from precore RNA and secreted from infected hepatocytes. HBeAg plays an essential role in HBV persistence and immune modulation (see Figure 38.2, Table 38.1).

Table 38.1 Old biomarkers for hepatitis B virus infection

Biomarker	Description	Function	Clinical utility
HBsAg	Envelope protein derived from episomal cccDNA and/or integrated DNA	Marker of acute or chronic HBV infection • Acute HB – transient HBsAg elevation • Chronic HB – HBsAg persistently elevated >6 mo Levels correlate with cccDNA transcription	• Diagnosis of HBV infection on initial presentation • Prediction of vertical transmission in pregnant women • Identification of patients for withdrawal of NA therapy • Prediction of treatment response in CHB • Prediction of relapse risk • Determine frequency of monitoring for inactive infections • Assess risk for seroconversion in immunosuppressed patients
HBV DNA	HBV viral genome	Marker of viral replication	• Diagnosis of HBV infection on initial presentation • Diagnosis of occult infection (HBsAg-neg, HBV-positive) • Identification of acute infection during window period • Identification of CHB phase • Identification of CHB in patients with HBsAg mutants and false-negative HBsAg • Identifies patients benefiting from antiviral treatment • Monitoring response to NA therapy • Prediction of vertical transmission in pregnant females • Prediction of HBV HCC development (inc. with HBV <2000 IU/mL)
HBe Ag	Soluble nonstructural protein derived from precore mRNA and secreted by infected hepatocytes	Marker of infectivity and disease severity Responsible for infection persistence and chronicity Potent immunomodulator against HBcAg T-cell telorogen	• Prediction of therapeutic response • Identification of CHB phase
Anti-HBe	Immune response to HBeAg	Marker of immunity (natural or with vaccination)	• Diagnosis of HBV infectious phase on initial presentation • Identification of HBV flares (elevations in HBV DNA or ALT levels) • Monitoring for HBeAg seroconversion in HBeAg-positive patients on treatment
Anti-HBsAb	Immune response to HBsAg	Denotes immunity to HBV	• Assess for prior vaccination or seroclearance

(Continued)

Table 38.1 (Continued)

Biomarker	Description	Function	Clinical utility
Anti-HBc	Immune response to HBcAg	Marker of HBV exposure Levels mirror hepatic inflammation Possible predictor of HBeAg seroconversion and response to antiviral therapy	• Diagnosis of current or occult infection on initial presentation • Confirmation of risk of reactivation • If negative: identification of patients in need of HBV vaccination
HBV genotype	Genotypes A–H	Epidemiologic data on HBV	• Consideration for PEG-IFN treatment • Assess risk of HCC • Assess risk of FHF
Precore or BCP mutation	Mutation on precore or BCP sequence of HBV DNA	Allow for viral escape from immune control	• Assess risk of HCC • Assess risk of progressive disease

ALT, alanine aminotransferase; BCP, basal core promoter; CHB, chronic hepatitis B; FHF, fulminant hepatic failure; HBV, hepatitis B virus; HCC, hepatocellular carcinoma; IFN, interferon; NA, nucleoside analog.

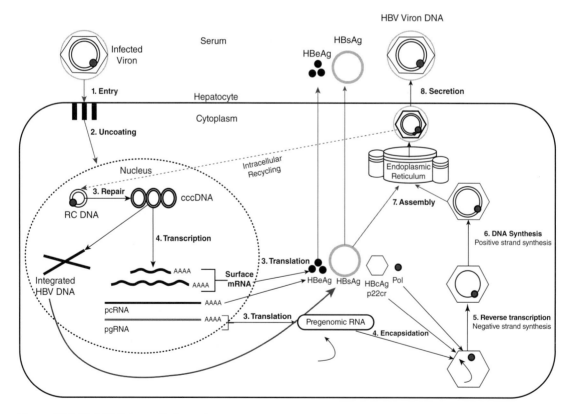

Figure 38.2 Hepatitis B virus replication cycle.

HBeAg characterizes the phases of CHB and is first detectable 6–12 weeks after HBV exposure (see Figure 38.1). HBeAg and its antibody (anti-HBe) are measured using immunoassays, but no quantitative assays are currently commercially available [5,8]. Seroconversion from HBeAg positivity to negativity marks an important transition in the natural course of HBV infection from highly infectious chronic HBeAg-negative disease or to inactive infection with low levels or undetectable HBV DNA. Spontaneous HBeAg loss or seroconversion occurs at an annual rate of 5–10% with antiviral therapy [9]. Precore and basal core promoter (BCP) mutations account for persistent viremia and active liver inflammation in HBeAg-negative patients. HBeAg seroconversion, provided it is accompanied by low HBV DNA levels, denotes better prognosis, making it a viable goal for current and future antiviral therapies. Measurements of the pc and core-related mutations are available via sequencing assays in commercial laboratories.

Hepatitis B core antigen and core-related antigen

Hepatitis B core-related antigen (HBcrAg) is a novel bio-marker for HBV infection that combines the quantification of three precore-derived proteins: hepatitis B core antigen (HBcAg), the structural nuclear capsid protein, HBeAg and the precore protein p22r found in DNA-free (empty) virion particles (see Figure 38.1). HBcrAg is measured via chemiluminescence which detects a single 149-amino acid sequence shared by its three constituents. Recent studies suggest HBcrAg may be a reliable marker for predicting spontaneous or treatment-induced HBeAg seroconversion [10] and a potential surrogate for cccDNA transcriptional activity [11–13]. Recent studies have also suggested that elevated HBcrAg levels predict HCC development in CHB [14]. As a result, HBcrAg may play a role in guiding NA treatment and predicting disease progression (see Table 38.2) and is being measured in all new drug development trials.

Table 38.2 New biomarkers for hepatitis B virus infection

Biomarker	Description	Function	Clinical utility
cccDNA	Intrahepatic transcriptional template for HBV Derived from rcDNA in the nucleus	Responsible for HBV infection persistence, chronicity and reactivation after withdrawl of NAs Quantified by liver biopsy Activity may correlate with disease progression	• None at this time
HBcrAg		Marker of viral replication Surrogate marker of cccDNA transcription Lower levels suggest more favorable disease progression	• Monitoring therapy outcomes • Prediction of HCC risk • Prediction of HBV reactivation with immunosuppresion • Prediction of HBeAg seroconversion with treatment
HBV RNA	Quantification of pgRNA levels and total serum HBV RNA	Surrogate marker of cccDNA transcription	
dsiDNA	Genomic DNA	Contributes to virion particles Recycled to reform cccDNA Integrated into host genome	• None at this time
Empty particles	Enveloped nucleocapsid without genome material	May play role on HCC development	• None at this time
Spliced DNA/ RNA	Truncated DNA/RNA formed during HBV replication	May contribute to HCC, poor response to interferon and liver disease	• None at this time

HBV, hepatitis B virus; HCC, hepatocellular carcinoma; NA, nucleoside analog.

Quantitative HBV RNA

Hepatitis B virus pregenomic RNAs (pgRNA) contained in hepatocyte cytoplasm (see Figure 38.2) are key intermediates that provide the template for polymerase (Pol), core proteins and reverse transcription. HBV RNA pgRNA is transcribed from cccDNA, so circulating levels reflect cccDNA virus transcriptional activity [8,15]. HBV RNA levels correlate with HBV DNA, serum HBsAg, alanine aminotransferase (ALT), and genetic variants [16,17]. NA treatment preferentially suppresses HBV DNA levels, making HBV RNA a potential biomarker for monitoring treatment response, with declining levels predicting seroconversion in HBeAg-positive patients and determining cccDNA activity in patients in general or those being treated with NA treatment [18,19] (see Table 38.2). The presence of pgRNA in patients with both HBsAg positivity and occult HBV infection which suggests pgRNA may contribute to HCC development [20].

Hepatitis B core antibody

Hepatitis B core antibody (anti-HBc) is a biomarker of HBV exposure and the presence of cccDNA and is seen in acute (IgM+) and chronic HBV infection (+ total anti-HBc and in some cases + anti-HB IgMc) (see Table 38.1). As the first antibody to appear after acute HBV infection, anti-HBc is a helpful biomarker for diagnosing occult infection, where HBsAg levels are undetectable but hepatitis B surface antibodies have not yet developed (see Figure 38.2). Higher anti-HBc titers predict increased rates of HBeAg seroconversion and reduced risk of relapse after discontinuation of NA treatment [8] as well as risk of HCC. Quantification of anti-HBc is useful for characterizing HBV exposure, differentiating infection from hepatitis, assessing vaccination need, and predicting reactivation, occult HBV infection, and treatment response. Anti-HBc has a false-positive rate of <2/1000.

Hepatitis B surface antibody

Hepatitis B surface antibody (anti-HBs) is a biomarker representing immune response to HBsAg achieved through vaccination if anti-HBc is negative. There is no such event as "natural" immunity and this term is now removed from our lexicon. Current assays detect anti-HBs not bound to SVPs or virion particles. Further studies are needed to better understand the role of anti-HBs in viral neutralization and immune control and test for HBsAg variants.

HBV genotypes and subtypes

To date, phylogenetic analyses have identified 10 HBV genotypes (A–J) with >8% genetic variation at the nucleotide level and more than 40 subtypes with 4–8% nucleotide divergence across the genome (Table 38.3) [21]. These genotypes and subtypes follow distinct geographic distributions and transmission routes and thus influence disease progression to HCC and treatment outcomes (Figure 38.3) [9,21,22]. Current guidelines recommend routine testing for HBV genotype only if PEG-interferon therapy is being considered, and there is risk for HCC, as higher likelihoods of HBsAg loss and HBeAg seroconversion are observed with A and B genotypes treated with PEG-interferon [21] and genotype C has a higher risk of HCC. Genotypes B and C are most prevalent in regions with high rates of vertical and perinatal transmission. According to recent studies published by the Hepatitis B Research Network, most chronic HBV infections in adults are genotype B (39%) and C (33%), and occur in persons born in Asia (67%) or Africa (11%). Studies investigating the relationship between genotype and risk of HCC development have yielded conflicting results, but two studies have suggested the possibility of increased incidence of HCC with genotype C [23]. There are two types of genotype A: A1 or Aa from Africa and Ae or A2 from Europe; distinction of these subtypes is a major research interest at this time.

Precore and basal core mutations

Precore and basal core promoter (BCP) mutations allow for viral escape from anti-HBe immune control of HBV, which may reduce the probability of HBsAg loss during long-term NA therapy [24]. In HBeAg-negative patients, these mutations promote viremia and hepatitis as evidenced by elevated HBV DNA levels and increased serum ALT [8]. A direct correlation is observed between infection chronicity, older patient age, and incidence of basal core mutations [8,25]. Double BCP mutations, especially in genotype C HBV, correlate with a 3.5-fold increased risk of HCC development due to upregulation of

Table 38.3 Characteristics of HBV genotypes

Genotypes	Subtypes	Origin/ geographic distribution	Clinical notes	Mutations/ recombinations	Predominant route of transmission	Response to antiviral therapy
A	A1 A2 A3	Africa Europe/North America Africa/Haiti	More likely to lose HBsAg than C and D A1 associated with aggressive liver disease	Higher frequency of BCP mutations than B and D	Parenteral or sexual	Responds better to interferon therapy than C and D
B	B1 B2 B3 B4 B5	Japan China Indonesia China Philippines Vietnam Cambodia France Inuits	Lower HBsAg than A and D More likely to lose HBsAg than C and D B1 associated with fulminant hepatitis	93% strains have recombination	Perinatal	Responds better to interferon therapy than C and D
C	C1 C2 C3 C4 C5–C12 C13–C16	Thailand Myanmar Vietnam Japan, China, Korea New Caledonia Polynesia Australian aborigines Philippines Indonesia	High replication capacity can result in more severe disease Slower progression to HBeAg seroconversion Lower HBsAg levels than A and D	Higher frequency of BCP mutations than B and D	Perinatal	
D	D1 D2 D3 D4 D5 D6	Middle East, Central Asia Europe, Lebanon Universal Pacific Islands, Papua New Guinea, Arctic Denes, India India Tunisia Nigeria	Early HBeAg seroconversion D3 often associated with OBI	High prevalence of precore mutations	Horizontal	
E	None	Africa, Western and Central			Horizontal	
F	F1 F2 F3 F4	Argentina, Costa Rica, El Salvador Alaska Nicaragua Venezuela Brazil Venezuela Colombia Argentina			Horizontal	
G	None	France, Germany, US		Two stop codons prevent HBeAg expression; requires another genotype, usually A, to establish CHB	Horizontal: sexual transmission in MSM	
H	None	Mexico, Japan, Nicaragua, USA	Often associated with OBI		Perinatal	
I	I1 I2	Vietnam, Laos, China Vietnam, Laos, India		Recombinant of A, C, G		
J (putative)		Japan/Borneo				

Source: Data compiled from Honer et al. [9], Kramvis [22], Sunbul [21].
BCP, basal core promoter; CHB, chronic hepatitis B; MSM, men who have sex with men; OBI, occult HBV infection.

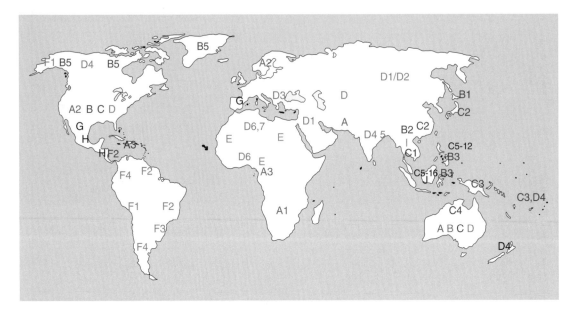

Figure 38.3 Worldwide distribution of hepatitis B virus genotypes.

pgRNA [8,26]. While routine testing for precore and BCP mutations is currently not recommended, it may become relevant as our understanding of HBV genetics becomes more nuanced.

Biomarkers associated with risk for progression

Chronic hepatitis B is a dynamic infection influenced by combination host and viral factors that dictate immunity, the emergency of mutants, and disease progression. Figure 38.2 delineates the five phases of chronic HBV infection, each defined by HBsAg status, HBV DNA level, HBeAg status, and ALT levels.

Future perspectives

Double-stranded linear DNA

Double-stranded linear DNA (dslDNA) is a minor genomic DNA formed through HBV RNA transcription. Once formed, it is secreted as a virion or recycled back into the nucleus where it undergoes integration into the host genome or reforms cccDNA. This means of viral integration contributes to HCC development through chromosomal

instability and mutagenesis [23]. Assays detecting dslDNA may therefore be a surrogate marker for integration and HCC development. Studies demonstrate higher dslDNA levels with cirrhosis, HCC, and antiviral therapy [27].

Spliced DNA/RNA

Truncated forms of RNA and DNA develop as a result of splicing during viral replication. Bayliss et al. demonstrated that spliced DNA and RNA sequences promote viral replication and may contribute to disease progression, HCC, and impaired response to interferon [28,29].

Empty particles

Empty enveloped nucleocapsids (HBsAg and HBcAg) are secreted in HBV replication along with virion particles (see Figure 38.2). The function of these particles remains unknown, given that they are unaffected by NA therapy and hence may estimate cccDNA transcriptional activity [30].

Gene expression

CCL4, IL-8, IFN-gamma, and FASLG represent genes of a cytokine-cytokine receptor that are downregulated in off-treatment remission. Through PBMC RNA analysis,

Kranidioti et al. suggested these genes could serve as biomarkers for predicting off-treatment remission in HBeAg-negative CHB patients [31].

Conclusion

Hepatitis B virus infection is complex and constantly evolving. Accurate diagnosis determining phases of HBV and stage of liver disease requires a consortium of biomarkers that provide key information on infectivity, treatment response, and disease progression. Newer biomarkers need to be further validated in larger cohorts but as new therapies emerge, they will play a vital role in diagnosing HBV, in drug development and in monitoring HBV infection on and off therapy, while they could potentially serve as endpoints in clinical trials.

References

1. Polaris Observatory Collaborators. Global prevalence, treatment, and prevention of hepatitis B virus infection in 2016: a modelling study. *Lancet Gastroenterology and Hepatology* 2018;3(6):383–403.
2. Stanaway JD, Flaxman A, Naghavi M et al. The global burden of viral hepatitis from 1990 to 2013: findings from the Global Burden of Disease Study 2013. *Lancet* 2016:388(10049):1081–1088.
3. Hsu YC, Mo L, Chang C et al. Association between serum level of hepatitis B surface antigen at end of entecavir therapy and risk of relapse in e antigen-negative patients. *Clinical Gastroenterology and Hepatology* 2016;14(10):1490–1498.e3.
4. Thompson AJ, Nguyen T, Iser D et al. Serum hepatitis B surface antigen and hepatitis B e antigen titers: disease phase influences correlation with viral load and intrahepatic hepatitis B virus markers. *Hepatology* 2010;51(6):1933–1944.
5. Hadziyannis SJ, Sevastianos V, Rapti I et al. Sustained responses and loss of HBsAg in HBeAg-negative patients with chronic hepatitis B who stop long-term treatment with adefovir. *Gastroenterology* 2012;143(3):629–636.e1.
6. Chen CJ, Yang H, Su J et al. Risk of hepatocellular carcinoma across a biological gradient of serum hepatitis B virus DNA level. *JAMA* 2006;295(1):65–73.
7. Allweiss L, Dandri M. The role of cccDNA in HBV maintenance. *Viruses* 2017;9(6):156.
8. Coffin CS., Zhou K, Terrault NA. New and old biomarkers for diagnosis and management of chronic hepatitis B virus infection. *Gastroenterology* 2019;156(2):355–368.e3.
9. Honer Zu Siederdissen C, Maasoumy B, Cornberg M. What is new on HBsAg and other diagnostic markers in HBV infection? *Best Practice and Research Clinical Gastroenterology* 2017;31(3):281–289.
10. Wang B, Carey I, Bruce M et al. HBsAg and HBcrAg as predictors of HBeAg seroconversion in HBeAg-positive patients treated with nucleos(t)ide analogues. *Journal of Viral Hepatitis* 2018;25(8):886–893.
11. Song G, Yang R, Rao H et al. Serum HBV core-related antigen is a good predictor for spontaneous HBeAg seroconversion in chronic hepatitis B patients. *Journal of Medical Virology* 2017;89(3):463–468.
12. Mak LY, Wong D, Cheung K et al. Review article: hepatitis B core-related antigen (HBcrAg): an emerging marker for chronic hepatitis B virus infection. *Alimentary Pharmacology and Therapeutics* 2018;47(1):43–54.
13. Wong DK, Seto W, Cheung K et al. Hepatitis B virus core-related antigen as a surrogate marker for covalently closed circular DNA. *Liver International* 2017;37(7):995–1001.
14. Tada T, Kumada T, Toyoda H et al. HBcrAg predicts hepatocellular carcinoma development: an analysis using time-dependent receiver operating characteristics. *Journal of Hepatology* 2016;65(1):48–56.
15. Giersch K, Allweiss L, Volz T et al. Serum HBV pgRNA as a clinical marker for cccDNA activity. *Journal of Hepatology* 2017;66(2):460–462.
16. van Bommel F. et al. Serum HBV RNA as a predictor of peginterferon alfa-2a response in patients with HBeAg-positive chronic hepatitis B. *Journal of Infectious Diseases* 2018:218(7):1066–1074.
17. Wang J, Yu T, Li G et al. Relationship between serum HBV-RNA levels and intrahepatic viral as well as histologic activity markers in entecavir-treated patients. *Journal of Hepatology* 2017; doi: 10.1016/j.jhep.2017.08.021.
18. Bömmel F, Bartens A, Mysickova A et al. Serum hepatitis B virus RNA levels as an early predictor of hepatitis B envelope antigen seroconversion during treatment with polymerase inhibitors. *Hepatology* 2015;61:66–76.
19. Jansen L, Kootstra N, van Dort K et al. Hepatitis B virus pregenomic RNA is present in virions in plasma and is associated with a response to pegylated interferon alfa-2a and nucleos(t)ide analogues. *Journal of Infectious Diseases* 2016;213(2):224–232.
20. Bai F, Yano Y, Fukumoto T et al. Quantification of pregenomic RNA and covalently closed circular DNA in hepatitis B virus-related hepatocellular carcinoma. *International Journal of Hepatology* 2013;2013:849290.
21. Sunbul M. Hepatitis B virus genotypes: global distribution and clinical importance. *World Journal of Gastroenterology* 2014;20(18):5427–5434.

22. Kramvis A. Genotypes and genetic variability of hepatitis B virus. *Intervirology* 2014;57(3–4):141–150.

23. Gaglio P, Singh S, Degertekin B et al. Impact of the hepatitis B virus genotype on pre- and post-liver transplantation outcomes. *Liver Transplantation* 2008;14(10):1420–1427.

24. Bayliss J, Yuen L, Rosenberg G et al. Deep sequencing shows that HBV basal core promoter and precore variants reduce the likelihood of HBsAg loss following tenofovir disoproxil fumarate therapy in HBeAg-positive chronic hepatitis B. *Gut* 2017;66(11):2013–2023.

25. Wu JF, Chiu Y, Chang K et al. Predictors of hepatitis B e antigen-negative hepatitis in chronic hepatitis B virus-infected patients from childhood to adulthood. *Hepatology* 2016;63(1):74–82.

26. Yang Z, Zhuang L, Lu Y et al. Naturally occurring basal core promoter A1762T/G1764A dual mutations increase the risk of HBV-related hepatocellular carcinoma: a meta-analysis. *Oncotarget* 2016;7(11):12525–12536.

27. Liu S, Zhou B, Valdes J et al. Serum hepatitis B virus RNA: a new potential biomarker for chronic hepatitis B virus infection. *Hepatology* 2019;69:1816–1827.

28. Bayliss J, Lim L, Thompson A et al. Hepatitis B virus splicing is enhanced prior to development of hepatocellular carcinoma. *Journal of Hepatology* 2013;59(5):1022–1028.

29. Jackson K, Locarnini S, Gish R. Diagnostics of hepatitis B virus: standard of care and investigational. *Clinical Liver Disease* 2018;12(1):5–11.

30. Hu J, Liu K. Complete and incomplete hepatitis B virus particles: formation, function, and application. *Viruses* 2017;9(3).

31. Kranidioti H, Manoloakopoulos S, Kontos G et al. Immunological biomarkers as indicators for outcome after discontinuation of nucleos(t)ide analogue therapy in patients with HBeAg negative chronic hepatitis B. *Journal of Viral Hepatitis* 2019;26:697–709.

PART IV
Ongoing Controversies

39 Is hepatocellular carcinoma risk impacted favorably or unfavorably by hepatitis C virus therapy with direct-acting antivirals?

Giuseppe Cabibbo, Calogero Cammà, and Antonio Craxì

Section of Gastroenterology and Hepatology, Dipartimento di Promozione della Salute, Materno Infantile, Medicina Interna e Specialistica di Eccellenza (PROMISE), University of Palermo, Palermo, Italy

LEARNING POINTS

- Cirrhosis is globally the strongest risk factor for HCC. HCV is a major risk factor in the Western world and Japan.
- DAAs have revolutionized the treatment of HCV infection, achieving high rates of sustained virologic response, in both compensated and decompensated cirrhosis, with high compliance to the therapy and a good safety profile.
- Despite some conflicting reports, use of DAAs improves outcomes in patients with HCV-related cirrhosis with or without HCC.

Hepatocellular carcinoma (HCC) is a major healthcare problem with an increasing incidence worldwide and a poor prognosis, and is the leading cause of mortality in patients with cirrhosis in the world [1]. Cirrhosis is the strongest risk factor for HCC, with hepatitis C virus (HCV) being a major risk factor in the Western world and Japan [2]. The prognosis for patients with cirrhosis due to HCV is driven by the progression towards hepatic decompensation and HCC, the latter being the leading cause of mortality in patients with compensated cirrhosis. In recent years, several studies of patients treated with interferon-based therapy have clearly documented that the risk for HCC was markedly lower in patients who achieved sustained virologic response (SVR) compared with those without an SVR [3].

In this context, the advent of the new direct-acting antivirals (DAAs) revolutionized the treatment of HCV infection, with very high rates (>90%) of SVR, very few contraindications, and low rate of adverse events [4]. There are no data from randomized controlled trials (RCTs) on the effect of HCV eradication by DAAs in patients with advanced or decompensated liver disease (with or without HCC), and in patients who were successfully treated for HCC. Moreover, RCTs comparing DAAs to no DAAs are not feasible, ethical or timely. Hence, the available data regarding HCC in these patients come from postmarketing surveillance, and mostly concern its occurrence (i.e., "*de novo*" HCC) or recurrence (relapse of previously cured HCC) during and after DAA treatment of patients with HCV cirrhosis.

This lack of data from RCTs is particularly relevant considering the recent alarm signal released about a potentially increased risk of early HCC recurrence in successfully treated patients who received DAA therapy, and increased risk of HCC occurrence with more aggressive tumor behavior after DAA treatment [5,6].

Hypothetically involved mechanisms regarding higher risk of HCC after DAA therapy focused on a loss of immune control owing to clearance of HCV-specific T-cells from the liver. Some researchers suggest that a rapid fall of antigenic load upon HCV eradication can promote a hyporesponsive state of memory helper T-cells and this new condition could have a role in the emergence of cancer events [7]. A recent study suggests that DAA-mediated

Clinical Dilemmas in Viral Liver Disease, Second Edition. Edited by Graham R. Foster and K. Rajender Reddy.
© 2020 John Wiley & Sons Ltd. Published 2020 by John Wiley & Sons Ltd.

increase of vascular endothelial growth factor (VEGF) favors HCC recurrence/occurrence in susceptible patients who already have abnormal activation in liver tissues of neo-angiogenetic pathways [8]. On the other hand, since DAA therapy is now the accepted standard of care in patients with HCV infection (mainly due to higher rate of SVR and its widely accepted effect on clinical outcomes such as decompensating events and all-cause mortality also in patients with advanced liver disease), RCTs comparing DAA to placebo are unethical and unfeasible.

The study of Conti et al. reported a high incidence (3.17% after 24 weeks of follow-up) of HCC after viral clearance [6]. Conversely, Kanwal et al. demonstrated, in a large retrospective cohort study that included 22 500 HCV patients treated with DAAs, an overall annual HCC incidence of 1.18% (95% confidence interval [CI] 1.04–1.32) [9]; interestingly, annual HCC incidence was markedly higher among patients who did not achieve SVR (3.45%; 95% CI 2.73–4.18) compared with those who did (0.90%; 95% CI 0.77–1.03).

Moreover, Calvaruso et al. collected data from a prospective study of 2249 consecutive patients with hepatitis C virus-associated cirrhosis (90.5% with Child–Pugh class A and 9.5% with Child--Pugh class B) treated with DAAs [10]. At one year after exposure to DAAs, HCC developed in 2.1% of patients with Child–Pugh class A with an SVR, 6.6% of patients with no SVR, 7.8% of patients with Child–Pugh class B with an SVR, and 12.4% of patients with no SVR (p<0.001 by log-rank test).

It is important to remember that the reported *de novo* occurrence rate after DAA therapy may be mainly due to the fact that patients with more advanced stages of cirrhosis (also in unselected Child–Pugh B class or with significant portal hypertension), who are at an intrinsically higher risk of cancer, can now have access to curative treatment. Conversely, when interferon/ribavirin was the only therapy option, treatment could be attempted only in well-compensated cirrhotic patients often without clinically significant portal hypertension, who are at lower risk of HCC.

Finally, the large metaanalysis conducted by Waziry et al., including 26 different studies (19 prospective, five retrospective, and two retrospective-prospective cohorts), achieved similar results in terms of HCC occurrence following SVR [11]: 1.14/199 per year [py] (95% CI 0.86–1.52) and 2.96/100 py (95% CI 5–29.58) in the interferon

and DAAs group respectively. Metaregression adjusting for study follow-up and age showed that DAA therapy was not associated with a higher HCC occurrence (relative risk [RR] 0.68; 95% CI 0.18–255; p=0.55).

Even if recent data from retrospective and prospective large cohort studies definitively clarified the benefit on reduction of HCC incident risk after SVR obtained with DAA, and that cirrhosis is the main driver of residual HCC risk after SVR [9,10], some doubts remain regarding the risk of HCC recurrence in successfully treated HCC, mainly because of methodologic limitations of the studies.

The clinical impact of DAA therapy on HCC recurrences is a controversial topic in which evidence is limited and sometimes contrasting, because these limitations are the results of different issues. First, as already mentioned, RCTs evaluating efficacy of DAA in patients successfully treated for HCC are lacking (and no longer feasible, ethical or timely); second, because observational studies are intrinsically affected by survivor treatment selection biases (i.e., misclassified or excluded immortal-time biases, as depicted in Figure 39.1), and all clinical practice data are characterized by a large number of methodologic weaknesses linked to this complex clinical context.

A retrospective analysis of 58 patients with prior HCC with complete response after resection, ablation or transarterial chemoembolization (TACE), and receiving antiviral therapy with DAA showed a radiologic tumor recurrence in 27.6% after a median follow-up of 5.7 months. No control group was included in this study [5]. Similarly, the study of Conti et al. evaluated recurrence of HCC after DAA therapy in 59 cirrhotic patients [6]. During the 24-week follow-up period, 17 (28.8%) patients showed HCC recurrences. Also in this study, no control group was included.

Conversely, data from three cohort studies including patients with chronic hepatitis C who were previously treated for HCC (HEPATHER study with 189 patients treated with DAA and 78 untreated patients; CirVir study with 13 patients treated with DAA and 66 untreated patients; and CUPILT study with 314 liver transplant recipients for HCC who were subsequently treated with DAA) showed no increase in HCC recurrence after DAA therapy compared to DAA-untreated patients [12].

Interestingly, recent studies have identified prior history of HCC recurrence as an independent predictor of HCC recurrence [13,14]; this result is particularly relevant as it

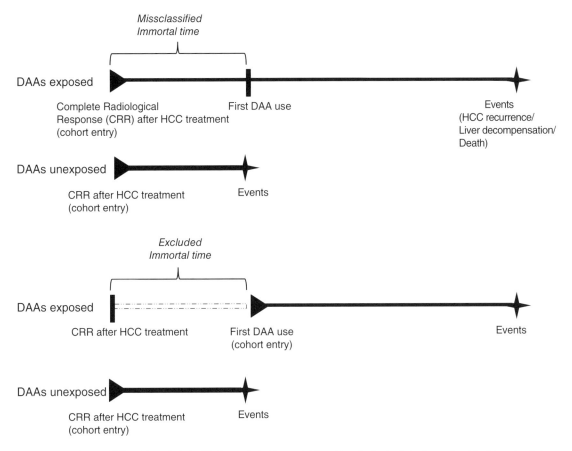

Figure 39.1 Immortal-time biases (misclassified or excluded immortal-time biases) of cohort studies on the risk of hepatocellular carcinoma (HCC) recurrences after direct-acting antiviral agents (DAAs).

underlines the wide heterogeneity of populations included in many studies.

Given the absence of RCTs with an untreated control arm (ethically unacceptable to design), a recently published metaanalysis of actuarial HCC survival and recurrence probabilities in patients with successfully treated HCC and compensated cirrhosis, without prior history of HCC recurrences, untreated for HCV [15], represents the benchmark reference control. This metaanalysis of 11 studies (701 patients) showed that pooled estimates of six-month, one-year and two-year recurrence probabilities were 7.4% (95% CI 4.0–10.0%), 20% (95% CI 12.7–27.4%), and 47% (95% CI 39.5–54.4%), respectively, while pooled estimates of three-year and five-year survival actuarial probabilities were 79.8% (95% CI 74.2–85.8%) and 58.6% (95% CI 51.1–67.1%).

So, how is it possible to definitively answer the question about a possible higher risk of HCC recurrence after DAA therapy? First, with cohort studies comparing DAA-untreated patients successfully treated for HCC with DAA-treated patients without history of recurrence; second, by metaanalysis of individual patient data, to better explore and explain heterogeneity of patients included in published studies. In the absence of the possibility of performing a RCT, propensity score methodology (propensity score matching and inverse probability treatment weighting [IPTW]) can be useful to compare DAA-treated and DAA-untreated patients and to substantiate the efficacy of DAA therapy in the improvement of significant clinical outcomes.

The impact of DAA treatment on overall survival was assessed for the first time in a multicenter prospective study conducted in a Italian cohort of patients at first diagnosis of early HCC who obtained a complete radiologic response after resection or ablation and were subsequently treated with DAAs [16]. DAA-treated patients (n = 163) were compared with a historical cohort of patients who did not receive treatment for HCV (n = 328) using propensity score matching and IPTW. Both the propensity score techniques showed that DAA treatment significantly improves overall survival, compared to no DAA treatment (hazard ratio [HR] 0.39; 95% CI 0.17–0.91; p=0.03, using propensity score matching). The risk for HCC recurrence was not significantly different between the two groups (HR 0.70; 95% CI 0.44–1.13; p=0.15), while a significant benefit of DAA treatment in reducing the risk of hepatic decompensation was observed (HR 0.32; 95% CI 0.13–0.84; p=0.02).

It has been speculated that the positive impact of DAAs on overall survival could be mediated by reduction of the risk for decompensation. The design of this study represents an attempt to emulate a randomized trial using observational data and for this purpose, authors mitigated the impact of time-related biases by performing time-dependent analyses and establishing a comparable index time for DAA-untreated patients. Both these approaches confirmed the positive impact of DAA therapy on overall survival.

Similarly, a large retrospective study conducted in North America on 793 patients who achieved complete response to HCC therapy compared DAA-treated (n = 304) and DAA-untreated patients (n = 489) using a propensity score model, showing that DAA therapy was not associated with HCC recurrence (HR 0.91, 95% CI 0.69–1.19) [17]. The authors addressed the issue of immortal-time bias using a landmark approach, confirming the same results and no differences were observed in HCC recurrence patterns between DAA-treated and DAA-untreated patients. These studies provided further evidence that DAA treatment after the achievement of complete radiologic response does not affect the risk for HCC recurrence that, although remaining high, is similar to that observed in DAA-untreated patients and that DAAs improve survival through the reduction of hepatic decompensation, which is the major driver of death in patients with successfully treated early HCC [18].

Another relevant point is related patients with viable HCC listed for liver transplant. In fact, some evidence has shown that in patients with decompensated cirrhosis and HCC, DAA treatment could improve liver function, reduce

risk of decompensation, and reduce waitlist dropout due to HCC progression or death [19,20].

Until that time, there is no evidence to avoid DAA treatment in patients without history of HCC, successfully treated for HCC, and listed for liver transplant (with or without HCC).

There is an urgent need for high-quality studies to evaluate benefit on clinical relevant outcomes of HCV eradication (risk of decompensation, HCC progression, and mortality) in patients with intermediate or advanced HCC on compensated cirrhosis.

References

1. European Association for the Study of the Liver. EASL Clinical Practice Guidelines: management of hepatocellular carcinoma. *Journal of Hepatology* 2018;69(1):182–236.
2. Torres HA, Shigle TL, Hammoudi N et al. The oncologic burden of hepatitis C virus infection: a clinical perspective. *CA Cancer Journal for Clinicians* 2017;67(5):411–431.
3. Morgan RL, Baack B, Smith BD, Yartel A, Pitasi M, Falck-Ytter Y. Eradication of hepatitis C virus infection and the development of hepatocellular carcinoma: a meta-analysis of observational studies. *Annals of Internal Medicine* 2013;158(5 Pt 1):329–337.
4. AASLD/IDSA HCV Guidance Panel. Hepatitis C guidance: AASLD-IDSA recommendations for testing, managing, and treating adults infected with hepatitis C virus. *Hepatology* 2015;62(3):932–954.
5. Reig M, Mariño Z, Perelló C et al. Unexpected high rate of early tumor recurrence in patients with HCV-related HCC undergoing interferon-free therapy. *Journal of Hepatology* 2016;65(4):719–726.
6. Conti F, Buonfiglioli F, Scuteri A et al. Early occurrence and recurrence of hepatocellular carcinoma in HCV-related cirrhosis treated with direct-acting antivirals. *Journal of Hepatology* 2016;65(4):727–733.
7. Dalai SK, Khoruzhenko S, Drake CG, Jie CC, Sadegh-Nasseri S. Resolution of infection promotes a state of dormancy and long survival of CD4 memory T cells. *Immunology and Cell Biology* 2011;89(8):870–881.
8. Faillaci F, Marzi L, Critelli R et al. Liver angiopoietin-2 is a key predictor of de novo or recurrent hepatocellular cancer after hepatitis C virus direct-acting antivirals. *Hepatology* 2018;68(3):1010–1024.
9. Kanwal F, Kramer J, Asch SM, Chayanupatkul M, Cao Y, El-Serag HB. Risk of hepatocellular cancer in HCV patients treated with direct-acting antiviral agents. *Gastroenterology* 2017;153(4):996–1005.e1.

10. Calvaruso V, Cabibbo G, Cacciola I et al., Rete Sicilia Selezione Terapia-HCV (RESIST-HCV). Incidence of hepatocellular carcinoma in patients with HCV-associated cirrhosis treated with direct-acting antiviral agents. *Gastroenterology* 2018;155(2):411–421.e4.

11. Waziry R, Hajarizadeh B, Grebely J et al. Hepatocellular carcinoma risk following direct-acting antiviral HCV therapy: a systematic review, meta-analyses, and meta-regression. *Journal of Hepatology* 2017;67(6):1204–1212.

12. ANRS Collaborative Study Group on Hepatocellular Carcinoma (ANRS CO22 HEPATHER, CO12 CirVir and CO23 CUPILT cohorts). Lack of evidence of an effect of direct-acting antivirals on the recurrence of hepatocellular carcinoma: data from three ANRS cohorts. *Journal of Hepatology* 2016;65(4):734–740.

13. Virlogeux V, Pradat P, Hartig-Lavie K et al. Direct-acting antiviral therapy decreases hepatocellular carcinoma recurrence rate in cirrhotic patients with chronic hepatitis C. *Liver International* 2017;37(8):1122–1127.

14. Cabibbo G, Petta S, Calvaruso V et al., Rete Sicilia Selezione Terapia-HCV (RESIST-HCV). Is early recurrence of hepatocellular carcinoma in HCV cirrhotic patients affected by treatment with direct-acting antivirals? A prospective multicentre study. *Alimentary and Pharmacology Therapeutics* 2017;46(7):688–695.

15. Cabibbo G, Petta S, Barbàra M et al., ITA.LI.CA Study Group. A meta-analysis of single HCV-untreated arm of studies evaluating outcomes after curative treatments of HCV-related hepatocellular carcinoma. *Liver International* 2017;37(8):1157–1166.

16. Cabibbo G, Celsa C, Calvaruso V et al. Direct-acting antivirals after successful treatment of early hepatocellular carcinoma improve survival in HCV-cirrhotic patients. *Journal of Hepatology* 2019;71:265–273.

17. Singal AG, Rich NE, Mehta N et al. Direct-acting antiviral therapy not associated with recurrence of hepatocellular carcinoma in a multicenter North American cohort study. *Gastroenterology* 2019;156(6):1683–1692.e1.

18. Cabibbo G, Petta S, Barbara M et al., Italian Liver Cancer (ITA.LI.CA) Study Group. Hepatic decompensation is the major driver of death in HCV-infected cirrhotic patients with successfully treated early hepatocellular carcinoma. *Journal of Hepatology* 2017;67(1):65–71.

19. Huang AC, Mehta N, Dodge JL, Yao FY, Terrault NA. Direct-acting antivirals do not increase the risk of hepatocellular carcinoma recurrence after local-regional therapy or liver transplant waitlist dropout. *Hepatology* 2018;68(2):449–461.

20. Belli LS, Berenguer M, Cortesi PA et al., European Liver and Intestine Association (ELITA). Delisting of liver transplant candidates with chronic hepatitis C after viral eradication: a European study. *Journal of Hepatology* 2016;65(3):524–531.

Global elimination of hepatitis C virus by 2030: the optimistic view

Gregory J. Dore and Marianne Martinello

The Kirby Institute, UNSW Sydney, Sydney, Australia

LEARNING POINTS

- The establishment of global HCV elimination 2030 targets has provided considerable impetus for national and international responses.

- Development of DAA therapy has generated the impetus for global HCV elimination, but primary prevention strategies, including high harm reduction coverage for people who inject drugs, are essential.

- Currently, 10 countries are considered on track to achieve HCV elimination targets by 2030, including both high-income and low- to middle-income countries.

- Strategies to enhance HCV screening and linkage to care are pivotal to the success of HCV elimination.

- Low-cost HCV diagnostics are as important as low-cost generic DAA therapy to global HCV elimination.

Introduction

Morbidity and mortality from infectious diseases, particularly acute infections, have progressively declined over the last century [1]. In recent decades, chronic infections have emerged as major global health threats, with annual deaths from HIV, tuberculosis, and chronic viral hepatitis (HBV and HCV) of 1.0 million, 1.2 million, and 1.3 million, respectively, evidence of their burden [2]. In recognition of this global disease burden, the United Nations Sustainable Development Goals proposed to "end the epidemics" of HIV, tuberculosis, and malaria, and "combat" viral hepatitis. In May 2016, the World Health Organization (WHO)

adopted the first global hepatitis strategy, setting the ambitious goal of "elimination of viral hepatitis as a public health threat" by 2030. HCV-specific targets included a 65% reduction in HCV-related mortality and an 80% reduction in HCV incidence (Table 40.1) [3,4].

Globally, around 70 million people were living with chronic HCV infection in 2016 [5]. Approximately 2 million new HCV infections occur annually, with injecting drug use and unsafe healthcare practices (including unsterile healthcare injection) the predominant modes of HCV transmission. Mortality from HCV-related cirrhosis and its complications, including hepatocellular carcinoma, is an estimated 475 000 deaths per year [6].

The development and availability of highly effective direct-acting antiviral agents (DAAs) have revolutionized HCV management and provide the therapeutic tools required to strive for elimination. In the absence of a vaccine, HCV elimination will require a combination of enhanced primary prevention activities and broad scale-up of DAA therapy (treatment as prevention). To achieve elimination, populations with high HCV prevalence and incidence will require targeted interventions. Despite major advances on the HCV therapeutic front, only 20% of people with chronic HCV are diagnosed, and around 5% have initiated HCV treatment.

In presenting the optimistic view of global HCV elimination, this chapter outlines the United Nations and WHO elimination targets, defines the epidemiologic concepts of *control*, *elimination*, and *eradication*, and discusses strategies required to achieve global HCV elimination. Examples of

Clinical Dilemmas in Viral Liver Disease, Second Edition. Edited by Graham R. Foster and K. Rajender Reddy.
© 2020 John Wiley & Sons Ltd. Published 2020 by John Wiley & Sons Ltd.

Table 40.1 World Health Organization HCV elimination targets

	2015 Baseline	2020 Target	2030 Target
Impact targets			
INCIDENCE	1 750 000	30% reduction 1 230 000	80% reduction <350 000
New cases of HCV infection			
MORTALITY	399 000	10% reduction 359 100	65% reduction 139 650
HCV-related deaths[a]			
Service delivery targets			
DIAGNOSIS	20%	30%	90%
Proportion diagnosed with HCV			
TREATMENT UPTAKE	7%	Not specified (3 million[b])	80% (cumulative)
Proportion with HCV diagnosed and initiated on treatment			
BLOOD SAFETY	97%	95%	100%
Donations screened with quality assurance			
INJECTION SAFETY	5%	0%	0%
Proportion of unsafe injections			
HARM REDUCTION	27	200	300
Number of sterile needles and syringes distributed per person who injects drugs per year			

[a] Death predominantly due to hepatocellular carcinoma and cirrhosis.
[b] Total cumulative HCV treatment uptake target by 2020.
Source: Compiled from references [3, 4,11].

successful national HCV strategies are presented, highlighting the facilitators and barriers to implementation of HCV elimination strategies. Elimination of HCV infection will require an enormous public health, political and economic commitment, but will have considerable potential benefits.

Infectious diseases elimination and HCV elimination as a global target

The holy grail of global infectious disease efforts is *eradication*, defined as *permanent reduction to zero of the worldwide incidence of infection* (Table 40.2) [7]. With only smallpox on the list of eradicated human infections, the prospect of adding HCV this century is remote. Epidemiological *elimination*, defined as *reduction to zero of the incidence of disease or infection in a defined geographical area*, is more achievable for HCV but presents considerable challenges, particularly without a highly effective vaccine on the horizon.

In striving for infectious disease elimination, three factors are of primary importance when considering biological and technical feasibility.

- The availability of an effective intervention (to disrupt transmission).
- The availability of practical, sensitive, and specific diagnostic tools.
- The role of humans in the life cycle of the pathogen (with no other vertebrate reservoir and no amplification in the environment).

In relation to HCV, effective therapeutic and prevention interventions are available to curb HCV transmission, HCV diagnostics are evolving to allow broader access and implementation, and infected humans are the exclusive reservoir of HCV in nature.

The DAA therapy era has transformed clinical management and provided great optimism for the global response. But, are global HCV elimination efforts realistic, particularly as HCV epidemiological *control* would have been more feasible? The WHO has clearly opted for HCV elimination, although an examination of the ambitious global viral hepatitis elimination 2030 targets indicates they are considerably less strict than the above epidemiologic

Table 40.2 Dahlem Workshop on the Eradication of Infectious Diseases

Epidemiologic term	Definition	Example(s)
Control	The reduction of disease incidence, prevalence, morbidity or mortality to a locally acceptable level as a result of deliberate efforts; continued intervention measures are required to maintain the reduction	Diarrheal diseases Schistosomiasis
Elimination of disease	Reduction to zero of the incidence of a specified disease in a defined geographical area as a result of deliberate efforts; continued intervention measures are required	Neonatal tetanus
Elimination of infection	Reduction to zero of the incidence of infection caused by a specific agent in a defined geographical area as a result of deliberate efforts; continued measures to prevent reestablishment of transmission are required	Measles Poliomyelitis
Eradication	Permanent reduction to zero of the worldwide incidence of infection caused by a specific agent as a result of deliberate efforts; intervention measures are no longer needed	Smallpox
Extinction	The specific infectious agent no longer exists in nature or in the laboratory	None

Source: Adapted from reference [7].

elimination definition. The use of *elimination* rather than *control* may simply relate to the enhanced aspirational element associated with the former term, and consistent with global efforts in relation to HBV, HIV, malaria, and tuberculosis.

Progress towards HCV elimination targets

At the end of 2017, 12 countries were considered "on track" to achieve WHO HCV elimination 2030 targets, including several high-income countries (Australia, France, Iceland, Italy, Japan, Netherlands, Spain, Switzerland, United Kingdom) and three low- to middle-income countries (Egypt, Georgia, Mongolia) (Table 40.3). In Egypt, the more than 1 million people treated since 2015 (of 6 million with chronic HCV) demonstrates what can be achieved in a low- to middle-income country setting with national leadership, low drug pricing, and development of an effective infrastructure for broad screening and delivery of therapy. An enormous task lies ahead to maintain this therapeutic momentum, through massive population-based HCV screening and linkage to care.

In many countries, declining DAA treatment numbers have followed the initial "warehouse" treatment effect. In Australia, 32 600 people with chronic HCV (of an estimated 227 000 total population) were treated in 2016 (Australian Government funding for DAA therapy commenced in March 2016), 21 400 treated in 2017, and 16 000 treated in 2018. Thus, around 70 000 people (30% of

chronic HCV population) have been treated since unrestricted DAA access began. Recent modeling indicates that a treatment level of around 14 000 per year in Australia will be required to achieve HCV elimination targets [8], although somewhat surprisingly, the 65% mortality reduction is more difficult than the 80% incidence reduction. The difficulty in achieving the mortality reduction target relates to the pre-DAA era mortality trajectory which was progressively increasing, with an expected further doubling by 2030 without DAA therapy. Thus, to turn around a rising mortality burden requires particularly high DAA uptake among those with more advanced disease, and probably reductions in liver-related comorbidity such as alcohol dependency.

The Australian success to date is related to several factors. Strong political leadership and national strategic development (National strategies since 2000, currently in the fifth National Hepatitis C Strategy), and well-established partnerships between government, clinical, academic, community and other stakeholders have been crucial. Centralized national independent assessment of new therapies (through the Pharmaceutical Benefits Advisory Committee) for Australian government subsidization together with robust price negotiations between the Australian government and the pharmaceutical industry were key to an internationally important unrestricted DAA program development for the period 2016–2020. Universal healthcare and strong harm reduction implementation were foundations for equity of access across socioeconomic

Table 40.3 Progress in policy and healthcare initiatives in countries on track to achieve the WHO 2030 HCV elimination targets

	Australia	France	Georgia	Italy	Spain	UK
National HCV strategy	✓	✓	✓	✓	✓	✓
National clinical guidelines for diagnosis and treatment of HCV	✓	✓	✓	✓	✓	✓
National expert advisory group	✓	✓	✓	✓	✓	✓
Mandatory blood donor screening	✓	✓	✓	✓	✓	✓
Harm reduction for PWID	✓	✓	✓	✓	✓	✓
Needle and syringe program	✓	✓	✓	✓	✓	✓
Opioid substitution therapy						
Publicly funded HCV screening	✓	✓	✓	✓	✓	✓
Government subsidized DAA therapy	✓	✓	✓	✓	✓	✓
DAA prescriber type	✓	✓	✓	✓	✓	✓
Specialist	✓	χ	χ	χ	χ	χ
General practitioner/primary care						

Source: Compiled from references [12–15].
DAA, direct-acting antiviral; PWID, people who inject drugs.

groups. The high initial DAA uptake, including among marginalized PWID populations [9], is testament to the importance of these foundations.

Mongolia, with a very high burden of HCV infection (HCV viremic prevalence >10%) and hepatocellular carcinoma among the general population, has demonstrated the impact of societal and political will in establishing an HCV elimination strategy in a low- to middle-income country (LMIC), with approximately 20 000 people having received DAA treatment (of an estimated 200 000 total population). With the publication of the Hepatitis Prevention, Control and Elimination Program 2016–2020, the Mongolian government allocated 232 billion Mongolian tögrög (approximately US$96 million) in funding, added HBV and HCV therapy to the national health insurance scheme (which covers most of the population) and petitioned for significant discounting in the cost of DAA therapy (generic sofosbuvir-ledipasvir, US$65).

Strategies required to enhance global HCV elimination efforts

Although HCV meets biological and technical criteria for potential HCV elimination, a successful elimination strategy must also consider contemporary economic, social, and political factors. Globally, financial, political, structural, and social barriers exist which complicate efforts to achieve HCV elimination in many countries and

regions. Challenges to HCV elimination include limited reliable epidemiologic data; inadequate HCV testing and resultant poor levels of diagnosis; limited access to care, treatment and harm reduction (particularly for PWID); a lack of HCV education and training for healthcare providers; continued healthcare-associated transmission (in LMIC); prevailing stigma and discrimination against people living with HCV and people at high risk of HCV; variable leadership and commitment from policy makers and governments; and financial barriers to testing, treatment, and care.

Clear momentum has developed internationally over the last three years since the launch of the WHO HCV elimination targets. Many countries have developed dedicated hepatitis C or viral hepatitis national strategies, a fundamental step towards elimination. Political will and advocacy are being developed and driven in many settings, and organizations such as UNITE – Parliamentarians Network to End HIV/AIDS, Viral Hepatitis and Tuberculosis are providing critical leadership. The mission of UNITE is to provide a global platform of current and former policy makers to raise awareness and advocate to end HIV/AIDS, viral hepatitis, and other infectious diseases as public health threats by 2030. These political and strategic developments, including enhanced leadership from the WHO, need to be strengthened.

Innovation, in the form of development of DAA therapy, has promoted the current optimism in the HCV sector.

The completion of DAA development pathways by the major pharmaceutical companies should not be an impediment to further innovation. Further therapeutic strategy development, including evaluation of shorter duration (4–6-week) DAA therapy, and exploration of technologies for delivery of long-acting antiviral therapy are essential. Global public and private sector investment is required to propel innovation, and organizations such as UNITAID will be pivotal to support and stimulate development of innovative therapeutic strategies. Innovation will also be crucial in the HCV diagnostic arena, to enable simplification of HCV screening and treatment monitoring through cheaper and more rapid tests that can be employed in centralized and decentralized point-of-care settings. HCV screening strategies will clearly need to be adapted to local epidemiology and budgetary considerations but the highly successful HCV screening programs in Egypt, Mongolia, and Georgia demonstrate what can be achieved in diverse settings.

Direct-acting antiviral therapy will play a key elimination role in relation to its treatment as prevention benefits, but strengthening of primary prevention strategies is even more crucial. Improvements have been made in recent years in global blood safety and infection control, but enhanced efforts are required. Harm reduction is appallingly inadequate globally, with only 1% of PWID living in countries with high coverage of needle syringe programs and opiate agonist therapy [10]. Pivotal will be harm reduction advances in countries with large PWID populations and suboptimal harm reduction, including the US, Russia, and China. Drug law reform is also essential to address issues of stigma, discrimination, and inequity in health service provision among many PWID populations.

Recent modeling indicates that global HCV elimination targets are achievable, but will require implementation of a comprehensive package of interventions. A combination of strategies to reduce risk of transmission through blood safety and infection control, PWID harm reduction, DAA treatment at diagnosis, and massive increases in screening are required. Importantly, several countries are pivotal to HCV elimination due to their large burden of infection, with successful implementation in China, India, Pakistan, and Egypt crucial to achieving global targets. Although the greatest contribution to HCV incidence reduction will come from blood safety and infection control measures, the modeling also indicates that PWID harm reduction gains are essential.

Reasons for optimism

The last three years have seen major strides in the global HCV response. Ongoing pharmaceutical company competition and advocacy have led to reductions in DAA pricing and parallel progressive removal of liver disease stage-based restrictions in many settings. Generic DAA production, coupled with many LMIC voluntary licenses and the occasional compulsory licence, should mean drug pricing is not a major impediment to achieving WHO HCV elimination targets.

Despite some setbacks, the overall trends are favorable in relation to globalism and public health responses. HCV elimination is an enormous challenge, but an optimistic approach to this challenge will bring considerable direct and indirect benefits. Development of simplified HCV treatment strategies, including primary care and community health-based models of care, will support the global health system reform agenda. The drive to engage with marginalized populations, including PWID and prisoners, in relation to HCV assessment and treatment has the potential to enhance harm reduction implementation and address the high levels of comorbidity in these populations.

Ultimately, optimism and progressive strategic development will prevail over pessimism and conservatism. The WHO HCV elimination targets may or may not be reached, but to strive to achieve these targets is the only way forward.

References

1. Lozano R, Naghavi M, Foreman K et al. Global and regional mortality from 235 causes of death for 20 age groups in 1990 and 2010: a systematic analysis for the Global Burden of Disease Study 2010. *Lancet* 2012;380(9859):2095–2128.
2. GBD 2016 Causes of Death Collaborators. Global, regional, and national age-sex specific mortality for 264 causes of death, 1980-2016: a systematic analysis for the Global Burden of Disease Study 2016. *Lancet* 2017;390(10100):1151–1210.
3. World Health Organization. Global Health Sector Strategy n Viral Hepatitis, 2016–2021. Geneva: World Health Organization, 2016.
4. United Nations General Assembly. Transforming Our World: the 2030 Agenda for Sustainable Development 2015. https://sustainabledevelopment.un.org/post2015/transformingourworld/publication

5. Blach S, Zeuzem S, Manns M et al. Global prevalence and genotype distribution of hepatitis C virus infection in 2015: a modelling study. *Lancet Gastroenterology and Hepatology* 2017;2(3):161–176.

6. Stanaway JD, Flaxman AD, Naghavi M et al. The global burden of viral hepatitis from 1990 to 2013: findings from the Global Burden of Disease Study 2013. *Lancet* 2016;388(10049):1081–1088.

7. Dowdle WR. The principles of disease elimination and eradication. *Bulletin of the World Health Organization* 1998;76 Suppl 2:22–25.

8. Kwon JA, Dore GJ, Grebely J et al. Australia on track to achieve WHO HCV elimination targets following rapid initial DAA treatment uptake: a modelling study. *Journal of Viral Hepatitis* 2019;26(1):83–92.

9. Iversen J, Dore GJ, Catlett B, Cunningham P, Grebely J, Maher L. Association between rapid utilisation of direct hepatitis C antivirals and decline in the prevalence of viremia among people who inject drugs in Australia. *Journal of Hepatology* 2019;70(1):33–9.

10. Grebely J, Larney S, Peacock A et al. Global, regional, and country-level estimates of hepatitis C infection among people who have recently injected drugs. *Addiction* 2019;114:150–166.

11. World Health Organization. Global Hepatitis Report 2017. Geneva: World Health Organization, 2017.

12. Centre for Disease Analysis, Polaris Observatory. http://cdafound.org/polaris-hepc-dashboard/

13. Hajarizadeh B, Grebely J, Matthews GV, Martinello M, Dore GJ. Uptake of direct-acting antiviral treatment for chronic hepatitis C in Australia. *Journal of Viral Hepatitis* 2018;25:640–648.

14. Dore GJ, Hajarizadeh B. Elimination of hepatitis C virus in Australia: Laying the foundation. *Infectious Disease Clinics of North America* 2018;32(2):269–279.

15. Nasrullah M, Sergeenko D, Gamkrelidze A, Averhoff F. HCV elimination – lessons learned from a small Eurasian country, Georgia. *Nature Reviews Gastroenterology and Hepatology* 2017;14:447.

Global elimination of hepatitis C virus by 2030: the pessimistic view

Thomas G. Cotter and Michael Charlton

Center for Liver Diseases, University of Chicago Medicine, Chicago, IL, USA

LEARNING POINTS

- The WHO has defined its HCV elimination targets as a 65% reduction in mortality (to less than 500 000 deaths per year) and an 80% reduction in incidence (to less than 1 million new infections per year) by 2030 from the 2015 baseline.

- While HCV infection meets criteria for elimination, current screening strategies globally are inadequate and resource allocation for screening and treatment is largely inadequate, particularly in resource-constrained countries.

- Globally, preventive strategies, although better with blood screening for HCV prior to transfusion, still need to be improved, to decrease the incidence of HCV, while treatments for chronic HCV are not widely available and affordable.

- True global elimination of HCV infection is not possible by 2030. Even the goals outlined by the WHO, which effectively amount to epidemiologic control, appear to be profoundly optimistic considering we are currently not on target for any of the aspects of the required multifaceted approach.

Introduction

It is estimated that 71 million individuals have hepatitis C virus (HCV) viremia worldwide, with the incidence still increasing [1]. If left untreated, chronic infection can lead to advanced liver disease with associated high morbidity and mortality rates from complications of decompensated disease, including hepatocellular carcinoma [2]. Since its molecular characterization by Michael Houghton and colleagues in 1988 [3], there have been remarkable advances in the diagnosis and treatment of HCV infection. Short-term oral pangenotypic direct-acting antiviral (DAA) therapy achieves sustained virologic response (SVR) in >95% of patients with HCV [2]. The observed effectiveness of DAA therapy has raised the theoretical possibility of HCV elimination. In this chapter we explore the headwinds faced in global HCV elimination efforts.

Like so many goals, achievability varies with the defined endpoint. The Dahlem Workshop on the Eradication of Infectious Diseases defined elimination as a reduction to zero of the incidence of infection in a geographical area as a result of deliberate efforts, with ongoing intervention measures required (e.g., measles) [4]. Control of infection is defined as the reduction of disease incidence, prevalence, morbidity, or mortality to a locally acceptable level [4]. The success of the DAA therapy instigated a commitment from all 194 member states of the World Health Organization (WHO) to eliminate HCV infection as a public health threat [5]. The WHO defined its HCV elimination targets as a 65% reduction in mortality (to less than 500 000 deaths per year) and an 80% reduction in incidence (to less than 1 million new infections per year) by 2030 from the 2015 baseline [5]. Even the lesser goals defined by the WHO, more in line with epidemiologic control considering the afore-mentioned accepted epidemiologic definitions, would represent an enormous worldwide health success if achieved.

Clinical Dilemmas in Viral Liver Disease, Second Edition. Edited by Graham R. Foster and K. Rajender Reddy
© 2020 John Wiley & Sons Ltd. Published 2020 by John Wiley & Sons Ltd.

On the surface, global HCV elimination would seem to be possible. HCV meets accepted criteria for disease elimination based on features of the infectious agents (reliably detected, and absence of a nonhuman reservoir), the magnitude of the health problem, and the effectiveness of interventions to prevent transmission and treat the disease [6]. Elimination of viral infectious diseases has, however, been a rarity with, hitherto, only one disease (smallpox) being eliminated globally. Importantly, smallpox has a highly effective vaccine, something HCV infection still lacks.

Achieving any meaningfully defined elimination of HCV will require a multifaceted approach, including identifying individuals with HCV infection, improving preventive services, and upscaling treatment programs. Unfortunately, there are impervious barriers to each of these domains, making it impossible for global elimination of HCV infection to be achieved by 2030; even the WHO goals to achieve epidemiologic control appear profoundly optimistic.

Underdiagnosis of HCV infection

One indicator of the likelihood of achieving HCV elimination is the effectiveness of current screening and treatment recommendations and policies. Of the 71 million individuals with HCV infection globally, only 14 million (20%) have been diagnosed [7]. Failure to diagnose HCV is thus a major hurdle in the elimination cascade, one which has prompted the World Hepatitis Alliance's rallying cry to "find the missing millions." The WHO has aimed for 90% diagnosed by 2030, which is the level where the benefits of DAAs will be fully reaped, according to a recent simulation modeling study [8].

As part of its initial attempts to address this shortcoming, the WHO recommended routine HCV testing of certain populations based on defined exposure risks or settings, and in populations with >5% seroprevalence of HCV antibody [9]. However, this approach has a number of limitations including lack of knowledge and/or time by physicians to assess for these risk factors, and reluctance of some patients to disclose risk factors. Recognizing these limitations, in 2012 the USA recommended one-time HCV testing for the 1945–1965 birth cohort or "baby boomers," after epidemiologic studies identified this cohort as having the highest prevalence of HCV (50% of all infections). This addition to the screening recommendations coincided with

a decrease of undiagnosed HCV in the US from 70% to 50% from 2012 to 2016 [10].

However, to meet the WHO goal of 90% diagnosed by 2030, the targeted rate of diagnosis needs to be 110 000 annually until 2020, 89 000 annually between 2020 and 2024, and >70 000 annually between 2025 and 2030 [11]. Achieving this will require extraordinary efforts, especially in the face of shifting demographics where increasing numbers of young adults now have HCV infection, outnumbering baby boomers in some US states [12]. Certainly, another change in the HCV screening recommendations will be required in the near future. One potential solution is the adoption of one-time HCV screening for all adults, akin to the current HIV recommendation. One-time HCV screening has been shown to be cost-effective in a recent health model [13]. Absent such a policy, WHO HCV elimination targets will not be achieved.

The US is the third leading country in the world for proportion of spending on essential services (which includes healthcare), with 22.6% of its total expenditure appropriated to these services [14]. There are 31 countries in the WHO which spend less than 5% of their total expenditure on essential services, including Mozambique at 1.8%, Bangladesh at 2.8%, Iraq at 1.7% and Venezuela at 3.1% [14]. Given the difficulties the US will have reaching the WHO goals, there is little hope for countries who allocate much lower financial resources to healthcare.

There are ongoing efforts to make cheaper and simpler screening assays available, such as point-of-care viral load fingerstick tests [15], but these are still not widely available on a global scale. Currently, Malta is the only country out of the 194 WHO members which is estimated to have diagnosis coverage at the WHO level [16]. Expecting all the other 193 countries, almost all of which are more populous and more complex geographically and demographically than Malta, to reach this high level of diagnosis coverage is ambitious, to say the least.

Inadequate prevention strategies

Considering the absence of an effective vaccine, the most critical tool in the elimination of smallpox infection, the primary prevention of HCV transmission is as important as treating those already infected in any HCV elimination strategy. The effect of prevention interventions on incidence of HCV infection is primarily dependent on local epidemiology. In general, lower income countries, such as Egypt, Mongolia, and Pakistan, benefit greatly from improvements in blood safety and infection control, while countries who have a large proportion of the HCV epidemic concentrated in people who inject drugs (PWIDs), such as the USA, Australia, and Spain, benefit more from interventions targeting this population.

In contrast to population or cohort screening, screening blood donors for HCV has been widely successful. There have been a number of initiatives, including the WHO Blood Transfusion Safety Program [17], which have helped to meet the 2020 performance targets for blood safety, with 97% of all blood donations globally now being screened for HCV [18]. Strenuous efforts are required to sustain this progress at the current level, particularly in low-income countries such as those in sub-Saharan Africa [19]. Despite this improvement, it is important to note that currently only 39% of countries worldwide operate hemovigilance systems [17].

Impressive improvements have also occurred in unsafe injections, with an 88% decrease in the proportion of injections administered with nonsterile equipment and an 83% decrease in HCV infection attributed to unsafe injections from 2000 to 2010 [20]. This progress was made essentially through a reduction in the reuse of injection devices. While substantial progress has been made, the Eastern Mediterranean region remains problematic, with 0.57 unsafe injections per person annually, while globally, 8% of injections continue to be given with unsterilized equipment [7]. Evidently, unsafe (often unnecessary) injections continue to be a major source of HCV infection and will hamper efforts to achieve the WHO's goal of an 80% reduction in incidence of HCV by 2030 [20].

With the notable improvements in blood safety and infection control, the successful elimination of HCV transmission is dependent on the effectiveness of HCV prevention among PWIDs. This is especially important considering that injection drug use is now the primary route of HCV transmission, with a 75% HCV antibody prevalence observed in PWIDs [21]. For this population, adequate access with high coverage (i.e., >100% of injections covered by a sterile needle) to opioid substitution therapy (OST) and needle exchange programs (NEPs) can reduce HCV transmission by up to 71% [22]. Although demonstrably effective, safe injection services are in short supply globally. In 2017, of 179 countries, only 93 and 86 countries reported having needle exchange and OST programs, respectively

[7]. Thirty-three sets of needles/syringes were distributed per PWID per year, which is far below the WHO targets of 200 and 300 distributions for 2020 and 2030, respectively [23]. As a specific example, the USA only provided 30 needles/syringes and only 19 OST treatments per PWID per year, despite a threefold increase in HCV incidence related to the opiate epidemic [23]. The Centers for Disease Control and Prevention (CDC) estimates that a sevenfold increase in NEPs, to 2200 NEPs, is required to serve the current number of PWIDs in the USA [24]. The resources and political will do not appear to be present in order to meet this increase.

Linkage to treatment services is an important concept, with full harm reduction (high-coverage NEPs + OST) shown to strengthen the effect of reducing HCV transmission to 79%, from 52% [25]. In addition, PWIDs can obtain testing and definitive HCV treatment when needed. Unfortunately, there are waiting lists at several NEPs, preventing many PWIDs from accessing treatment [26]. Additional populations, such as prisoners, require vastly improved access to these interventions considering that 26% of incarcerated persons have been infected with HCV [27]. This population currently has meager access to NEPs and OST.

A recently published simulation modeling study showed the WHO incidence elimination goal being met by 2032 after increasing coverage of full harm reduction to 40% (this was assuming other targets in diagnosis, prevention, and treatment were already met) [8]. However, only 1% of PWID live in countries with such high coverage of these services [23]. This highlights the remoteness of achieving the WHO's lofty elimination goals by 2030. In fact, if the efficacy of these harm reduction services is lower than the estimates in some settings [28], this "elimination" target will not be reached until after 2050. The required scaling up of harm reduction services by 2030 is not possible, especially when considering the volatility of political will and reliable sources of funding globally, both of which are vital for harm reduction services to succeed, as observed in the impressive Hepatitis C Action Plan program in Scotland [29].

Undertreatment of HCV infection

As part of its elimination strategy, the goal of the WHO is 80% treatment rate by 2030 [5]. Firstly, it is important to acknowledge that the treatment of only those already in care will not translate into substantial reductions in HCV deaths or incidence, and identifying the "missing millions" is essential in order to see the full benefit of treatment. While highly effective DAA therapy is available, accessibility remains an issue [2]. The current treatment rate is extremely low, with only 7% of those diagnosed with HCV having received treatment. According to the Global Hepatitis Report 2017, only 1.1 million HCV patients were on treatment in the year 2015 [30], and in 2016, only 1.76 million additional HCV patients received treatment [31].

The reason for the profound undertreatment of patients is more than just the cost, although this remains the primary issue. As an example, while costs per treatment course have markedly decreased in the USA from $84 000–$96 000 to about $25 000 [32], there are still 12 states which continue to deny HCV treatment until patients develop severe liver fibrosis [33]. Patients

covered by Medicaid experience increased rates of treatment denial and have restrictions on who can prescribe DAA therapy. Restrictions based on recent drug use result in the inability to cure those with the highest risk for transmission. Restricting treatment to only those with advanced fibrosis ignores the morbidity associated with chronic infection, including fatigue, and the extrahepatic complications, such as lymphoma [34]. In addition, HCV cure before the development of advanced fibrosis eliminates the risk of future liver cancer and obviates the need for ongoing HCC screening. For all these reasons, treatment of HCV, regardless of stage, is the best strategy, with cost-effective analyses clearly showing the cost-benefit of this strategy [35]. The simplicity of current DAA therapy allows primary care providers (PCPs) to move into the primary position for treatment, which has helped with accessibility.

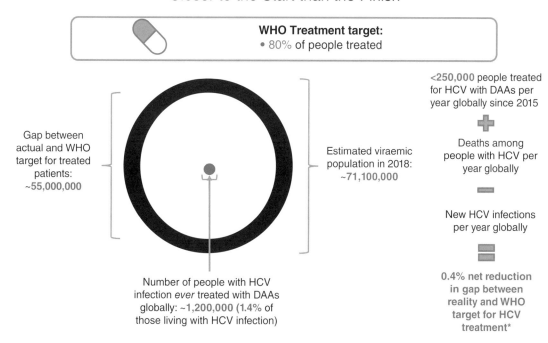

Figure 41.1 The global race to eliminate HCV: closer to the start than the finish. *Source*: Blach S et al. *Lancet Gastroenterology and Hepatology* 2017;2:161–176; WHO. Hepatitis C – Fact Sheet, updated October 2017. www.who.int/mediacentre/factsheets/fs164/en/; Polaris Observatory. http://polarisobservatory.org/polaris/hepC.htm.*Hill et al. *Journal of Virus Eradication* 2017;3(3):117–123.

Approved DAAs have been included in the WHO's Model List of Essential Medications to facilitate high-level drug price negotiations in countries that have national drug plans, and as a result over 100 countries now have access to generic medicines for $200 or less per curative treatment [7]. For example, Egypt has received a 99% price reduction. Even at these lower costs, middle- to low-income countries with a high prevalence of HCV infection still have difficulty increasing their treatment rates. Of HCV-infected persons, 62% live in countries where generic HCV medications are available [7]. However, in 2016, only 10 countries (Australia, France, Germany, Iceland, Spain, the Netherlands, Egypt, Qatar, Japan, and the USA) had treated 7% of their HCV-infected population and 44 countries had treated <1%. As a result, in 2017, the global population of HCV-infected persons decreased by only 300 000 (0.4%) persons, to an estimated 69.55 million [36]. The prevalence is *increasing* in sub-Saharan Africa and Eastern Europe. Far higher rates of DAA treatment are required for worldwide elimination of HCV (Figure 41.1). Considering these factors, it is highly unlikely that the WHO goals for treatment rate will be met.

As an extension of HCV treatment, there is the subset population of PWID who are high priority because of both the high burden of infection and the potential to transmit to others. The success of treating PWIDs is well established, as evidenced by the 94% SVR rate observed in the SIMPLIFY trial [37]. Moreover, treatment outcomes for PWID are comparable to those for other HCV-infected persons, and the risk of reinfection is low (0.0–6.4/100 person-years) [38]. Targeted treatment as prevention approaches among PWID need to be done in the context of enhanced harm reduction interventions. As outlined in the preceding section, the required scaling up of harm reduction services which provide a vital linkage to treatment is unlikely to occur by 2030.

Conclusion

True global elimination of HCV infection is not possible by 2030. Even the goals outlined by the WHO, which effectively amount to epidemiologic control, appear to be profoundly optimistic considering we are currently not on target for any of the aspects of the required multifaceted approach.

References

1. Polaris Observatory HCV Collaborators. Global prevalence and genotype distribution of hepatitis C virus infection in 2015: a modelling study. *Lancet Gastroenterology and Hepatology* 2017;2:161–176.
2. AASLD-IDSA Guidance Panel. Hepatitis C guidance: AASLD-IDSA recommendations for testing, managing, and treating adults infected with hepatitis C virus. *Hepatology* 2015;62:932–954.
3. Houghton M. The long and winding road leading to the identification of the hepatitis C virus. *Journal of Hepatology* 2009;51:939–948.
4. Dowdle WR. The Eradication of Infectious Diseases: Report of the Dahlem Workshop on the Eradication of Infections Diseases. Chichester: John Wiley & Sons, 1998.
5. World Health Organization. Global Health Sector Strategy on Viral Hepatitis 2016–2021. https://apps.who.int/iris/bitstream/handle/10665/246177/WHO-HIV-2016.06-eng.pdf?sequence=1
6. Centers for Disease Control and Prevention. The principles of disease elimination/eradication. In: Global Disease Elimination and Eradication as Public Health Strategies. www.cdc.gov/mmwr/pdf/other/mm48SU01.pdf
7. Hutin YJ, Bulterys M, Hirnschall GO. How far are we from viral hepatitis elimination service coverage targets? *Journal of the International AIDS Society* 2018;21 Suppl 2:e25050.
8. Heffernan A, Cooke GS, Nayagam S et al. Scaling up prevention and treatment towards the elimination of hepatitis C: a global mathematical model. *Lancet* 2019;393:1319–1329.
9. World Health Organization. Guidelines on Hepatitis B and C Testing. Geneva: World Health Organization. http://apps.who.int/iris/bitstream/handle/10665/254621/9789241549981-eng.pdf;jsessionid.47D22C07727811EA
10. Barocas JA, Wang J, White LF et al. Hepatitis C testing increased among baby boomers following the 2012 change to CDC testing recommendations. *Health Affairs* 2017;36:2142–2150.
11. National Academies of Sciences, Engineering, and Medicine, Health and Medicine Division, Board on Population Health and Public Health Practice, et al. A National Strategy for the Elimination of Hepatitis B and C: Phase Two Report. Washington, DC: National Academies of Science 2017
12. Morse A, Barritt ASt, Jhaveri R. Individual state hepatitis C data supports expanding screening beyond baby boomers to all adults. *Gastroenterology* 2018;154:1850–1851 e2.
13. Eckman MH, Ward JW, Sherman KE. Cost effectiveness of universal screening for hepatitis C virus infection in the era of direct-acting, pangenotypic treatment regimens. *Clinical Gastroenterology and Hepatology* 2019;17:930–939.
14. World Health Organization. World Health Statistics 2018: Monitoring Health for the SDGs. https://apps.who.int/iris/

bitstream/handle/10665/272596/9789241565585-eng.pdf?ua=1

15. Grebely J, Lamoury FMJ, Hajarizadeh B et al. Evaluation of the Xpert HCV Viral Load point-of-care assay from vene-puncture-collected and finger-stick capillary whole-blood samples: a cohort study. *Lancet Gastroenterology and Hepatology* 2017;2:514–520.

16. European Union HCV Collaboration. Hepatitis C virus prevalence and level of intervention required to achieve the WHO targets for elimination in the European Union by 2030: a modelling study. *Lancet Gastroenterology and Hepatology* 2017;2:325–336.

17. World Health Organization. Blood Transfusion Safety. www.who.int/bloodsafety/en/

18. World Health Organization. Global Status Report on Blood Safety and Availability 2016. https://apps.who.int/iris/bitstream/handle/10665/254987/9789241565431-eng.pdf?sequence=1

19. Tagny CT, Mbanya D, Tapko JB et al. Blood safety in Sub-Saharan Africa: a multi-factorial problem. *Transfusion* 2008;48:1256–1261.

20. Pepin J, Abou Chakra CN, Pepin E et al. Evolution of the global burden of viral infections from unsafe medical injec-tions, 2000–2010. *PLoS One* 2014;9:e99677.

21. Tseng FC, O'Brien TR, Zhang M et al. Seroprevalence of hepatitis C virus and hepatitis B virus among San Francisco injection drug users, 1998 to 2000. *Hepatology* 2007;46:666–671.

22. Platt L, Sweeney S, Ward Z et al. Assessing the impact and cost-effectiveness of needle and syringe provision and opioid substitution therapy on hepatitis C transmission among peo-ple who inject drugs in the UK: an analysis of pooled data sets and economic modelling. Southampton (UK), 2017. https://discovery.dundee.ac.uk/en/publications/assessing-the-impact-and-cost-effectiveness-of-needle-and-syringe

23. Larney S, Peacock A, Leung J et al. Global, regional, and country-level coverage of interventions to prevent and man-age HIV and hepatitis C among people who inject drugs: a systematic review. *Lancet Global Health* 2017;5:e1208–e1220.

24. Canary L, Hariri S, Campbell C et al. Geographic disparities in access to syringe services programs among young persons with hepatitis C virus infection in the United States. *Clinical Infectious Diseases* 2017;65:514–517.

25. Turner KM, Hutchinson S, Vickerman P et al. The impact of needle and syringe provision and opiate substitution therapy on the incidence of hepatitis C virus in injecting drug users: pooling of UK evidence. *Addiction* 2011;106:1978–1988.

26. Sigmon SC, Meyer C, Hruska B et al. Bridging waitlist delays with interim buprenorphine treatment: initial feasibility. *Addictive Behaviors* 2015;51:136–142.

27. Larney S, Kopinski H, Beckwith CG et al. Incidence and prevalence of hepatitis C in prisons and other closed set-tings: results of a systematic review and meta-analysis. *Hepatology* 2013;58:1215–1224.

28. Platt L, Minozzi S, Reed J et al. Needle syringe programmes and opioid substitution therapy for preventing hepatitis C transmission in people who inject drugs. *Cochrane Database of Systemaic Reviews* 2017;9:CD012021.

29. Palmateer NE, Taylor A, Goldberg DJ et al. Rapid decline in HCV incidence among people who inject drugs associated with national scale-up in coverage of a combination of harm reduction interventions. *PLoS One* 2014;9:e104515.

30. World Health Organization. Global Hepatitis Report 2017. https://apps.who.int/iris/bitstream/handle/10665/255016/9789241565455-eng.pdf?sequence=1

31. World Health Organization. Progress Report on Access to Hepatitis C treatment, Focus on Overcoming Barriers in Low and Middle Income Countries. http://apps.who.int/iris/bitstream/10665/260445/1/WHO-CDS-HIV-18.4-eng.pdf?ua=1.

32. Chhatwal J, He T, Hur C et al. Direct-acting antiviral agents for patients with hepatitis C virus genotype 1 infection are cost-saving. *Clinical Gastroenterology and Hepatology* 2017;15:827–837 e8.

33. Harvard University, Center for Health Law and Policy Innovation. Hepatitis C: State of Medicaid Access 2017 National Summary Report. www.chlpi.org/health_library/hepatitis-c-state-medicaid-access-2017-national-summary-report/

34. Younossi ZM, Stepanova M, Henry L et al. Association of work productivity with clinical and patient-reported factors in patients infected with hepatitis C virus. *Journal of Viral Hepatitis* 2016;23:623–630.

35. Chhatwal J, Kanwal F, Roberts MS et al. Cost-effectiveness and budget impact of hepatitis C virus treatment with sofos-buvir and ledipasvir in the United States. *Annals of Internal Medicine* 2015;162:397–406.

36. Hill AM, Nath S, Simmons B. The road to elimination of hepatitis C: analysis of cures versus new infections in 91 countries. *Journal of Virus Eradication* 2017;3:117–123.

37. Grebely J, Dalgard O, Conway B et al. Sofosbuvir and velpa-tasvir for hepatitis C virus infection in people with recent injection drug use (SIMPLIFY): an open-label, single-arm, phase 4, multicentre trial. *Lancet Gastroenterology and Hepatology* 2018;3:153–161.

38. Midgard H, Weir A, Palmateer N et al. HCV epidemiology in high-risk groups and the risk of reinfection. *Journal of Hepatology* 2016;65:S33–S45.

Index

Abbott ARCHITECT 43
abdominal ultrasound 15
acoustic radiation force impulse imaging 4, 10, 11
acute hepatitis B infection 145–8
   antiviral therapy 146–8
   rationale for treatment 145–6
   viral kinetics 146
acute hepatitis C infection 29–32
   definition 29–30
   early antiviral therapy 31–2
   risk factors for progression to chronic disease 30
   spontaneous resolution 30
   symptoms 29–30
   treatment response rates 30–1
adenoviral vectors 210
adipokines 60
adjuvants 172–3
alanine aminotransferase (ALT)
   normal levels 151
   postpartum flares in HBV carrier mothers 161–2
   posttreatment flares 178
alpha-fetoprotein 16
aluminum hydroxide (alum) 172–3
American Association for the Study of Liver Disease (AASLD)
   guidelines
   HBeAg-positive chronic infection treatment 158
   HCV/HBV coinfection 186
   hepatocellular carcinoma surveillance 15, 16
   liver biopsy 11, 12
   normal ALT levels 151
   tenofovir disoproxil fumarate in pregnancy and
     breastfeeding 161, 162

American Association for the Study of Liver Disease/Infectious
   Disease Society of America (AASLD/IDSA) guidelines
   HBV vaccination, pre-HCV antiviral therapy 83
   HCV screening 41
   HCV testing, management, and treatment 42, 44–5, 66
   HCV treatment in children 96
   liver biopsy 11
   screening in pregnancy 94
amiodarone 87, 99, 101
amlodipine 87
anticoagulants 91
antiepileptic drugs 91
anti-HBc 226
anti-HBe 225
anti-HBs 226
antiplatelets 91
antiretrovirals 89
antivirals
   acute HBV infection 146–8
   pretreatment liver disease severity assessment 4, 6
   prevention of chronic infection in acute HBV
     infection 147–8
   prophylaxis in pregnancy 161
   safety in pregnancy and breastfeeding 162
   see also direct-acting antiviral therapy
apixaban 91
ASCEND study 205
Asian-Pacific Association for the Study of the Liver (APASL)
   guidelines
   HBeAg-positive chronic infection treatment 158
   hepatocellular carcinoma surveillance 15
   liver biopsy 12

Clinical Dilemmas in Viral Liver Disease, Second Edition. Edited by Graham R. Foster and K. Rajender Reddy.
© 2020 John Wiley & Sons Ltd. Published 2020 by John Wiley & Sons Ltd.

ASO4 173
aspirin 91
AST to platelet ratio index (APRI) 4, 6, 10, 152–3
ASTRAL-4 study 37, 45
atazanavir 103
atorvastatin 102
Australia, HCV elimination strategy 240–1
autovaccination 176

B-cell vaccines 210
basal core promoter mutations 225, 226, 228
Baveno VI criteria 7
BE3A score 113
bictegravir 89
bioequivalence 67
blood donor screening 246
brain abnormalities 55–6
breast cancer resistance protein (BCRP) 86, 87, 88, 101, 102
breastfeeding, antiviral safety 162
buprenorphine 87, 92
burden of hepatitis 19–24
buyers' clubs 67, 69–70

C-EDGE CO-STAR study 79
carbamazepine 87, 90
cardiac transplantation 134
carfentanil 92
CD8+ T-cells 176
cell-free DNA 16
CHAMPS study 123
chemotherapy
    HBV reactivation 153
    HEV infection 190
children
    HBV treatment 164–7
    HCV treatment 94–6
chimeric hepatitis C virus 75
chronic kidney disease 48–51, 98, 141
ciclosporin 88, 89, 102
cirrhosis
    decompensated 37, 38, 97–8, 112–13, 114–15, 141
    HBV in children 164
    HCV/HBV coinfection 182, 183
    hepatocellular carcinoma 233
    injecting drug users 78
CirVir study 234
clopidogrel 91
cobicistat 89, 103
cognitive impairment 55–6

complete task-shifting 205–6
compulsory license 67
computed tomography 15–16, 17
contingency management 122–3
contraceptives 92, 102
counseling 109
covalently closed circular DNA 222
CpG 173
CUPILT study 234
cytochrome P450 enzymes 86, 88, 89, 92, 98, 101, 102

dabigatran 87, 88, 91, 101, 102
daclatasvir 37, 49, 91, 101, 103
darunavir 89, 102
dasabuvir 36, 37, 49, 88, 91, 92, 102, 103
decompensated cirrhosis 37, 38, 97–8, 112–13, 114–15, 141
default effect 127
depression 55, 56–7
digoxin 87, 101
direct-acting antiviral therapy 36–9
    children 95–6
    chronic kidney disease 48–51, 98, 141
    decompensated liver disease 38, 97–8, 112–13, 115, 141
    drug–drug interactions 86–92, 98–103, 129, 135
    early treatment of HCV 31–2
    Egyptian model of care 217–18
    generic 66–71, 248
    HBV reactivation 82–5
    HCV/HBV coinfection 183, 184–6, 187
    health-related quality of life 56–7
    hepatocellular carcinoma risk 119, 233–6
    history of hepatocellular carcinoma 119
    injecting drug users 79–80, 91–2, 108
    metabolism 48–9
    obesity 61
    pangenotypic 37–8, 44–5, 49, 95–6, 115
    pharmacology 87–9
    posttransplant 37, 113–14, 135, 141
    pretransplant 112–13, 118
    real-life effectiveness 138–41
    safety issues 97–103
    salvage regimen 37–9
    side effects 97
    waitlist patients (bridge therapy/locoablation) 119
direct-acting oral anticoagulants 91
discrimination 109, 218
dolutegravir 89, 103
double-stranded linear DNA 228
dried blood spot 43
drug–drug interactions 86–92, 98–103, 129, 135

edoxaban 102
education, injecting drug users 109
efavirenz 89, 103
Egypt, model of care 217–18
elbasvir 36, 49, 88, 102, 103
elimination of hepatitis C virus 238–42, 244–8
    definition 239, 244
    high-prevalence, low-income countries 216–19
    WHO targets 208–9, 239, 244
empty particles 228
end of treatment response 107
entecavir 153, 165, 166
eradication 239
ERCHIVES study 51
ethical issues, HCV-positive organ donors 135–6
ethinylestradiol-containing contraceptives 92, 102
etravirine 89, 103
European Association for the Study of the Liver (EASL) guidelines
    acute HBV therapy 148
    HBeAg-positive chronic infection treatment 158
    HCV diagnosis, management, and treatment 42, 44–5, 66, 103
    HCV/HBV coinfection 186
    hepatocellular carcinoma surveillance 15
    liver biopsy 11, 12
    pre-antiviral liver disease assessment 4, 6
    tenofovir disoproxil fumarate in pregnancy and
        breastfeeding 161, 162
European Liver Fibrosis Study Group panel (ELF) 10
EXPANDER study 133–4
EXPEDITION 4 and 5 studies 49

fatigue 55, 57
FENDrix® 173
fentanyl 92
Fibroscan® 4
fibrosis see liver fibrosis
Fibrosis-4 (FIB-4) 4, 6, 152–3
FibroSpect II® 10
FibroSure® 10
FibroTest® 4, 10
fulminant hepatitis 145, 147, 148
functional cure 175, 220, 222

GALAD 17
gene expression 228–9
glecaprevir 89, 91, 92
glecaprevir/pibrentasvir 37, 38–9, 45, 49, 88–9, 90, 95–6,
    102, 103
grazoprevir 89, 92
grazoprevir/elbasvir 36, 49, 88, 102, 103

harm reduction 79, 108, 242, 246
HBeAg-negative infection 150–4, 177–8, 180, 222
HBeAg-positive infection 156–9, 161, 178, 222
    children 166–7
health-related quality of life 54–7
healthcare worker exposure 31, 32
heart transplantation 134
Hepascore® 10
HEPATHER study 234
hepatitis B core antibody 226
hepatitis B core-related antigen (HBcrAg) 225
    inactive carriers 152
hepatitis B e antigen (HBeAg) 222, 225
hepatitis B surface antibody 226
hepatitis B surface antigen (HBsAg) 178, 222
    inactive carriers 152
hepatitis B vaccination
    adjuvants 172–3
    breakthrough events 171
    doubling vaccine dose 171–2
    impact of 20, 160–1
    intradermal injection 172
    low (hypo-) responders 170
    nonresponders 169–74
    pre-HCV antiviral therapy 83
    repeat immunization 171–2
hepatitis B virus DNA
    inactive carriers 151
    quantitative testing 222
hepatitis B virus infection
    acute infection management 145–8
    antivirals 146–8
    children 164–7
    diagnostics 220–9
    estimates of disease burden 19–24
    functional cure 175, 220, 222
    genotypes and subtypes 226
    HBeAg-negative patients 150–4, 177–8, 180, 222
    HBeAg-positive (immune tolerant) patients 156–9, 161,
        166–7, 178, 222
    HCV coinfection 182–7
    hepatocellular carcinoma risk 157–8, 226
    inactive carrier state 150–4, 167
    liver biopsy 12
    natural history of virus 220
    phases of chronic disease 156
    pregnancy 160–2
    preventing chronic infection in acute HBV 147–8
    progression to chronicity 145
    reactivation during HCV coinfection treatment 184, 185–6

reactivation in inactive carriers 153, 167
reactivation while on direct-acting antiviral therapy 82–5
sterilizing cure 220
stopping therapy 175–80
hepatitis B virus RNA 226
hepatitis C vaccines 208–14
    B-cell vaccines 210
    T-cell vaccines 210
hepatitis C virus core antigen test 43, 45
hepatitis C virus infection
    acute infection treatment 29–32
    advanced liver disease 112–15
    children 94–6
    chimeric HCV 75
    decompensated cirrhosis 112–13, 114–15, 141
    diagnostic testing 43–4
    direct-acting antiviral therapy *see* direct-acting antiviral
        therapy
    early antiviral therapy in acute cases 31–2
    elimination 208–9, 216–19, 238–42, 244–8
    endpoint of therapy 42
    estimates of disease burden 19–24
    guidelines for diagnosis, management, and treatment
        monitoring 42, 44–5, 66, 103
    HBV coinfection 182–7
    HBV reactivation 82–5
    HBV vaccination 83
    health-related quality of life 54–7
    healthcare worker exposure 31, 32
    hepatocellular carcinoma risk 233–6
    hepatocellular carcinoma treatment 117–20
    HIV co-infection 102–3
    incentives for patients 122–4
    injecting drug users 30, 31, 78–80, 106–10, 125
    liver biopsy 12
    models of care 80, 217–18
    multiple genotypes 74–6
    obesity 59–63
    opioid epidemic 30, 78–9
    organ donors 115, 132–6
    postexposure prophylaxis 32
    postorthotopic liver transplant 37
    prevention strategies 245–6
    prison population 124, 125–30
    real-life therapy effectiveness 138–41
    renal disease 48–51
    ribavirin therapy 35–9, 95
    risk factors for acute to chronic progression 30
    screening 41, 42–3, 94, 218–19, 245, 246
    simplified management algorithm 42–5

    spontaneous resolution 30
    symptoms of acute infection 29–30
    task-shifting of treatment 203–6
    treatment response in acute relative to chronic infection 30–1
    underdiagnosis 245
    undertreatment 246–8
hepatitis E virus infection 189–91
hepatitis E virus vaccines 193–9
hepatocellular carcinoma
    cirrhosis 233
    HBeAg-positive chronic infection 157–8
    HBV genotype 226
    HBV inactive carriers 153
    HCV/HBV coinfection 182, 183, 186
    HCV in children 95
    HCV treatment 117–20
    liver biopsy 12
    liver stiffness 7
    risk stratification 17
    risk with direct-acting antiviral therapy 119, 233–6
    screening 15–18
    sustained virologic response 15, 117, 233, 234
Heplisav B® 173
HEV 239 vaccine 194–6
HIV
    HCV coinfection 102–3
    HEV coinfection 191
    task-shifting programs 205
human challenge models 211

immunostimulatory DNA sequences 173
immunosuppression
    HBV reactivation 153
    HEV infection 190
    HEV vaccine 198
inactive carrier state 150–4, 167
incentives for patients 122–4
infection control 216
Infectious Disease Society of America (IDSA) guidelines *see*
        American Association for the Study of Liver Disease/
        Infectious Disease Society of America (AASLD/IDSA)
        guidelines
informed consent 127–8
injecting drug users 106–10, 125
    acute hepatitis C infection 30, 31
    care provision 79, 80, 108–9
    challenges of HCV 78–80
    cirrhosis identification 78
    counseling 109
    criminalization of drug use 109, 125

injecting drug users (*cont'd*)
  direct-acting antiviral therapy 79–80, 91–2, 108
  education 109
  harm reduction 79, 108, 242, 246
  incentives for patients 122–3
  needle and syringe programs 79, 108, 242, 246
  opioid substitution therapy 79, 91, 92, 108, 242, 246
  posttreatment surveillance 109
  reinfection 79–80, 108, 109, 110
  risk factors for HCV acquisition 107
  screening 109
  targeted strategies 109
  treatment as prevention 31, 79, 110, 248
injections, unsafe 246
insulin resistance 60
interferons
  acute HBV infection 146
  HBV treatment in children 165–6
  obesity 60–1
  ribavirin and 36
  see also pegylated-interferon
inverse probability treatment weighting 235–6

kidney transplantation 133–4

labelling 55
lamivudine
  acute HBV infection 146–7, 148
  HBV reactivation prevention 153
  HBV treatment in children 165, 166
  pregnancy and breastfeeding 161, 162
ledipasvir 36, 37, 38, 49, 87, 89, 95, 101, 103, 185
leptin 60
liver biopsy 9–13
  alternatives 10–11
  endoscopic ultrasound-guided 9
  guidelines 11–12
  hepatocellular carcinoma diagnosis 12
  limitations 9
  pre-antiviral treatment 6
liver fibrosis
  HBV in children 164
  HBV inactive carriers 152–3
  injecting drug users 78
  liver stiffness measurement 3, 4, 6–7, 10–11
  monitoring disease progression 7
  monitoring regression 6–7
  noninvasive markers 3–7
  obese patients 60, 61–2
  SAFE approach 11
  serum markers 3, 4, 6–7, 10

Liver Imaging Reporting and Data System (LI-RADS) 12
liver stiffness 3, 4, 6–7, 10–11
liver transplantation
  efficacy and safety of treatment after 113–14, 141
  efficacy and safety of treatment before 112–13, 118
  HCV+ donors 115, 134
  multiple HCV genotypes 79–80
  posttransplant direct-acting antiviral therapy 37, 113–14,
    135, 141
lopinavir 102
lung transplantation 133–4

magnetic resonance elastography 4, 10, 11
magnetic resonance imaging 15–16, 17
maraviroc 103
MELD purgatory 115, 118
methadone 92
mild cognitive impairment 55–6
modafinil 88, 99, 101, 102
models of care 80, 217–18
Mongolia, HCV elimination strategy 241
mortality rates 20, 22

needle and syringe programs 79, 108, 242, 246
nevirapine 103
nonalcoholic fatty liver disease 59, 60
nonalcoholic steatohepatitis 59, 60

obesity 59–63
occupational exposure 31, 32
ombitasvir 36, 37, 49, 88, 91, 92, 102, 103
omeprazole 89
operational delivery networks 124, 126, 129
opioid epidemic 30, 78–9
opioid substitution therapy 79, 91, 92, 108, 242, 246
opt-out testing 126, 127–8
OraQuick HCV Rapid Antibody Test Kit 43
organ donors 115, 132–6
Organ Procurement and Transplant Network (OPTN) 12
organic anion transporting protein (OATP) 86, 87, 88, 89,
    101, 102
Ortho ELISA 43
outbreaks, hepatitis E 198–9
oxcarbazepine 102

P-glycoprotein 86, 87, 88, 89, 98, 101, 102
paritaprevir 89
paritaprevir/ombitasvir/dasabuvir (+ritonavir) 36, 37, 49, 88,
    91, 92, 102
partial task-shifting 204–5
peer mentors 123

pegylated-interferon
    HBV inactive carriers 154
    HBV treatment in children 165
    HCV/HBV coinfection 182–3, 184, 186
    HEV infection 191
    ribavirin and 36
phenobarbital 90
phenytoin 91
pibrentasvir 37, 38–9, 45, 49, 88–9, 90, 95–6, 102, 103
point-of-care HCV RNA test 43
point shear wave elastography 4
portal hypertension 7
postexposure prophylaxis 32
prasugrel 91
precore mutations 225, 226, 228
pregnancy
    HBV 160–2
    HCV screening 94
    HEV infection 189
    HEV vaccine 196
prequalified products 67
pre-S1/pre-S2/S vaccine 173
prisoners
    HCV treatment 125–30
    incentivizing testing and treatment 124
    screening 109, 126–30
progestogen-only contraceptives 92, 102
programmed cell death protein-1 176
Project ECHO 204–5
propensity score matching 235–6
proton pump inhibitors 87, 89–91, 101, 102, 141

quality of life 54–7
quasi-species 74
quetiapine 102

raltegravir 89, 103
rapid diagnostic tests 42–3
reactivation of HBV
    during HCV coinfection treatment 184, 185–6
    in inactive carriers 153, 167
    while on direct-acting antiviral therapy 82–5
recombinant 56 kDa vaccine 194
REDMPTION-1 study 70
reinfection 79–80, 108, 109, 110
renal disease 48–51, 98, 141
resistance-associated substitutions 31, 37
REVEAL study 158
ribavirin
    decompensated liver disease 37
    HCV 35–9, 95

    HCV/HBV coinfection 182–3, 184, 186
    HEV 191
rifabutin 99
rifampicin 87
rifapentine 99
rilpivirine 103
rituximab, HBV reactivation 153
ritonavir 49, 88, 89, 91, 92, 102, 103
rivaroxaban 91
rosuvastatin 87, 88, 101, 102
RUBY-1 and -2 studies 49

SAFE approach 11
SAGE recommendations 196–9
St John's wort 87
Sci-B-Vac® 173
screening
    blood donors 246
    economics of HCV screening 218–19
    HCV infection 41, 42–3, 94, 245, 246
    hepatocellular carcinoma 15–18
    incentive use 124
    injecting drug users 109
    pregnancy 94
    prisoners 109, 126–30
    universal versus targeted 125
SD Bioline HCV 43
serotonin system 57
serum markers
    hepatocellular carcinoma surveillance and risk
        stratification 16–17
    liver fibrosis 3, 4, 6–7, 10
SHARED study 44
shear-wave elastography (2D) 4, 10
simeprevir 49
SIMPLIFY study 79, 248
simvastatin 102
skipping HCV genotype 44
sofosbuvir 36, 99, 103
    renal safety 50–1
sofosbuvir/daclatasvir 37
sofosbuvir/ledipasvir 36, 37, 49, 87, 89, 95, 185
sofosbuvir/ledipasvir/ribavirin 37, 38
sofosbuvir/ledipasvir/voxilaprevir 49
sofosbuvir/ribavirin 36
sofosbuvir/velpatasvir 37, 38, 44–5, 49, 56, 87–8, 89–90, 95–6
sofosbuvir/velpatasvir/voxilaprevir 37, 38, 88, 89, 90, 91, 103
spliced DNA/RNA 228
statins 87, 88, 101, 102
sterilizing cure 220
stigma 109

suppressor of cytokine signalling (SOCS) family 60
sustained virologic response (SVR) 48, 107
  children 95
  generic direct-acting antivirals 68–9, 70
  HCV/HBV coinfection 183–4, 185
  health-related quality of life 56
  hepatocellular carcinoma risk 15, 117, 233, 234
  HEV infection 191
  incentivized patients 123
  liver stiffness 6–7
  obesity 60–1
  posttransplant 113–14, 115
  real-life therapy 138–41
  task-shifting 204, 205, 206
  treatment as prevention 79
synthetic opioids 92

T-cell exhaustion 176
T-cell vaccines 210
tacrolimus 102
task-shifting 203–6
telbivudine 161, 162
tenofovir alafenamide 89
tenofovir disoproxil fumarate
  drug–drug interactions 89, 103
  HBV reactivation prevention 153
  HBV treatment in children 165, 166
  pregnancy and breastfeeding 161, 162
THINKER study 133
ticagrelor 91, 102
TNF-alpha 60
training
  Egyptian model of care 217
  prison HCV testing 127, 128, 129
  task-shifting 204, 205–6

transient elastography 4, 10–11
  HBV inactive carriers 153
  obesity 60
transplantation
  HCV-positive organs 115, 132–6
  HEV infection 190–1
  HEV vaccine for recipients 198
  see also liver transplantation
travel-associated hepatitis E 198
treatment as prevention 31, 79, 110, 248
2-D shear-wave elastography 4, 10

UNITE 241
unsafe injections 246
USHER study 134

vaccine adjuvants 172–3
velpatasvir 37, 38, 44–5, 49, 56, 87–8, 89–90, 91, 95–6, 101–2, 103
viral recurrence 107–8
viral relapse 108
visceral fat 59–60
voluntary license 67
voxilaprevir 37, 38, 49, 88, 89, 90, 91, 102, 103

"warehouse" treatment effects 240–1
warfarin 91
WHO
  HCV elimination targets 208–9, 239, 244
  HCV screening recommendations 245
  HCV treatment guidelines 66
  prequalified products 67
  SAGE recommendations for HEV vaccine 196–9

Xpert HCV Viral Load assay 43